New Frontiers in Gastrointestinal Surgery

New Frontiers in Gastrointestinal Surgery

Edited by Benson Scott

hayle
medical

New York

Hayle Medical,
750 Third Avenue, 9ᵗʰ Floor,
New York, NY 10017, USA

Visit us on the World Wide Web at:
www.haylemedical.com

ISBN: 978-1-63241-612-4

Cataloging-in-Publication Data

New frontiers in gastrointestinal surgery / edited by Benson Scott.
    p. cm.
Includes bibliographical references and index.
ISBN 978-1-63241-612-4
1. Gastrointestinal system--Surgery. 2. Digestive organs--Surgery. I. Scott, Benson.
RD540 .N49 2019
617.4--dc23

Table of Contents

Preface

Gastrointestinal surgery, also known as digestive system surgery can be classified into two parts, i.e., upper gastrointestinal surgery and lower gastrointestinal surgery. Upper gastrointestinal surgery (GI) is a practice of surgery which is concerned with the upper parts of the gastrointestinal tract. The tasks performed by an upper GI surgeon include esophagectomy, liver resection and pancreaticoduodenectomy. Lower gastrointestinal surgery, also known as lower GI surgery is a practice of surgery concerned with colorectal surgery as well as surgery of the small intestine. A lower GI surgeon usually deals with colectomy and low or ultralow resections for rectal cancer. This book contains some path-breaking studies related to gastrointestinal surgery. It discusses the fundamental as well as modern approaches of gastrointestinal surgery. This book includes contributions of experts and doctors which will provide innovative insights to readers.

This book has been the outcome of endless efforts put in by authors and researchers on various issues and topics within the field. The book is a comprehensive collection of significant researches that are addressed in a variety of chapters. It will surely enhance the knowledge of the field among readers across the globe.

It gives us an immense pleasure to thank our researchers and authors for their efforts to submit their piece of writing before the deadlines. Finally in the end, I would like to thank my family and colleagues who have been a great source of inspiration and support.

Editor

Severe gastric variceal haemorrhage due to splenic artery thrombosis and consecutive arterial bypass

Klaus T von Trotha[1*], Marcel Binnebösel[1], Son Truong[1], Florian F Behrendt[2], Hermann E Wasmuth[3], Ulf P Neumann[1] and Marc Jansen[4]

Abstract

Background: Upper gastrointestinal haemorrhage is mainly caused by ulcers. Gastric varicosis due to portal hypertension can also be held responsible for upper gastrointestinal bleeding. Portal hypertension causes the development of a collateral circulation from the portal to the caval venous system resulting in development of oesophageal and gastric fundus varices. Those may also be held responsible for upper gastrointestinal haemorrhage.

Case presentation: In this study, we describe the case of a 69-year-old male with recurrent severe upper gastrointestinal bleeding caused by arterial submucosal collaterals due to idiopathic splenic artery thrombosis. The diagnosis was secured using endoscopic duplex ultrasound and angiography. The patient was successfully treated with a laparoscopic splenectomy and complete dissection of the short gastric arteries, resulting in the collapse of the submucosal arteries in the gastric wall. Follow-up gastroscopy was performed on the 12th postoperative week and showed no signs of bleeding and a significant reduction in the arterial blood flow within the gastric wall. Subsequent follow-up after 6 months also showed no further gastrointestinal bleeding as well as subjective good quality of life for the patient.

Conclusion: Submucosal arterial collaterals must be excluded by endosonography via endoscopy in case of recurrent upper gastrointestinal bleeding. Laparoscopic splenectomy provides adequate treatment in preventing any recurrent bleeding, if gastric arterial collaterals are caused by splenic artery thrombosis.

Keywords: Splenic artery thrombosis, upper gastrointestinal bleeding, laparoscopy, splenectomy, duplex ultra sound

Background

Among the most common causes of upper gastrointestinal bleeding are ulcers of the duodenum or stomach, accounting for approximately 50% of all cases. These are followed by erosions of the duodenum or stomach, varicosis of the oesophagus or gastric fundus, and reflux disease [1]. It has been shown that 4/5 of all ulcers are located on the lesser curvature of the stomach, while more atypical localisations include corpus, fundus, and greater curvature of the stomach.

Gastric varicosis is often the result of portal hypertension in the liver. Such portal hypertension is caused by simultaneous increases in the portal vascular territory, the so-called "backward flow", as well as increased arterial blood flow within the splanchnic vascular territory,

the "forward flow". This results in the development of a collateral circulation from the portal to the caval venous system. It is these portal gastric oesophageal collaterals that cause the oesophageal and gastric fundus varices. Indeed, up to 60% of all patients with liver cirrhosis experience bleeding episodes from oesophageal or corpus-/fundus varicosis bleeding [1].

In this study, we present a rare case of severe upper gastrointestinal haemorrhage caused by arterial collaterals to the spleen after thrombosis of the splenic artery. Symptoms, diagnosis, and treatment, including follow-up, are presented.

Case presentation

A 69-year-old patient was admitted for care due to recurrent upper gastrointestinal bleeding. The patient had previously received treated for similar symptoms two years prior at another facility. Upper gastrointestinal

---

* Correspondence: kvontrotha@ukaachen.de
[1]Department of Surgery, University Hospital of the RWTH Aachen, Germany
Full list of author information is available at the end of the article

endoscopy revealed bleeding next to a varicose shaped submucosal vessel located at the fundus of the stomach (Figure 1). The bleeding could be successfully stilled with an injection of N-butyl-2-cyanoacrylate/Lipiodol and subsequent clipping.

Further investigation, using computed tomography (CT) and conventional angiography revealed the cause of the prominent varicose shaped vessels, namely thrombosis of the splenic artery (Figure 2). Surprisingly, conventional angiography of the celiac trunk was able to demonstrate collateral vessels via the left gastric artery to the spleen. Furthermore, selective angiography of the superior mesenteric artery showed collateral vessels to the caudal portion of the spleen. In order to verify the nature of these unexpected arterial collaterals via the submucosal vessels at the gastric fundus and the reversed blood flow, a CT scan was employed, and revealed the presence of Lipiodol within the arterial collaterals as well as in the vessels of the upper portion of the spleen. Lipiodol had been injected in a mixture with N-butyl- 2-cyanoacrylate during the treatment of the gastrointestinal bleeding (Figure 3). As a complication of the therapy, the adjacent splenic tissue demonstrated signs of infarction, most likely caused by the N-butyl- 2-cyanoacrylate.

Computed tomography also showed a slight increase in liver vascularisation as indicative of possible cirrhotic remodelling. To eliminate the possibility of cirrhotic liver remodelling, a fibroscan was conducted to measure liver stiffness. The result yielded a mean score of 4.2 kPa, and thereby excluded the possibility of significant fibrosis.

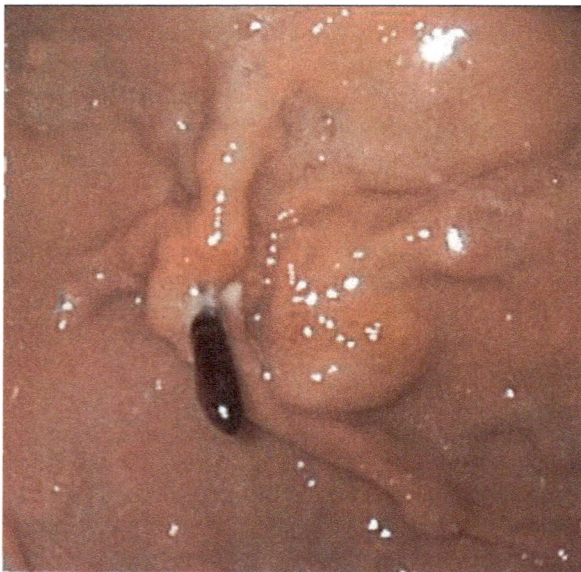

Figure 2 Angiography of the the coeliac trunc (1) showing the common hepatic artery (2) and the left gastric artery with multiple collateral vessels (3). The splenic artery as third branch is missing. Residual of N-butyl-2-cyanoacrylate lipiodol injection (4) can be seen.

Also of importance was the fact there were no signs of oesophageal or gastric venous varicosis. Abdominal ultrasound was also able to safely exclude any signs of liver cirrhosis, including ascites or splenomegaly.

In order to prove that the submucosal vessels were indeed arterial collaterals, a gastrointestinal endoscopy of the stomach using color-duplex ultrasound was performed. Multiple arterial vessels, but no venous collaterals, could be identified in the gastric fundus (Figure 4).

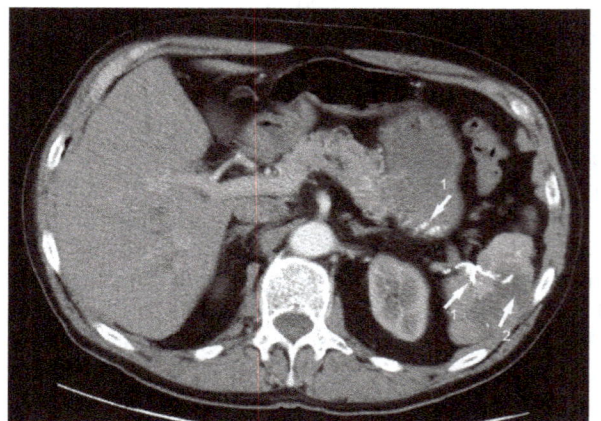

Figure 1 The upper gastrointestinal endoscopy showed preoperative thick submucous varices along a small ulcer, one clip in situ.

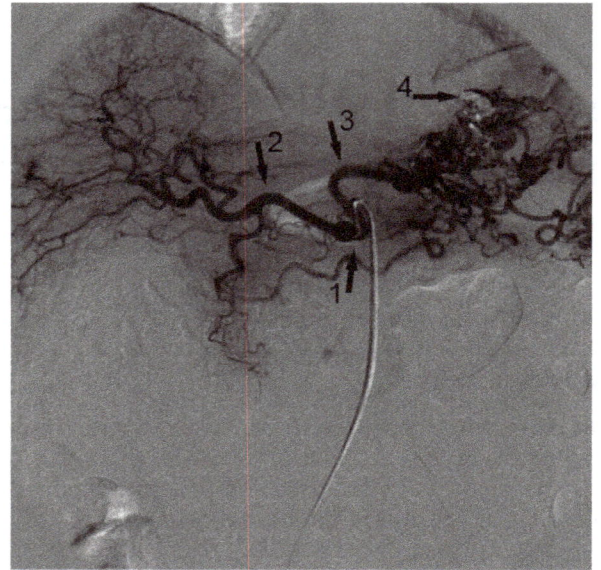

Figure 3 Axial contrast enhanced CT scan of the upper abdomen showing lipiodol in the arterial collaterals of the stomach running to the spleen (1). Furthermore, CT revealed an infarction of splenic tissue adjacent to these vessels (2).

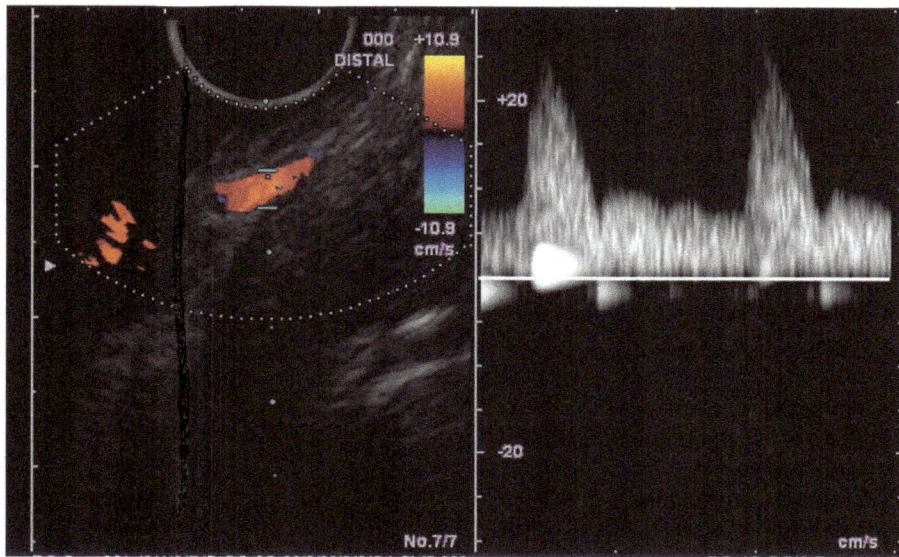

Figure 4 Endoscopic colour duplex sonography showing arterial flow on the apparently gastric varices.

The examination results, in combination with a medical history of splenic artery thrombosis, suggested that the varicose shaped vessels did not originate from cirrhosis, but were in fact symptomatic collaterals caused by the thrombosis.

Pancreatitis and blunt abdominal trauma are among the known causes of splenic artery thrombosis [2,3]. However, both could be excluded given the patient's medical history. Additionally, a cardiovascular origin could be ruled out. In order to further elucidate its origin, thrombophilia diagnostic was performed. Here, no relevant anomalies were detected (Protein C (function: 107% (n: 70-149%), Protein S function: 72% (n: 75-130%), Protein S (quant.) 86% (n: 75-140%), Protein S (quant.) 97% (n: 72-150%), APC-Resistance 2.4 (n: > 2.0)). Analysis of specific clotting factors showed that factor XIII was within the normal range (80% n: 70-140%), while factor VIII was slightly elevated at x > 164% (n: 70-140%). Testing for factor V Leiden thrombophilia as well as the prothrombin G20210A-Mutation also proved unremarkable.

In order to reduce the arterial blood flow via the gastric collaterals, a laparoscopic splenectomy was performed to prevent further bleeding. Two weeks prior to the operation a triple vaccination (pneumococcus, mengingococcus, h. influenzae) was administered. No technical difficulties occurred, and the entire surgical course could be completed without complication. Blood loss was held at a minimum, and the patient could be extubated immediately postoperatively and remained in the intensive care unit for one night. The patient experienced no major complications and was discharged on the seventh postoperative day.

In the course of the follow-up 12 weeks after surgery, an upper gastrointestinal endoscopy was performed twice. Both showed a significant reduction in submucosal arterial collaterals. Endoscopic duplex ultrasound detected only a minimal residual arterial signal. The patient showed good quality of life after a 6 month follow-up and presented with no further gastrointestinal bleeding.

Discussion and conclusion

Upper gastrointestinal bleeding are most commonly caused by either ulcers of various origin (50%) or gastric or oesophageal varices (20%). A large percentage of such duodenal and peptic ulcers are caused by helicobacter pylori induced gastroduodenitis, while only 20% are caused by nonsteroidal antiphlogistics [4,5] In this case, helicobacter pylori colonisation of the mucosa was not responsible for the development of an ulcer. Usually, the gastric bleeding due to ulcers is caused by erosion of the submucosal venous or arterial vessels. The most common location for such arterial bleeding is in the postpyloric region, due to erosion of the gastroduodenal artery. Though our patient presented with a small ulcer at the gastric fundus, it was unable to explain the cause of the varicose malformation.

Venous varices are often a symptom of portal hypertension, usually caused by liver cirrhosis [6,7]. In this case, venous blood flow is restricted through the portal vein and is redirected via venous collaterals to the right atrium. Such porto-caval collaterals are made noticeable through oesophageal and gastric varicosis, caput medusae, as well as rectal varicosis. Patients with gastric varicosis due to portal hypertension and ulcers bear a high risk of bleeding [8]. Arterial collaterals, as seen in this case, are generally not due to portal hypertension. Further excluding such a possible origin in our patient, a clinically relevant portal hypertension was ruled out using fibroscan, abdominal ultrasound, and computed tomography.

Splenic artery collaterals with gastric funcal varices as well as their possible complications have, until now, rarely been described [9-11]. The full pathomechanism remains unclear but thrombosis of the splenic artery can cause arterial collaterals via the route described. In addition, submucosal collaterals have been reported in patients with a congenital absence of the splenic artery [12,13].

In contrast, coiling of the splenic artery is a common procedure employed in the treatment of hypersplenism, otherwise known as the 'splenic artery steal syndrome,' in patients before and after liver transplantation. This procedure has been performed in cases where perfusion of the transplant is reduced and liver function impaired, or in order to improve liver perfusion prior to operation. While post-interventional abscesses or splenic infarct have been described and require splenectomy, gastric arterial collaterals have not been reported up till now, which underscores the rare nature of the present case [14,15].

N-butyl-2-cyanoacrylate injection for the treatment of gastric bleeding causes thrombosis of the renal vein [16], splenic artery occlusion [17] as well as portal vein thrombosis [18]. Because the varicose collaterals were clearly visible in the first gastroscopy, where N-butyl-2-cyanoacrylate injection was performed, we can safely assume that N-butyl-2-cyanoacrylate injection was not responsible for the splenic artery thrombosis. Blood sampling and thrombophilia diagnostic showed only a slight increase in factor VIII (approximately 164% n: 70-140). Increased factor VIII levels have previously been related to an increased risk for venous thromboembolism, especially in patients with cirrhosis and cancer [19,20] and low shear conditions [21], not though, for thromboembolism within the arterial circulation.

During the operation, massive collateral vessels via the short gastric arteries to the spleen were clearly visible (Figure 5). In addition, the cranial portion of the spleen showed signs of reduced perfusion. The collaterals via the short gastric arteries, as well as the main vessels of the spleen, were successfully ligated and cut during the laparoscopic procedure.

The cause for the thrombosis remains unclear, yet angiography has shown that the collaterals were sufficient to provide blood flow for the remaining spleen. Splenectomy was able to effectively reduce the collateral blood flow via the gastric arteries. This result was confirmed in the follow-up gastroscopy, which showed only remnants of the original varicosis. As such, we were able to conclude that thrombosis of the splenic artery was due to malformation of gastric submucosal arterial collaterals.

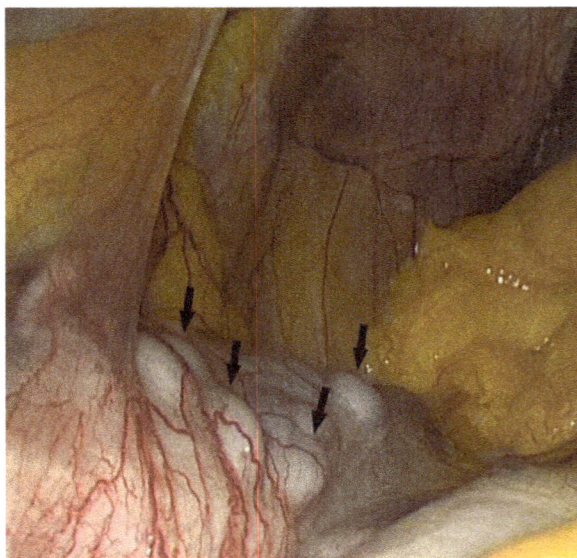

Figure 5 Intraoperative situation showing the thick arterial collaterals along the gastric fundus.

In the case of recurrent upper gastrointestinal bleedings from varicose-like structures, submucosal arterial collaterals must be excluded by endosonography via endoscopy. Should further ambiguity exist, further diagnostic, such as angiography and CT scan, are warranted.

If gastric submucous arterial collaterals can be shown, for example due to splenic artery thrombosis, laparoscopic splenectomy provides adequate treatment in preventing any recurrent bleeding.

The findings and procedures described in this paper were presented in video form at the 127th Congress of the German Society for Surgery on April 20-23, 2010 in Berlin, Germany.

Permissions

None of the material has been previously published.

Author details

[1]Department of Surgery, University Hospital of the RWTH Aachen, Germany. [2]Department of Diagnostic Radiology, University Hospital of the RWTH Aachen, Germany. [3]Department of Medicine III, University Hospital of the RWTH Aachen, Germany. [4]Department of Surgery, HELIOS Hospital Emil von Behring Berlin, Germany.

Authors' contributions

KT drafted and finalized the manuscript, prepared the figures, MB reviewed the manuscript and prepared the figures, FB prepared and provided

radiologic figures and report, UN critically reviewed the manuscript and has given final approve for publication, HW and ST performed gastrointestinal endoscopy, duplex sonography of the stomach as well as the followup controls, MJ and KT performed the operation.
All authors read and approved the final manuscript.

Competing interests
The authors declare that they have no competing interests.

References
1. van Leerdam ME: **Epidemiology of acute upper gastrointestinal bleeding.** *Best Pract Res Clin Gastroenterol* 2008, **22**:209-224.
2. Dror S, Dani BZ, Ur M, Yoram K: **Spontaneous thrombosis of a splenic pseudoaneurysm after blunt abdominal trauma.** *J Trauma* 2002, **53**:383-385.
3. Gow KW, Murphy JJ, Blair GK, Stringer DA, Culham JA, Fraser GC: **Splanchnic artery pseudo-aneurysms secondary to blunt abdominal trauma in children.** *J Pediatr Surg* 1996, **31**:812-815.
4. Kalra BS, Chaturvedi S, Tayal V, Gupta U: **Evaluation of gastric tolerability, antinociceptive and antiinflammatory activity of combination NSAIDs in rats.** *Indian J Dent Res* 2009, **20**:418-422.
5. Redeen S, Petersson F, Kechagias S, Mardh E, Borch K: **Natural history of chronic gastritis in a population-based cohort.** *Scand J Gastroenterol* 2010, **45((5))**:540-9.
6. Garcia-Tsao G, Lim JK: **Management and treatment of patients with cirrhosis and portal hypertension: recommendations from the Department of Veterans Affairs Hepatitis C Resource Center Program and the National Hepatitis C Program.** *Am J Gastroenterol* 2009, **104**:1802-1829.
7. Moore KP, Aithal GP: **Guidelines on the management of ascites in cirrhosis.** *Gut* 2006, **55(Suppl 6)**:vi1-12.
8. Navarro VJ, Garcia-Tsao G: **Variceal hemorrhage.** *Crit Care Clin* 1995, **11**:391-414.
9. Baron PW, Sindram D, Suhocki P, Webb DD, Clavien PA: **Upper gastrointestinal bleeding from gastric submucosal arterial collaterals secondary to splenic artery occlusion: treatment by splenectomy and partial gastric devascularization.** *Am J Gastroenterol* 2000, **95**:3003-3004.
10. Cyrany J, Kopacova M, Rejchrt S, Jirkovsky V, Al-Tashi M, Bures J: **Gastric arterial bleeding secondary to chronic occlusion of the splenic artery (with video).** *Gastrointest Endosc* 2010, **71**:1335.
11. Mnatzakanian G, Smaggus A, Wang CS, Common AA, Jeejeebhoy KN: **Splenic artery collaterals masquerading as gastric fundal varices on endoscopy: a sticky situation.** *Gastrointest Endosc* 2008, **67**:751-755.
12. Durrans D, Fawcitt RA, Taylor TV: **Congenital absence of the splenic artery associated with major gastric bleeding in adolescence.** *Br J Surg* 1985, **72**:456-457.
13. Spriggs DW: **Congenital absence of the splenic artery.** *Cardiovasc Intervent Radiol* 1984, **7**:303-305.
14. Mogl MT, Nussler NC, Presser SJ, Podrabsky P, Denecke T, Grieser C, Neuhaus P, Guckelberger O: **Evolving experience with prevention and treatment of splenic artery syndrome after orthotopic liver transplantation.** *Transpl Int* 2010.
15. Vogl TJ, Pegios W, Balzer JO, Lobo M, Neuhaus P: **[Arterial steal syndrome in patients after liver transplantation: transarterial embolization of the splenic and gastroduodenal arteries].** *Rofo* 2001, **173**:908-913.
16. Vincent M, Lerat F, Trogrlic S, Laurent V, Feray C, Dupas B: **[Left renal vein thrombosis following sclerotherapy for gastric varices].** *J Radiol* 2009, **90**:745-746.
17. Yu LK, Hsu CW, Tseng JH, Liu NJ, Sheen IS: **Splenic infarction complicated by splenic artery occlusion after N-butyl-2-cyanoacrylate injection for gastric varices: case report.** *Gastrointest Endosc* 2005, **61**:343-345.
18. Amouroux C, Cervoni JP, Delabrousse E, Koch S, Thevenot T, Di M V: **[Portal vein thrombosis after cyanoacrylate injection therapy in bleeding gastric varices].** *Gastroenterol Clin Biol* 2009, **33**:205-207.
19. Vormittag R, Simanek R, Ay C, Dunkler D, Quehenberger P, Marosi C, Zielinski C, Pabinger I: **High factor VIII levels independently predict venous thromboembolism in cancer patients: the cancer and thrombosis study.** *Arterioscler Thromb Vasc Biol* 2009, **29**:2176-2181.
20. Tripodi A, Primignani M, Chantarangkul V, Dell'Era A, Clerici M, de FR, Colombo M, Mannucci PM: **An imbalance of pro- vs anti-coagulation factors in plasma from patients with cirrhosis.** *Gastroenterology* 2009, **137**:2105-2111.
21. Sugita C, Yamashita A, Moriguchi-Goto S, Furukoji E, Takahashi M, Harada A, Soeda T, Kitazawa T, Hattori K, Tamura S, Asada Y: **Factor VIII contributes to platelet-fibrin thrombus formation via thrombin generation under low shear conditions.** *Thromb Res* 2009, **124**:601-607.

Does recurrent laryngeal nerve lymph node metastasis really affect the prognosis in node-positive patients with squamous cell carcinoma of the middle thoracic esophagus?

Jie Wu[1]*, Qi-Xun Chen[1], Xing-Ming Zhou[1], Wei-Ming Mao[1] and Mark J Krasna[2]

Abstract

Background: Recurrent laryngeal nerve (RLN) lymph node metastasis used to be shown a predictor for poor prognosis in esophageal squamous cell carcinoma. The purpose of this study was to evaluate the prognostic impact of RLN node metastasis and the number of metastatic lymph nodes in node-positive patients with squamous cell carcinoma of middle thoracic esophagus.

Methods: A cohort of 235 patients who underwent curative surgery for squamous cell carcinoma of middle thoracic esophagus was investigated. The prognostic impact was evaluated by univariate and multivariate analyses.

Results: Lymph node metastasis was found in 133 patients. Among them, 81 had metastatic RLN nodes, and 52 had at least one positive node but no RLN nodal involvement. The most significant difference in survival was detected between patients with metastatic lymph nodes below and above a cutoff value of six ($P < 0.001$). Multivariate analysis revealed that the number of metastatic lymph nodes was a significant factor associated with overall survival ($P < 0.001$), but RLN lymph node metastasis was not ($P = 0.865$).

Conclusions: RLN Lymph node metastasis is not, but the number of metastatic nodes is a prognostic predictor in node-positive patients with squamous cell carcinoma of the middle thoracic esophagus.

Keywords: Esophageal cancer, Lymph node metastasis, Recurrent laryngeal nerve, Squamous cell carcinoma

Background

In esophageal cancer, lymph node metastasis most likely occurs on neck, mediastinum and abdomen. Recurrent laryngeal nerve (RLN) lymph node is located at the cervical base continuous to the upper mediastinum, which is one of the most common sites of lymph node metastasis in thoracic esophageal squamous cell carcinoma [1-4]. The clinical significance of RLN node metastasis in surgical treatment of thoracic esophageal squamous cell carcinoma has been discussed previously. Early metastasis [2,5], initial metastasis [6,7], and even micrometastasis [7] of esophageal squamous cell carcinoma often occur in RLN nodes. In addition,

nodal involvement in RLN has been regarded as an indication for three-field lymphadenectomy in the surgical treatment of esophageal cancer [4,8-10]. More importantly, RLN node metastasis has been shown to be a strong predictor of poor prognosis in thoracic esophageal squamous cell carcinoma [3,11].

However, some studies showed that the site of nodal involvement was not associated with the prognosis of thoracic esophageal squamous cell carcinoma, and the number of metastatic lymph nodes had a greater prognostic significance in thoracic esophageal squamous cell carcinoma [12-14]. These results are contradictory to the findings mentioned above that RLN node metastasis is an unfavorable prognostic factor in thoracic esophageal squamous cell carcinoma. To evaluate the outcome of curative esophagectomy treatment, as well as the prognostic impacts of RLN node metastasis and the

* Correspondence: wujiephd729@126.com
[1]Department of Thoarcic Surgery, Zhejinang Cancer Hospital, 38 Guangji Road, Hangzhou 310022, China
Full list of author information is available at the end of the article

number of metastatic lymph nodes, in this study, we analyzed a cohort of patients with squamous cell carcinoma of the middle esophagus admitted in our institution.

Methods
Patients
Three hundred and twenty six patients with squamous cell carcinoma of the middle thoracic esophagus were surgically treated at the Department of Thoracic Surgery of Zhejiang Cancer Hospital, Hangzhou, China from January 2003 to December 2009. Among these patients, 26 patients with R1 (microscopic residual disease) or R2 (macroscopic residual disease) resections, 48 patients receiving preoperative therapy (chemotherapy and/or radiotherapy), 8 patients with histories of gastric cancer, 5 patients with synchronous cancers (gastric cancer or laryngeal cancer) and 4 patients with non-squamous cell carcinoma of the middle thoracic esophagus were excluded. The records of the remaining 235 patients with curative esophagectomy were retrospectively reviewed. Written informed consents were obtained from all patients before surgery. The Institutional Review Board of Zhejiang Cancer Hospital approved the study and the need for individual patient consent was waived.

The cohort of patients included 194 males and 41 females with an average age of 58 ranging from 37 to 79 years old. Preoperative evaluation included endoscopy with biopsy, barium swallow examination, computerized tomography of the chest and upper abdomen, and ultrasound of the neck. Pulmonary and cardiac function tests were routinely performed to assess medical operability. Histological diagnosis of each of the patients was established before treatment. Tumor location, grade, and stage were defined according to the 7th edition of UICC TNM classification [15]. Recurrent laryngeal nerve palsy and the presence of clinical supraclavicular or cervical nodal involvement were considered a contraindication for surgery.

In our institution, two types of lymphadenectomy were performed for esophageal cancer depending on the operators' surgical preference. Four surgeons performed 2-field lymphadenectomy, while 2 performed 3-field lymphadenecotmy as a chief operator.

Surgical procedure
A transthoracic esophagectomy was performed for each of the 235 patients with either a 2-field or a 3-field lymphadenectomy. The surgical procedure of esophagectomy with 2-field lymphadenectomy was described previously [16]. In principle, this procedure consisted of esophagectomy with total mediastinal lymphadenectomy through a right thoracotomy, and upper abdominal lymphadenectomy through an upper median laparotomy. Total mediastinal lymphadenctomy was performed according to the classification defined by the International Society for Diseases of the Esophagus (ISDE) [17]. The extent of lymphadenectomy involved dissection of the bilateral RLNs, paratracheal, brachiocephalic artery,

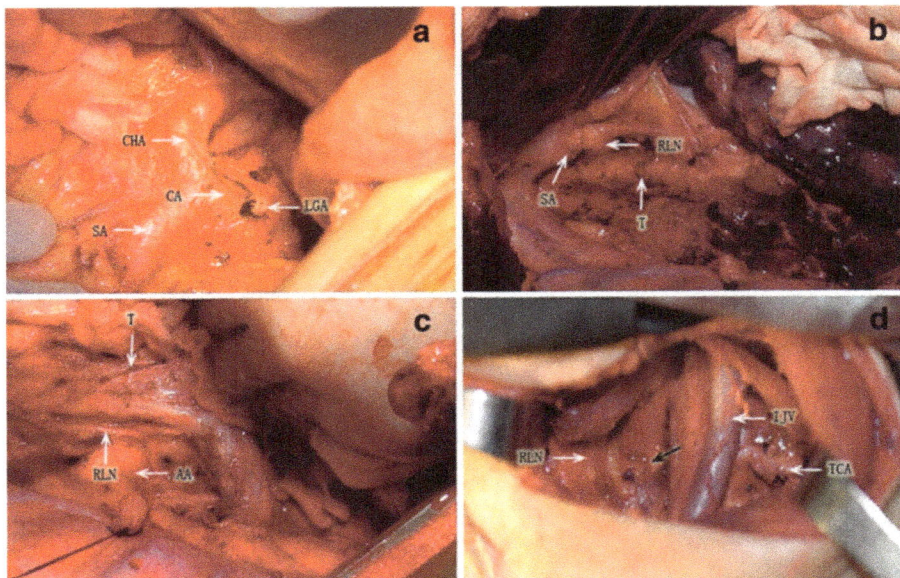

Figure 1 Lymphadenectomy for esophageal carcinoma. (a) Upper abdominal field. CA: celiac artery, CHA: common hepatic artery, SA: splenic artery, LGA: left gastric artery. **(b)** Right upper mediastinal field. SA: subclavian artery, RLN: (right) recurrent laryngeal nerve, T: trachea. **(c)** Left upper mediastinal field. RLN: (left) recurrent laryngeal nerve, AA: aotic arch, T: trachea. **(d)** Left cervical field: TCA: transverse cervical artery. IJV: internal jugular vein, RLN: (left) recurrent laryngeal nerve, black arrow: anastomotic site.

paraesophageal, and infraaortic arch nodes, in addition to the middle and lower mediastinal nodes. Upper abdominal lymphadenectomy was performed to include the paracardial, lesser curvature, left gastric, common hepatic, celiac, and splenic nodes. The 3-field lymphadenectomy included cervical lymphadenectomy of the paraesophageal, deep cervical, and supraclavicular nodes in addition to 2-field lymphadenectomy performed through a collar cervical incision. Esophageal anastomosis was performed in the neck for each patient (Figure 1). Gastrointestinal continuity reconstruction was achieved by stomach bypass in 233 patients and by colon conduit in 2 patients. After surgery, the anatomical location of the removed nodes were labeled by the operating surgeon, and then histologically examined with hematoxylin and eosin staining.

Follow-up

Complete follow-up information was available for all patients. Survival time was defined as the period from the date of surgery till death (including surgical related death and non-cancer related death) or the most recent follow-up in March 2013. The duration of follow-up ranged from 1 month to 131 months (average 45 months, median 37 months). One hundred and sixty four patients died, and the remaining 71 were still alive at the last contact.

Statistical analysis

Survival curves were constructed using Kaplan-Meier method [18], and log-rank test was used to determine significance [19]. To confirm the optimal cutoff value for the number of metastatic lymph nodes, the Cox proportional hazard model was used to compare survival rates between the groups with fewer and more metastatic lymph nodes [20]. The number of metastatic lymph nodes with the highest χ^2 value was regarded as the optimal cutoff level. The influence of each clinicopathological variable on survival was assessed using Cox proportional hazard model. A P value of less than 0.05 was considered statistically significant.

Results

Clinicopatholgoical features

Clinicopathological features of the patients are summarized in Table 1. Of the 235 patients, 159 underwent 2-field and 76 underwent 3-field lymphadenectomy. The majority of patients had T3 disease (157 patients, 67%). Among the 8 patients with T4 tumors, invasions to the lungs were diagnosed in 3 patients, and invasions to the pericardia were diagnosed in 5 patients. A total of 102 patients had no lymph node metastases (43%), and 133 patients had lymph node metastases (57%). Mediastinal and abdominal lymph node metastases were found in

Table 1 Clinicopathological features of the 235 patients with squamous cell carcinoma of the middle thoracic esophagus

Variables	No. (%)
Age (years)	
< 60	132 (56)
≥ 60	103 (44)
Sex	
Male	194 (83)
Female	41 (17)
Differentiation	
G1	49 (21)
G2	143 (61)
G3	43 (18)
T category	
T1	32 (14)
T2	38 (16)
T3	157 (67)
T4	8 (3)
Node status	
N0	102 (43)
N1	57 (24)
N2	49 (21)
N3	27 (11)
Positive (N+)	133 (57)
RLN -	52 (22)
RLN +	81 (35)
Lymphatic and venous invasion	
No	190 (81)
Yes	45 (19)
Intramural metastasis	
No	220 (94)
Yes	15 (6)
Adjuvant therapy	
No	179 (76)
Yes	56 (24)
Lymphadenectomy type	
2-field	159 (68)
3-field	76 (32)

124 (53%) and 46 (20%) patients respectively. Cervical lymph node metastases were found in 23 of 76 (30%) patients who underwent 3-field lymphadenectomy. Of the 133 patients with nodal involvement, 81 (61%) had metastatic RLN nodes and 52 (39%) had at least one positive node but no RLN nodal involvement. The minority of patients (56 patients, 24%) received adjuvant therapy postoperatively.

Table 2 Cutoff values for the number of metastatic lymph nodes analyzed by Cox proportional hazard model

Cut-off values	χ^2	Hazards ratio (95% CI)	P value
1 vs. ≥2	2.758	1.457 (0.932-2.278)	0.099
2≤ vs. ≥3	5.706	1.599 (1.084-2.359)	0.018
3≤ vs. ≥4	4.042	1.486 (1.008-2.191)	0.046
4≤ vs. ≥5	8.854	1.804 (1.209-2.692)	0.004
5≤ vs. ≥6	19.610	2.542 (1.658-3.898)	<0.001
6≤ vs. ≥7	20.903	2.820 (1.774-4.482)	<0.001
7≤ vs. ≥8	15.544	2.269 (1.597-4.330)	<0.001
8≤ vs. ≥9	6.543	2.070 (1.171-3.660)	0.012
9≤ vs. ≥10	6.696	2.189 (1.191-4.023)	0.012
10≤ vs. ≥11	2.698	1.766 (0.888-3.514)	0.105

The number of metastatic lymph nodes and its stratification

The number of metastatic lymph nodes of the 133 patients ranged from 1 to 32, with a mean of 4.4 and a median of 3. The Cox proportional hazards regression model revealed that the most significant difference in survival was identified with a cutoff value of six metastatic lymph nodes, yielding a χ^2 value of 20.903, a

hazard ratio of 2.820, and a 95% confidence interval of 1.774-4.482 (Table 2).

Survival

The median survival for all patients was 37 months, and the 1-, 3- and 5-year survival rates were 79%, 51%, and 39%, respectively. The Kaplan-Meier curves constructed using the optimal values for the number of metastatic lymph nodes are shown in Figure 2. The median survival time of patients without lymph node metastasis, with ≤ 6 metastatic lymph nodes, and with ≥ 7 metastatic lymph nodes were 83, 30 and 11 months, respectively. There were significant differences between patients without lymph node metastasis and with ≤ 6 metastatic lymph nodes ($P < 0.001$), between patients without lymph node metastasis and with ≥ 7 metastatic lymph nodes ($P < 0.001$), and between patients with ≤ 6 metastatic lymph nodes and with ≥ 7 metastatic lymph nodes ($P < 0.001$).

Survival curves based on lymph node status are shown in Figure 3. The median survival time of node-negative patients, node-positive patients without RLN nodal involvement and RLN node-positive patients were 83, 24 and 24 months, respectively. There were significant differences between node-negative patients and RLN

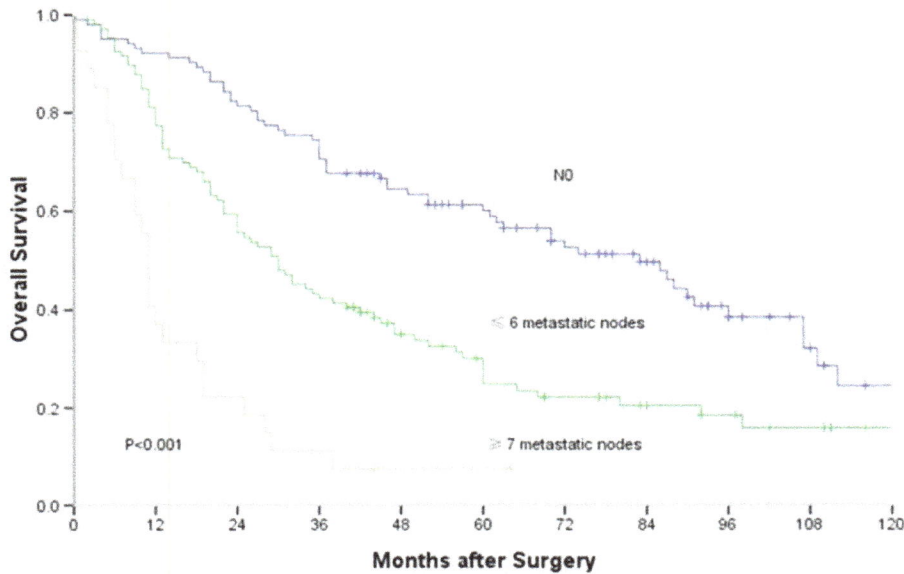

Patients at risk											
N0	102	94	83	72	61	51	39	29	15	9	5
≤ 6 nodes +	106	82	59	45	29	19	15	10	8	5	1
≥ 7 nodes +	27	10	6	3	1	1	0	0	0	0	0

Figure 2 Survival curves of patients with various number of metastatic nodes (without lymph node metastasis vs. with ≤ 6 metastatic nodes, $P < 0.001$; with ≤ 6 metastatic nodes vs. with ≥ 7 metastatic nodes, $P < 0.001$; without lymph node metastasis vs. with ≥ 7 metastatic nodes, $P < 0.001$).

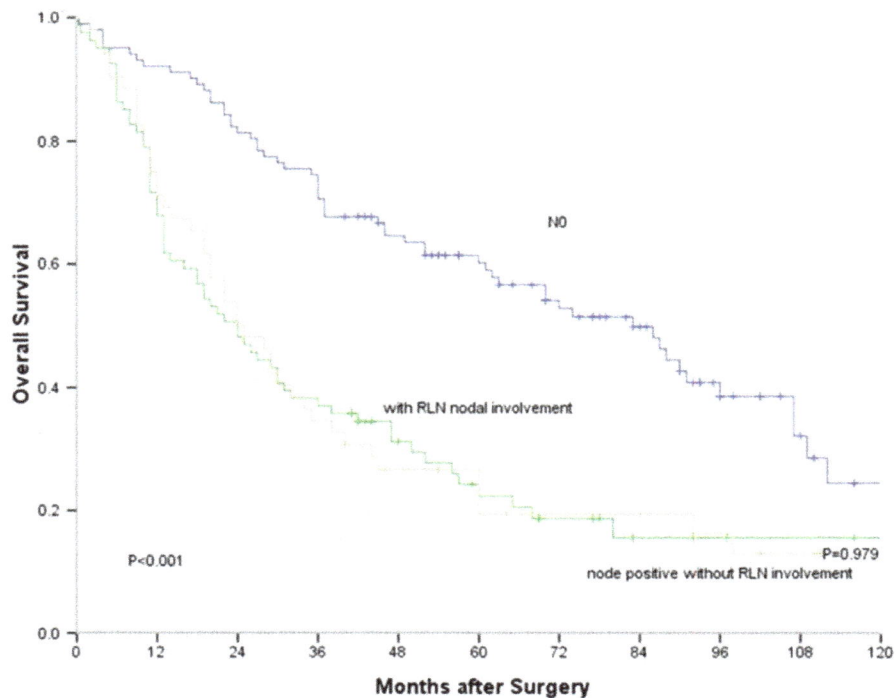

Figure 3 Survival curves of patients with different RLN node status (without lymph node metastasis vs. with RLN nodal involvement, $P < 0.001$; without lymph node metastasis vs. node-positive without RLN nodal involvement, $P < 0.001$; with RLN nodal involvement vs. node-positive without RLN nodal involvement, $P = 0.979$).

node-positive patients ($P < 0.001$), and between node-negative patients and node-positive patients without RLN nodal involvement ($P < 0.001$). There was no significant difference between RLN node-positive patients and node-positive patients without RLN nodal involvement ($P = 0.979$).

Furthermore, the difference in survival time of patients with ≤ 6 metastatic lymph nodes was insignificant between RLN node-positive patients and node-positive patients without RLN nodal involvement. Similarly, the difference in survival between the two groups mentioned above and patients with ≥ 7 metastatic lymph nodes was also insignificant ($P = 0.804$) ($P = 0.143$) (Figure 4).

In addition, survival curves based on N stages according to the 7th edition of UICC TNM classification are shown in Figure 5. The median survival time of N0, N1, N2, and N3 patients were 83, 32, 24, and 11 months respectively. There was a significant difference in survival time among all these patients ($P < 0.001$). However, the difference in survival time was insignificant between N1 and N2 patients ($P = 0.869$).

Univariate and multivariate analyses for clinicopathological variables

In a univariate analysis for survival, T category ($P < 0.001$), node status ($P < 0.001$), lymphatic and venous invasion ($P = 0.001$), intramural metastasis ($P = 0.009$) and adjuvant therapy ($P = 0.034$) were significantly associated with overall survival (Table 3). Because three methods (N stage, number of metastatic nodes, RLN node metastasis) were used in stratifying N status, three Cox models were constructed to avoid problems with the presence of multicollinearity. As shown in Table 4, the number of positive nodes ($P < 0.001$) were identified as a significant factor associated with overall survival, while RLN node metastasis was not a prognostic predicator ($P = 0.865$). In a model with stratification by N stage, N2 stage was insignificantly associated with overall survival ($P = 0.722$).

RLN node status and the type of lymphadenectomy

In the 81 patients with RLN node metastasis, the difference in survival rate was insignificant between 2-field and 3-field lymphadenectomy ($P = 0.843$). In the other

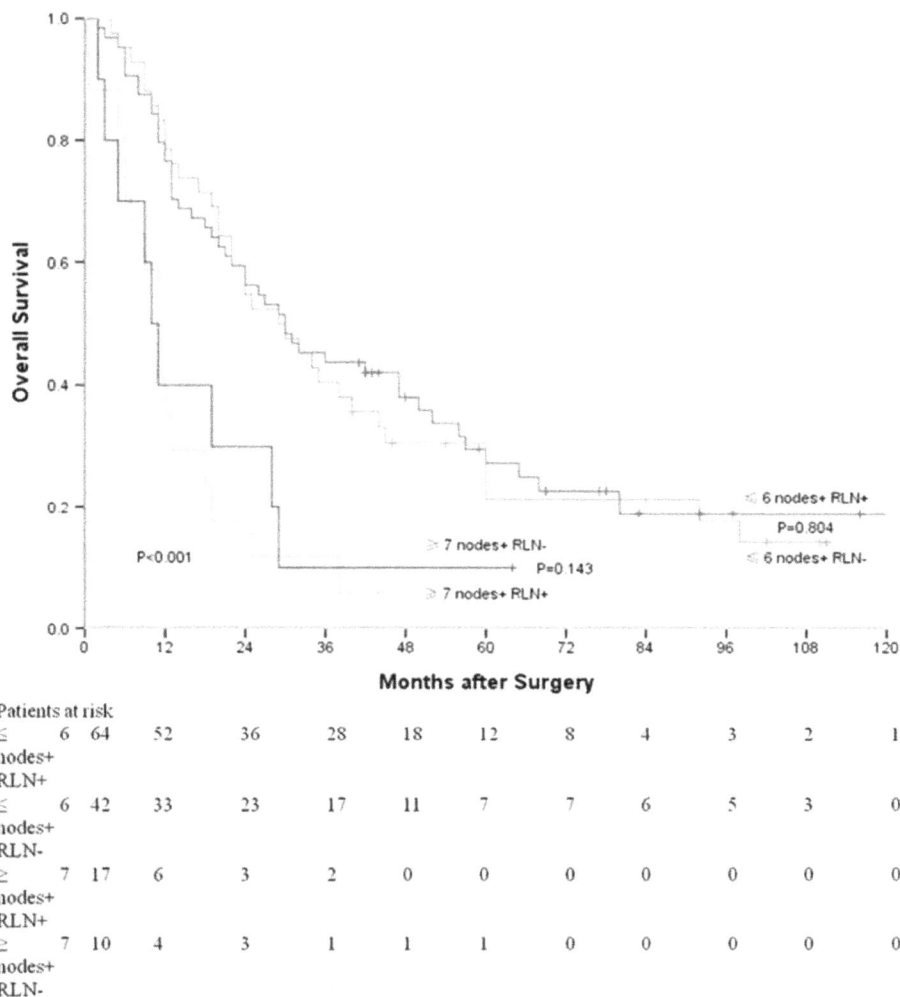

Figure 4 Survival curves of patients with various number of metastatic nodes and different recurrent laryngeal nerve node status (≤ 6 nodes + RLN + vs. ≤ 6 nodes + RLN-, P = 0.928; ≥ 7 nodes + RLN- vs. ≥ 7 nodes + RLN+, P = 0.520).

154 patients without RLN node metastasis, survival rate did not differ significantly between 2-field and 3-field lymphadenectomy ($P = 0.661$).

Discussion

Here we demonstrated that the presence of RLN node metastasis was not a prognostic predicator in node-positive patients with squamous cell carcinoma of the middle thoracic esophagus. A previous report including 55 patients with esophageal squamous cell carcinoma who underwent esophagectomy with 2-field lymphdenectomy showed that RLN node metastasis was the strongest prognostic predicator [11]. That report was more heterogeneous in term of tumor site: tumors were located below and above the carina in 40 and 15 patients, respectively [11]. Different tumor sites might lead to different frequencies of lymph node metastasis. In that report, frequencies of RLN node metastasis was 18% in all patients (10/55) and 26% (10/34) in node-positive patients [11]. While in our study, the frequencies of RLN node metastasis were 34% (81/235) in all patients and 62% (81/133) in node-positive patients. More importantly, Authors only performed univariate analysis, but did not perform multivariate analysis in that cohort [11]. Dealing with data this way may cause confounding effect that influenced the interpretation of results. There was another report on clinical outcomes of 106 patients with esophageal squamous cell carcinoma who underwent 3-field lymphadenectomy [3]. Univariate and multivariate analyses indicated that RLN node metastasis was the most unfavorable prognostic factor [3]. In that series, 10, 67 and 29 patients had tumors located in the upper, middle and lower thoracic esophagus, respectively. Although RLN node metastasis occurred

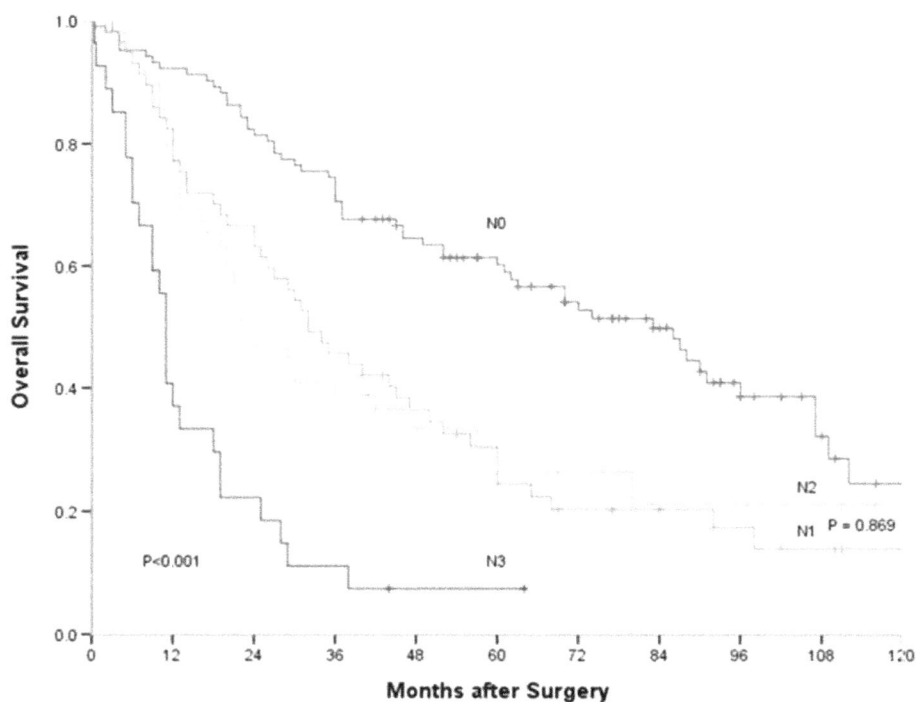

Figure 5 Survival curves of patients with different N stages (N0 vs. N1, *P* < 0.001; N0 vs. N2, *P* < 0.001; N0 vs. N3, *P* < 0.001; N1 vs. N2, *P* = 0.869; N1 vs. N3, *P* < 0.001; N2 vs. N3, *P* < 0.001).

in 60 of 78 (77%) node-positive patients, the report did not state how many patients with lesions in the middle thoracic esophagus had RLN node metastasis. Furthermore, the factor of the number of metastatic lymph nodes was not included in the analysis [3].

Among various possible prognostic predicator of esophageal carcinoma, the importance of number of metastatic nodes has been widely recognized [1,10,11,13,21]. Patients with a large number of metastatic nodes had a lower average survival rate than those with less metastatic nodes. Stratification of the number of metastatic nodes varied in different reports (for example, 1–3 vs ≥ 4 [11,13], 1–4 vs ≥ 5 [10], 1–5 vs ≥ 6 [21], and 1–7 vs ≥ 8 [1]). Our report showed that the survival rate decreased with an increasing number of metastatic nodes, and that the optimal cutoff value was between 1–6 and ≥ 7 metastatic nodes. On the other hand, there was little evidence supporting that the site of metastatic nodes influenced the prognosis of esophageal carcinoma [14,22,23]. For example, celiac node metastasis, which was regarded as M1 disease in the past, did not mean

poor prognosis in node-positive patients with esophageal cancer [22,23]. It was found that for middle and lower thoracic esophageal carcinoma, survival of patients with celiac node metastasis did not differ from those with left gastric node metastasis [23]. The 7th edition of TNM staging system also has redefined a regional node of esophageal cancer as any periesophageal lymph nodes from cervical nodes to celiac nodes; yet N staging has already been subclassfied according to the number of metastatic nodes [15].

The frequency of RLN node metastasis was reported between 20% and 50% in patients with squamous cell carcinoma of the upper and middle thoracic esophagus [1,2,4,8]. In our institution, upper thoracic tumor is routinely treated with radiotherapy-dominated multidisciplinary therapy. Some authors pointed out that RLN was the initial metastatic site (including micrometastatic site) in esophageal squamous cell carcinoma [6,7]. Others found that the histology of RLN node was characterized by large cortical area without anthracosis and hyalinization, which suggests a high filtration activity [5]. All

Table 3 Univariate analysis of 235 patients with squamous cell carcinoma of the middle thoracic esophagus

Variables	No. of patients	Survival (%) 1y 3y 5y	Median survival time (months)	P value
Age (years)				0.771
< 60	132	78 52 40	37	
≥ 60	103	81 51 37	42	
Sex				0.206
Male	194	79 50 38	36	
Female	41	71 59 43	60	
Differentiation				0.080
G1	49	88 55 49	45	
G2	143	81 53 40	42	
G3	43	65 40 36	24	
T category				<0.001*
T1/T2	70	91 71 62	86	
T3/T4	165	74 42 29	29	
Node status				<0.001*
N0	102	92 71 60	83	
N1	57	77 46 24	32	
N2	49	78 39 26	24	
N3	27	37 11 7	11	
Node status				<0.001*
N0	102	92 71 60	83	
N + RLN-	52	71 35 19	24	
N + RLN+	81	68 37 22	24	
Node status				<0.001*
N0	102	92 71 60	83	
≤ 6 positive nodes (N+)	106	77 43 25	30	
≥ 7 positive nodes (N+)	27	37 11 7	11	
Lymphatic and venous invasion				<0.001*
No	190	82 56 42	44	
Yes	45	67 31 23	22	
Intramural metastasis				0.009*
No	220	81 53 40	42	
Yes	15	60 20 20	18	
Adjuvant therapy				0.034*
No	179	79 53 44	46	
Yes	56	79 45 19	25	
Lymphadenectomy type				0.271
2-field	159	80 54 41	45	
3-field	76	78 45 35	33	

*Variables were also used for multivariate analysis.

Table 4 Multivariate analysis for 133 node-positive patients with squamous cell carcinoma of the middle thoracic esophagus

Variables	Hazard ratio	95% CI	P value
Model 1			
N1	1.000 (reference)		
N2	1.084	0.696-1.688	0.722
N3	3.135	1.877-5.236	<0.001
Model 2			
N + RLN-	1.000		0.865
N + RLN+	1.035	0.693-1.548	
Model 3			
≤ 6 positive nodes (N+)	1.000 (reference)		<0.001
≥ 7 positive nodes (N+)	3.022	1.888-4.837	

these features of RLN nodes need to be further investigated. Some authors found that the prognoses of patients with RLN node metastasis was better in the three-field lymphadenectomy group than in the two-field lymphadenectomy group, while in patients without RLN node metastasis, there was no significant differences in survival between these two groups [8]. Their results could not be duplicated in this study. It should be noted that the features of patients in that study including age, tumor location and disease stage, differed between patients with RLN node metastasis and those without RLN node metastasis [8]. These differences between patients groups could cause biased results. Frequency of cervical nodal metastasis (30%) in this report was similar to previous reported. Significant associations between RLN node metastasis and cervical node metastasis in esophageal squamous cell carcinoma were emphasized by many authors, and they firmly believed that 3-field lymphadenectomy was indicated if RLN node metastasis happens [4,8-10]. But there is lack of high-level evidence supporting 3-field lymphadenectomy in terms of long-term survival [13,24,25]. Instead it is certain that increased postoperative morbidity and impaired long-term quality of life are associated with 3-field lymphdenectomy [24,25]. Although 3-field lymphadenectomy might offer survival benefit for selected patients with esophageal cancer, the controversy over the optimal extent of lymphadenectomy still exists [25,26]. For a majority of patients there would be no arguments about performing two-field lymphadenectomy to offer a balance between benefits and risks. In addition, the emphasis of three-field lymphadenectomy lies more in RLN lymphadenectomy than in cervical lymphadenectomy [24]. In this study, 3-filed lymphadenetomy did not show its survival benefits compared with 2-field lymphadenectomy, but RLN node metastasis also did not portend a worse prognosis in node-positive patients. Thus lymphadenectomy including dissection of RLN nodes is strongly supported.

Several potential shortcomings of the present study are worth mentioning. This retrospective study from a single institution suffers from the typical biases associated with such studies. The choice of surgical procedures depended on surgeons' preference without strict criteria. It is likewise unavoidable that lymphadenectomy was performed in more or less different extent by different surgeons. In addition, there was no set standard for patients to receive adjuvant therapy. As shown in the result of the univariate analysis, patients with adjuvant therapy had worse survival than those without adjuvant therapy. The majority of patients with adjuvant therapy had a large number of metastatic nodes (data not shown). However, this series was proved to be homogenous in clinical variables including tumor site and pathologic type. Further multi-institutional studies with larger sample size are needed to confirm these results.

Conclusions

RLN lymph node metastasis is not a prognostic predictor in node-positive patients with squamous cell carcinoma of the middle thoracic esophagus. However, the number of metastatic nodes is a key prognostic predictor. Systemic lymphadenectomy including dissection of RLN nodes is therefore necessary for these patients.

Competing interests
The authors have no conflicts of interest to disclose.

Authors' contributions
JW conceived this study, collected data, performed analysis and drafted the manuscript. QXC participated in study design, literature search and coordination. JW, QXC, XMZ and WMM participated in the treatment of these patients. MJK performed data analysis and helped to draft the manuscript. All authors read and approve the final manuscript.

Acknowledgements
This work was supported in part by a grant from the Health Bureau of Zhejiang Province, China (No. 2008B029).

Author details
[1]Department of Thoarcic Surgery, Zhejinang Cancer Hospital, 38 Guangji Road, Hangzhou 310022, China. [2]Meridian Cancer Care, Jersey Shore University Medical Center, Neptune, New Jersey, USA.

References
1. Akiyama H, Tsurumaru M, Udagawa H, Kajiyama Y: Radical lymph node dissection for cancer of the thoracic esophagus. Ann Surg 1994, 220:364–373.
2. Matsubara T, Ueda M, Nagao N, Takahashi T, Nakajima T, Nishi M: Cervicothoracic approach for total mesoesophageal dissection in cancer of the thoracic esophagus. J Am Coll Surg 1998, 187:238–245.
3. Baba M, Aikou T, Yoshinaka H, Natsugoe S, Fukumoto T, Shimazu H, Akazawa K: Long-term results of subtotal esophagectomy with three-field lymphadenectomy for carcinoma of the thoracic esophagus. Ann Surg 1994, 219:310–316.
4. Sato F, Shimada Y, Li Z, Kano M, Watanabe G, Maeda M, Kawabe A, Kaganoi J, Itami A, Nagatani S, Imamura M: Paratracheal lymph node metastasis is associated with cervical lymph node metastasis in patients with thoracic esophageal squamous cell carcinoma. Ann Surg Oncol 2002, 9:65–70.
5. Mizutani M, Murakami G, Nawata S, Hitrai I, Kimura W: Anatomy of right recurrent nerve node: why does early metastasis of esophageal cancer occur in it? Surg Radiol Anat 2006, 28:333–338.
6. Matsubara T, Ueda M, Kaisaki S, Kuroda J, Uchida C, Kokudo N, Takahashi T, Nakajima T, Yanagisawa A: Localization of initial lymph node metastasis from carcinoma of the thoracic esophagus. Cancer 2000, 89:1869–1873.
7. Natsugoe S, Matsumoto M, Okumura H, Nakashima S, Higashi H, Uenosono Y, Ehi K, Ishigami S, Takao S, Aikou T: Initial metastatic, including micrometastatic, sites of lymph nodes in esophageal squamous cell carcinoma. J Surg Oncol 2005, 89:6–11.
8. Shiozaki H, Yano M, Tsujinaka T, Inoue M, Tamura S, Doki Y, Yasuda T, Fujiwara Y, Monden M: Lymph node metastasis along the recurrent nerve chain is an indication for cervical lymph node dissection in thoracic esophageal cancer. Dis Esophagus 2001, 14:191–196.
9. Nagatani S, Shimada Y, Kondo M, Kaganoi J, Maeda M, Watanabe G, Imamura M: A strategy for determining which thoracic esophageal cancer patients should undergo cervical lymph node dissection. Ann Thorac Surg 2005, 80:1881–1886.
10. Tabira Y, Yasunaga M, Tanaka M, Nakano K, Sakaguchi T, Nagamoto N, Ogi S, Kitamura N: Recurrent nerve nodal involvement is associated with cervical nodal metastasis in thoracic esophageal carcinoma. J Am Coll Surg 2000, 191:232–237.
11. Malassagne B, Tiret E, Duprez D, Coste J, De Sigalony JP, Parc R: Prognostic Value of thoracic recurrent nerve nodal involvement in esophageal squamous cell carcinoma. J Am Coll Surg 1997, 185:244–249.
12. Shimada H, Okazumi S, Matsubara H, Nabeya Y, Shiratori T, Shimizu T, Shuto K, Hayashi H, Ochiai T: Impact of the number and extent of positive lymph nodes in 200 patients with thoracic esophageal squamous cell carcinoma after three-field lymph node dissection. World J Surg 2006, 30:1441–1449.
13. Lin CS, Chang SC, Wei YH, Chou TY, Wu YC, Lin HC, Wang LS, Hsu WH: Prognostic variables in thoracic esophageal squamous cell carcinoma. Ann Thorac Surg 2009, 87:1056–1065.
14. Kunisaki C, Makino H, Kimura J, Oshima T, Fujii S, Takagawa R, Kosaka T, Ono HA, Akiyama H: Impact of lymph-node metastasis site in patients with thoracic esophageal cancer. J Surg Oncol 2010, 101:36–42.
15. Rice TW, Blackstone EH, Rusch VW: 7th edition of the AJCC cancer staging manual: Esophagus and esophagogastric junction. Ann Surg Oncol 2010, 17:1721–1724.
16. Wu J, Chai Y, Zhou XM, Chen QX, Yan FL: Ivor Lewis subtotal esophagectomy with two-field lymphadenectomy for squamous cell carcinoma of the lower thoracic esophagus. World J Gastroenterol 2008, 14:5084–5089.
17. Bumm R, Wong J: More or less surgery for esophageal cancer: extent of lymphadenectomy for squamous cell carcinoma: how much is necessary? Dis Esophagus 1994, 7:151–155.
18. Kaplan EL, Meier P: Nonparametric estimation from incomplete observations. J Am Stat Assoc 1958, 53:457–481.
19. Peto R, Pike MC, Armitage P, Breslow NE, Cox DR, Howard SV, Mantel N, McPherson K, Peto J, Smith PG: Design and analysis of randomized clinical trials requiring prolonged observation of each patient. II. analysis and examples. Br J Cancer 1977, 35:1–39.
20. Cox DR: Statistical significance tests. Br J Clin Pharmacol 1982, 14:325–331.
21. Bollschweiler E, Baldus SE, Schröder W, Schneider PM, Hölscher AH: Staging of esophageal carcinoma: length of tumor and number of involved regional lymph nodes. Are these independent prognostic factors? J Surg Oncol 2006, 94:355–363.
22. Schomas DA, Quevedo JF, Donahue JM, Nichols FC 3rd, Romero Y, Miller RC: The prognostic importance of pathologically involved celiac node metastases in node-positive patients with carcinoma of the distal esophagus or gastroesophageal junction: a surgical series from the Mayo Clinic. Dis Esophagus 2010, 23:232–239.

23. Seto Y, Fukuda T, Yamada K, Matsubara T, Hiki N, Fukunaga T, Oyama S, Yamaguchi T, Nakajima T, Kato Y: Celiac lymph nodes: distant or regional for thoracic esophageal carcinoma? *Dis Esophagus* 2008, 21:704–707.

24. Law S, Wong J: Two-field dissection is enough for esophageal cancer. *Dis Esophagus* 2001, 14:98–103.

25. Mariette C, Piessen G: Oesophageal cancer: how radical should surgery be? *Eu J Surg Oncol* 2012, 38:210–203.

26. Jamieson GG, Lamb PJ, Thompson SK: The role of lymphadenectomy in esophageal cancer. *Ann Surg* 2009, 250:206–209.

Feasibility of capsule endoscopy in elderly patients with obscure gastrointestinal bleeding

G Orlando[4], IM Luppino[1], MA Lerose[4], R Gervasi[4], B Amato[2], G Silecchia[3], A Puzziello[4*]

Abstract

Background: Anemia is the most common hematologic abnormality in older populations. Furthermore, iron deficiency anemia is common and merits investigation and treatment, as it usually results from chronic occult bleeding from the gastrointestinal tract. In view of a wide use of capsule endoscopy as a diagnostic procedure for occult gastrointestinal bleeding and of the growth of aging population, we performed a literature review about the feasibility of capsule endoscopy in the elderly.

Methods: We conducted a literature search in the PubMed database in July 2012, and all English-language publications on capsule endoscopy in elderly patients since 2005 were retrieved. The potential original articles mainly focused on obscure gastrointestinal bleeding were all identified and full texts were obtained and reviewed for further hand data retrieving.

Results: We retrieved only six papers based on different primary end-points. Four were retrospective non randomized studies and two were prospective non randomized studies. In the end 65, 70, 80 and 85 years were used as an age cut-off. All studies evaluate the diagnostic yield of capsule endoscopy in iron deficiency anemia. Only three studies assess the feasibility of capsule examination of the elderly.

Conclusions: Iron deficiency anemia in the elderly with or without obscure gastrointestinal bleeding is the major indication for capsule endoscopy after a negative esophago-gastro-duodenoscopy and colonoscopy. It is safe and effective to identify a small bowel pathology without a great discomfort for the elderly. Inability to swallow the capsule, battery failure before capsule reaches the cecum, and capsule retention are some of the important problems associated with capsule endoscopy in elderly as well as in younger patients.

Introduction

Anemia is the most common hematologic abnormality in older populations. Furthermore, iron deficiency anemia is common and merits investigation and treatment, as it usually results from chronic occult bleeding from the gastrointestinal tract. The incidence of gastrointestinal bleeding in patients over the age of 80 is high, over 350 cases per 100000 person-years [1]. Furthermore about 20% of the elderly have a negative upper and lower gastrointestinal endoscopy and two-thirds of theme have a lesion in the small bowel [2].

On the other hand, capsule endoscopy (CE) has developed an important role in the investigation of patients with obscure gastrointestinal bleeding (OGB) when upper endoscopy, push enteroscopy, colonoscopy, and barium contrast radiography of the small bowel are negative. CE is becoming so commonly used in practice and accepted by patients due to its noninvasive technique, compared with double-balloon endoscopy, that some authors also demonstrated its feasibility in patients who have undergone small-bowel resection for benign or malignant disease [3]. In view of a wide use of CE as a diagnostic procedure for

* Correspondence: puzziello@unicz.it
[4]Endocrinosurgery Unit, Dept of Medical and Surgical Sciences, University Magna Graecia, Catanzaro, Italy
Full list of author information is available at the end of the article

OGB and of the growth of an aging population we performed a literature review on the utility and safety of CE in the elderly with obscure gastrointestinal bleeding. A second end-point of our study aims to confirm the spectrum of small bowel pathologies in this age group as a dominant cause of OGB.

Therefore, we performed this review of global literature to provide current state-of-the-art data on the number and type of CE-related publications, the indications, the diagnostic yield, the completion, and retention rates in evaluating OGB in the elderly.

Material and methods

The literature search was conducted in the PubMed database in July 2012, and all English-language publications on CE since 2005 were retrieved. The search terms that we selected were "video capsule endoscopy OR capsule endoscopy OR wireless capsule endoscopy OR capsule endoscope OR video capsule endoscope AND elderly OR older adult" which were mainly based on the official thesaurus (MeSH). All initial search results were reviewed by title and abstracts. Then, the potential original articles mainly focusing on obscure gastrointestinal bleeding were all identified, and full texts were obtained and reviewed for further hand data retrieving.

We selected only six papers with different primary endpoints. Four were retrospective non randomized studies and two were prospective non randomized studies. In the end 65, 70, 80 and 85 (oldest old) years were used as an age cut-off. All studies also evaluate the diagnostic yield of capsule endoscopy in iron deficiency anemia and more frequent CE findings in different age groups. Only three studies specifically assess the feasibility of capsule examination in the elderly with respect to bowel preparation, complete examination, patient's compliance, transit time and capsule retention. Capsule retention was defined as a capsule endoscope remaining in the digestive tract for a minimum of 2 weeks or one that required directed intervention or therapy to aid its passage.

Results

Bowel preparation

Two studies [4,5] report a trend for poorer small bowel preparation in patient aged >65 years. This difference reached statistical significance in the proximal (p < 0.046) and in the distal (p < 0.048) half of CE small bowel transit time in respect to patients aged < 65 yr (5), and mainly in patients aged >80 years (Table 1) [4].

Study discomfort

Only one study specifically reports a marked discomfort in age group (> 80 years) (p < 0,0001) with respect to the younger group. Furthermore, in the age group (> 80

Table 1 Incomplete bowel preparation rate (modified from Tsibouris et al.)

	> 80 years	< 80 years	P value
Incomplete bowel preparation	17% (25/145)	3% (13/470)	< 0,0001

years) 58% of patients found capsule endoscopy study very tiresome and difficult compared to 8% in the younger group (p< 0.0001) [4].

Complete examination

Complete examination is defined as capsule passing through the ileocecal valve or into the colon in the images during its working time and capsule being excreted in 2 weeks, regardless of technical failure or poor small-bowel preparation. Two studies only report a rate of capsule not reaching the cecum of 6% and 7.5%. Two others randomized studies demonstrate that the percentage of patients in which the capsule reached the terminal ileum did not differ between aged and younger groups. ($p_1 = 0.78$; $p_2 = 0.51$) [4,5]. A prospective non randomized study also reports no difference in small bowel transit time (p > 0.78).

Capsule endoscopy findings

The diagnostic yield of CE for the suspected bleeding source in all patients with OGB has been reported to range from 38% to 93%. The small bowel is the most likely source of bleeding in patients with continuing blood loss and negative upper and lower gastrointestinal endoscopies. No significant difference was found between the different age groups with regards to either the detection rate (p>0.05) or diagnostic rate (p>0.05), while there was significant difference ($P < 10^{-3}$) in CE study findings among different age groups. Angiodysplasia was the most prevalent finding (43.6%) in patient > 65 years, with a growing rate in patients > 80 years. Tsibouris et al. report in fact an 80% rate of angiodysplasia in aged group (median age 82.7 yr) with respect to the younger group (median age 63.4 yr) (p<0.0001).

Discussion

In our study, we found no differences between the aged group and younger group with regard to the probability of completing the small bowel study and small bowel transit time. The p value for differences in the detection and diagnostic rates between the different age groups was non-significant, which suggests that CE examination has good detection and diagnostic capacity for OGB in individuals of various ages. The only relevant report was the poorer small bowel preparation in the elderly that could increase small bowel transit time and make video-capture worse. In the patient > 80 years with an iron deficiency anemia with or without OGB and negative upper endoscopy and colonoscopy the CE should have a high chance to reveal vascular anomalies. In fact diagnostic yield of CE in the evaluation of unexplained iron deficiency anemia progressively increases with advancing age and is highest among patients over 85 years of age (the oldest). This may be explained due to the fact that ASA, NSAIDs, and warfarin usage is more in older adults compared to younger patients.

Conclusions

Since the first brief communication published in Nature in 2000 [6] introducing capsule endoscopy, CE has been so widely used in clinical practice that, although it is a useful tool for evaluating small bowel disease, some authors also demonstrated the utility and safety in patients who have undergone small-bowel resection for benign or malignant disease [3].

Nevertheless the most common indication remains the evaluation of OGB when upper endoscopy, push enteroscopy, colonoscopy, and barium contrast radiography of the small bowel are negative [7,8]. There is very little in the published literature on the use of CE in OGB in the elderly that data on contraindications and limitations are sparse. On the other hand as the population is rapidly ageing, it is expected that more elderly patients will undergo CE studies for various indications.

Although CE is a useful tool for evaluating smallbowel disease, it is impossible to view the entire small bowel in all patients because some capsules have not passed the ileo-cecal valve before battery exhaustion for various reasons. More randomized studies are necessary to examine if ageing affects either CE completion rate or the quality of bowel preparation, which are the two factors compromising the performance of CE and the small bowel transit time.

Ultimately, very few patients over the age of 80 have been included in capsule endoscopy studies, so it has been difficult to draw safe conclusions for this age group. Furthermore the selected studies took a different age cut off, using 65 years rather than 80 or 85 years (oldest old).

The main disadvantages of CE include capsule retention, false-negative results, and the lack of means for tissue proof or therapeutic intervention [9,10]. All patients in the aged group with suspected small bowel stenosis (previous history of incomplete ileus, prior abdominal operation) should receive a patency capsule before the capsule endoscopy examination as some authors suggest [4].

In conclusion, the use of CE can be considered another useful tool for the physician in the evaluation of OGB among the elderly, but other randomized studies are necessary to specifically evaluate in homogeneous age groups possible complications and contraindications.

Acknowledgements
This article has been published as part of *BMC Surgery* Volume 12 Supplement 1, 2012: Selected articles from the XXV National Congress of the Italian Society of Geriatric Surgery. The full contents of the supplement are available online at http://www.biomedcentral.com/bmcsurg/supplements/12/S1.

Author details
[1]Gastroenterology and Endoscopy Unit, T. Campanella Oncological Foundation, Catanzaro, Italy. [2]General Surgery Unit, Dept of General Surgery, Geriatric and Endoscopy, University Federico II, Naples, Italy. [3]General Surgery Unit, Dept of Medical and Surgical Biotechnology and Sciences, University la Sapienza, Roma, Italy. [4]Endocrinosurgery Unit, Dept of Medical and Surgical Sciences, University Magna Graecia, Catanzaro, Italy.

Authors' contributions
GO: conception and design, interpretation of data, given final approval of the version to be published; IML: acquisition of data, drafting the manuscript, given final approval of the version to be published; MAL: acquisition of data, drafting the manuscript, given final approval of the version to be published; RG: acquisition of data, drafting the manuscript, given final approval of the version to be published; BA: acquisition of data, drafting the manuscript, given final approval of the version to be published; GS: acquisition of data, interpretation of data, given final approval of the version to be published; AP: conception and design, critical revision, given final approval of the version to be published.

Competing interests
The authors declare that they have no competing interests.

References
1. Lanas A, García-Rodríguez LA, Polo-Tomás M, Ponce M, Alonso-Abreu I, Perez-Aisa MA, Perez-Gisbert J, Bujanda L, Castro M, Muñoz M, Rodrigo L, Calvet X, Del-Pino D, Garcia S: Time trends and impact of upper and lower gastrointestinal bleeding and perforation in clinical practice. *Am J Gastroenterol* 2009, **104**:1633-41.
2. American Gastroenterological Association medical position statement: evaluation and management of occult and obscure gastrointestinal bleeding. *Gastroenterology* 2000, **118**:197-200.
3. De Palma GD, Rega M, Puzziello A, Aprea G, Ciacci C, Castiglione F, Ciamarra P, Persico M, Patrone F, Mastantuono L, Persico G: Capsule endoscopy is safe and effective after small-bowel resection. *Gastrointest Endosc* 2004, **60**:135-8.
4. Tsibouris P, Kalantzis C, Apostolopoulos P, Alexandrakis G, Mavrogianni P, Kalantzis N: Capsule endoscopy findings in patients with occult or overt bleeding older than 80 years. *Digestive Endoscopy* 2012, **24**:154-158.
5. Papadopoulos AA, Triantafyllou K, Kalantzis C, Adamopoulos A, Ladas D, Kalli T, Apostolopoulos P, Kalantzis N, Ladas SD: Effects of Ageing on Small Bowel Video-Capsule Endoscopy Examination. *Am J Gastroenterol* 2008, **103**:2474-80.
6. Iddan G, Meron G, Glukhovsky A, Swain P: Wireless capsule endoscopy. *Nature* 2000, **405**:417.
7. Sidhu R, McAlindon ME: Age should not be a barrier to performing capsule endoscopy in the elderly with anaemia. *Dig Dis Sci* 2011, **56**:2497-8.
8. Shyung LR, Lin SC, Chang WH, Wang HY, Chu CH, Wang TE, Shih SC: Capsule endoscopy in elderly patients with obscure gastrointestinal bleeding: retrospective analysis of 152 cases. *Int J Gerontol* 2010, **4**:1.
9. Muhammad A, Pitchumoni CS: Evaluation of iron deficiency anemia in older adults: the role of wireless capsule endoscopy. *J Clin Gastroenterol* 2009, **43**:627-31.
10. Zhang BL, Chen C, Li YM: Capsule endoscopy examination identifies different leading causes of obscure gastrointestinal bleeding in patients of different ages. *Turk J Gastroenterol* 2012, **23**:220-225.

Gastric outlet obstruction at Bugando Medical Centre in Northwestern Tanzania: a prospective review of 184 cases

Hyasinta Jaka[1,2†], Mabula D Mchembe[3†], Peter F Rambau[4†] and Phillipo L Chalya[5*]

Abstract

Background: Gastric outlet obstruction poses diagnostic and therapeutic challenges to general surgeons practicing in resource-limited countries. There is a paucity of published data on this subject in our setting. This study was undertaken to highlight the etiological spectrum and treatment outcome of gastric outlet obstruction in our setting and to identify prognostic factors for morbidity and mortality.

Methods: This was a descriptive prospective study which was conducted at Bugando Medical Centre between March 2009 and February 2013. All patients with a clinical diagnosis of gastric outlet obstruction were, after informed consent for the study, consecutively enrolled into the study. Statistical data analysis was done using SPSS computer software version 17.0.

Results: A total of 184 patients were studied. More than two-third of patients were males. Patients with malignant gastric outlet obstruction were older than those of benign type. This difference was statistically significant (p < 0.001). Gastric cancer was the commonest malignant cause of gastric outlet obstruction where as peptic ulcer disease was the commonest benign cause. In children, the commonest cause of gastric outlet obstruction was congenital pyloric stenosis (13.0%). Non-bilious vomiting (100%) and weight loss (93.5%) were the most frequent symptoms. Eighteen (9.8%) patients were HIV positive with the median CD 4+ count of 282 cells/μl. A total of 168 (91.3%) patients underwent surgery. Of these, gastro-jejunostomy (61.9%) was the most common surgical procedure performed. The complication rate was 32.1 % mainly surgical site infections (38.2%). The median hospital stay and mortality rate were 14 days and 18.5% respectively. The presence of postoperative complication was the main predictor of hospital stay (p = 0.002), whereas the age > 60 years, co-existing medical illness, malignant cause, HIV positivity, low CD 4 count (<200 cells/μl), high ASA class and presence of surgical site infection significantly predicted mortality (p< 0.001). The follow up of patients was generally poor as more than 60% of patients were lost to follow up.

Conclusion: Gastric outlet obstruction in our setting is more prevalent in males and the cause is mostly malignant. The majority of patients present late with poor general condition. Early recognition of the diagnosis, aggressive resuscitation and early institution of surgical management is of paramount importance if morbidity and mortality associated with gastric outlet obstruction are to be avoided.

Keywords: Gastric outlet obstruction, Etiological spectrum, Treatment, Outcome, Tanzania

* Correspondence: drphillipoleo@yahoo.com
†Equal contributors
[5]Department of Surgery, Catholic University of Health and Allied Sciences-Bugando, Mwanza, Tanzania
Full list of author information is available at the end of the article

Background

Gastric Outlet Obstruction implies complete or incomplete obstruction of the distal stomach, pylorus or proximal duodenum [1]. This may occur as an obstructing mass lesion, external compression or as a result of obstruction from acute edema, chronic scarring and fibrosis or a combination of both [1,2]. Gastric outlet obstruction is not a single entity; it is the clinical and pathophysiological consequence of any disease process that produces a mechanical impediment to gastric emptying [3].

Globally, the incidence of gastric outlet obstruction has been reported to be less than 5% in patients with peptic ulcer disease, which is the leading benign cause of the problem, whereas the incidence of gastric outlet obstruction in patients with peripancreatic malignancy, the most common malignant etiology, has been reported as 15-20% [3-5].

Gastric Outlet Obstruction may be caused by a heterogeneous group of diseases that include both benign and malignant conditions [1,6]. In children, the condition is commonly caused by pyloric stenosis which refers to a narrowing of the pylorus, the opening from the stomach into the small intestine. In adults, mechanical obstruction due to ulcers, tumors or gastric polyps are common causes of gastric outlet obstruction [7]. In the past, when peptic ulcer disease was more prevalent, benign causes were the most common; however, one review shows that only 37% of patients with gastric outlet obstruction have benign disease and the remaining patients have obstruction secondary to malignancy [3-5].

The management of gastric outlet obstruction poses diagnostic and therapeutic challenges to general surgeons practicing in resource-limited countries. Late presentation of the disease coupled with lack of modern diagnostic and therapeutic facilities are among the hallmarks of the disease in developing countries [6]. The outcome of treatment of gastric outlet obstruction may be poor especially in developing countries where advanced diagnostic and therapeutic facilities are not readily available in most centers [6,7].

Gastric outlet obstruction is usually a preterminal event in patients with advanced malignancies of the stomach, pancreas, and duodenum. Surgery is associated with a high complication rate, and relatively high morbidity and mortality rates, due to poor nutrition and general status or progressing tumor infiltration in these patients [8]. The use of self-expandable metal stents to treat gastric outlet obstructions have been demonstrated to be an effective alternative to surgical bypass with lower morbidity and mortality rates, shorter hospitalization, and a lower cost of the overall treatment [9,10]. However, these facilities are not usually available in most centers in developing countries including Tanzania,

Despite increase in the number of admissions of these patients in our setting, no clinical study has been done to analyze this problem. This study was undertaken to highlight the etiological spectrum and treatment outcome of gastric outlet obstruction in our setting and to identify prognostic factors for morbidity and mortality.

Methods

Study design and setting

Between March 2009 and February 2013, a descriptive prospective study involving all patients with a clinical diagnosis of gastric outlet obstruction was conducted at Bugando Medical Centre. Bugando Medical Centre is located in Mwanza city along the shore of Lake Victoria in the northwestern part of Tanzania. It is a tertiary care and teaching hospital for the Catholic University of Health and Allied Sciences-Bugando (CUHAS-Bugando) and other paramedics and has a bed capacity of 1000. Bugando Medical Centre is one of the four largest referral hospitals in the country and serves as a referral centre for tertiary specialist care for a catchment population of approximately 13 million people.

Study population

All patients with a clinical diagnosis of gastric outlet obstruction seen at Bugando Medical Centre during the study period were consecutively included into the study. Patients with gastroparesis without any mechanical obstruction or a previously known cancer were excluded from the study. Patients who failed to consent for HIV testing were also excluded from the study. The diagnosis of gastric outlet obstruction was based on clinical presentation, an upper gastrointestinal barium study, and/or an inability during upper endoscopy to intubate the second portion of the duodenum.

Preoperatively, all the patients recruited into the study had intravenous fluids to correct fluid and electrolyte deficits; nasogastric suction; urethral catheterization and broad-spectrum antibiotic coverage. They had preoperative anaesthetic assessment using the American Society of Anesthetists (ASA) classification [11]. Adequate hydration was indicated by an hourly urine output of 30 ml/hour.

Relevant preoperative laboratory investigations included complete blood count, hemoglobin levels, serum albumin, serum electrolytes, urea and creatinine, HIV testing (using Tanzania HIV Rapid Test Algorithm) [12] and CD 4+ count (using FACS or FACSCALIBUR from BD Biosciences USA). Imaging investigations included plain abdominal x-rays, barium studies, abdominal ultrasound and Computerized tomography scan. The diagnosis of gastric outlet obstruction was confirmed by upper gastrointestinal endoscopy and intra-operative finding.

Intra-operatively, all patients, under general anesthesia were subjected to exploratory laparotomy through midline incision. At operation, the diagnosis of gastric outlet obstruction was made by noting a cicatrized first part of duodenum or pylorus with a dilated and thick-walled stomach. The type of surgical procedure was done according to whether the cause of gastric outlet obstruction was benign or malignant. The operations were performed either by a consultant surgeon or a senior resident under the direct supervision of a consultant surgeon.

Biopsy was taken from either a mass of peripyloric lymph nodes or any gastric mass for histological examination. Intraoperative tissue biopsy was taken for histopathological studies; a portion of the tissue was fixed in 10 per cent formalin; routine processing was done as per standard operative procedures and stained with haemotoxylin and eosin.

Postoperatively patients were kept nil orally till return of bowl sounds and at that time nasogastric tubes were removed. Intravenous antibiotics were used for up to three day and continue with oral antibiotics. The postoperative outcome was monitored; patients in ASA classes IV and V were admitted into intensive care unit after surgery. Data on each patient were entered into a questionnaire prepared for the study. The study variables included socio-demographic (i.e. age and sex, level of education, occupation and area of residence), clinical presentation, HIV status, laboratory, radiological and endoscopic findings, ASA classification, operative findings and surgical procedure performed. The variables studied in the postoperative period were postoperative complications, hospital stay and mortality. Patients were followed up for a period of twelve months or till death whichever is earlier.

Statistical analysis

The statistical analysis was performed using statistical package for social sciences (SPSS) version 17.0 for Windows (SPSS, Chicago IL, U.S.A). The median and ranges were calculated for continuous variables whereas proportions and frequency tables were used to summarize categorical variables. Continuous variables were categorized. Chi-square (χ2) test were used to test for the significance of association between the independent (predictor) and dependent (outcome) variables in the categorical variables. The level of significance was considered as $P < 0.05$. Multivariate logistic regression analysis was used to determine predictor variables that predict the outcome.

Ethical consideration

Ethical approval to conduct the study was obtained from the Catholic University of Health and Allied Sciences-Bugando/Bugando Medical Center joint institutional ethic review committee before the commencement of the study.

Patients were required to sign a written informed consent for the study and for HIV testing.

Results

Patient's characteristics

During the study period, a total of 184 patients of gastric outlet obstruction were enrolled. The age of patients at presentation ranged from 2 weeks to 78 years with a median age of 46 years. The modal age group in children was 0 – 10 years (median 2 weeks) and in adult it was 51–60 (median 52 years). Patients aged ten years and below accounted for 33 (17.3%) patients (Figure 1). Of these, 26 (78.8%) patients were aged below two months. The median age of patients with benign causes was 34 years (range 2 weeks to 46 years), while that of malignant causes was 56 years (range 42 to 78 years). The difference in age distribution of the benign and malignant disease was statistically significant ($P < 0.001$). There were 122 (66.3%) males and 62 (33.7%) were females with a male to female ratio of 2: 1. Both the benign and malignant gastric outlet obstruction was found to be more commonly amongst the males than females. The male to female ratio for benign gastric outlet obstruction was 1.2: 1, while it was 3.2: 1 for the malignant gastric outlet obstruction. This difference was statistically significant ($P < 0.001$). The majority of patients, 156 (84.8%) came from the rural areas located a considerable distance from the study area and more than 80% of them were unemployed. Most of our patients, 149 (81.0%) had either primary or no formal education and the vast majority of them, 175 (95.1%) had no identifiable health insurance.

Etiological spectrum of gastric outlet obstruction

The etiology of gastric outlet obstruction was benign in 82 (44.6%) cases, whereas 102 (55.4%) patients had

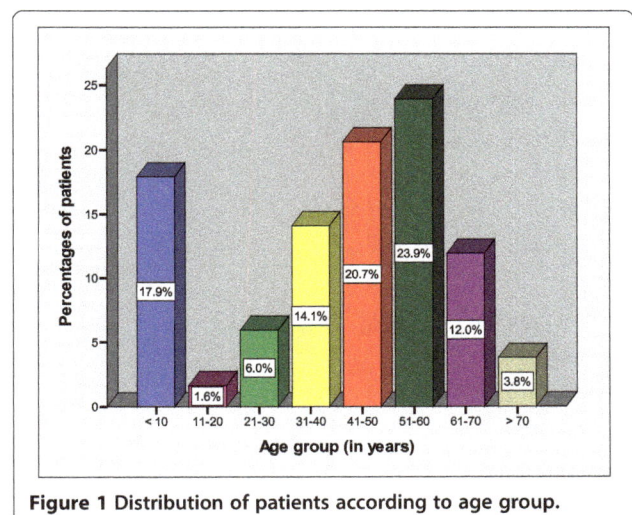

Figure 1 Distribution of patients according to age group.

malignant cause. Peptic ulcer disease was the commonest cause among the benign group in 28.2% of patients, whereas the commonest cause among the malignant group was gastric cancer in 42.9% of patients. In children, the commonest cause of gastric outlet obstruction was pyloric stenosis accounting for 13.0% of cases (Table 1).

Clinical presentation of patients with gastric outlet obstruction

The duration of illness ranged from 1 week to 8 years with a median duration of 6 months respectively. The time interval between symptom onset and diagnosis was often more than 6 months in the majority of patients (148, 80.4%). The clinical presentation of gastric outlet obstruction is shown in Table 2. Previous history of peptic ulcer disease was reported in 35 (19.0%) patients. Patients with a previous history of peptic ulcer disease had had symptoms for durations ranging from six months to 10 years (median 2 years) and all of them were not on regular anti-ulcer therapy. History of alcohol and smoking was reported in 104 (56.5%) and 67 (36.4%) patients respectively.

In this study, nine (4.9%) patients had associated comorbid illness namely tuberculosis in 3 patients and hypertension, diabetes mellitus and sickle cell disease in 2 patients each respectively. Eighteen (9.8%) patients were HIV positive. Of these, 5 (27.8%) patients were known cases on ant-retroviral therapy (ARV) and the remaining 13 (72.2%) patients were newly diagnosed patients.

Table 1 Distribution of patients according to causes of gastric outlet obstruction

Causes of gastric outlet obstruction	Number of patients	Percentage
Benign causes	**82**	**44.6**
• Peptic ulcers	52	28.3
• Hypertrophic pyloric stenosis	24	13.0
• Gastric polyp	2	1.1
• Caustic ingestion	2	1.1
• Iatrogenic	1	0.5
• Gastric/duodenal tuberculosis	1	0.5
• Prepyloric web	1	0.5
Malignant causes	**102**	**55.4**
• Gastric cancer	79	42.9
• Carcinoma pancreas	16	8.7
• Periampullary Ca	3	1.6
• Cholangiocarcinoma	3	1.6
• Duodenal carcinoma	1	0.5

Table 2 Distribution of patients according to clinical presentation

Clinical presentation	Frequency	Percentage
Non-bilious vomiting	184	100
Weight loss	172	93.5
Succession splash	144	78.3
Bloating/epigastric fullness,	104	56.5
Epigastric pain	104	56.5
Dehydration	101	54.9
Epigastric mass	46	25.0
Shock	23	12.5

Investigations among patients with gastric outlet obstruction

One hundred thirty-two (71.7%) of the patients had plain abdominal x-ray films available for review and demonstrated gastric air-fluid levels in 102 (77.3%) patients. Barium meal and follow through performed in 47 (25.5%) revealed an enlarged stomach and pyloroduodenal stenosis in 42 (89.4%) patients. Upper gastrointestinal endoscopy (oesophagogastroduodenoscopy) performed in 154 (83.7%) revealed positive results in all patients (100%) and this was diagnostic. Abdominal ultrasound and Computerized tomography (CT) scan performed in 89 (48.4%) and 18 (9.8%) patients demonstrated positive results in 82 (92.1%) and 18 (100%) patients respectively. Complete Blood Count, Hemoglobin levels and ESR were done in all patients. More than eighty percent of the patients had Hemoglobin levels less than 10.0 gm/dl and ESR in the first hour was found ranging between 12–148 mm. Serum electrolytes performed in all patients revealed *hypokalemic hypochloremic metabolic alkalosis* in 106 (57.6%) patients. Serum albumin done in 126 (68.5%) patients revealed hypoalbuminaemia in 108 (58.7%) patients. HIV status was known in all patients and revealed positive results in 18 (9.8%) patients. CD 4+ count among HIV positive patients was available in only 15 patients and ranged from 102 cells/μl to 745 cells/μl with the median CD 4+ count of 282 cells/μl. A total of eight (44.4%) HIV positive patients had CD4+ count below 200 cells/μl and the remaining 10 (55.6%) patients had CD4+ count of ≥200 cells/μl.

Pre-operative anaesthetic assessment and admission patterns

All patients who were scheduled for operation (168) were assessed pre-operatively using the American Society of Anesthetists (ASA) pre-operative grading (Table 3). The majority of patients had ASA class II accounting for 33.7% of cases (Figure 2). A high ASA class was found to be an independent predictor of mortality (p = 0.003).

Table 3 American Society of Anesthetists (ASA) classification

ASA class	Description
I	Healthy individual with no systemic disease
II	Mild systemic disease not limiting activity
III	Severe systemic disease that limits activity but is not incapacitating
IV	Incapacitating systemic disease which is constantly life threatening
V	Moribund, not expected to survive 24 hours with or without operation

Note: E is added to the class when the case is an emergency e.g. IIE refers to ASA class scheduled for emergency surgery.

Table 4 Distribution of patients according to type of surgical procedure (N= 168)

Type of surgical procedure	Frequency	Percentage
Gastro-jejunostomy	104	61.9
Ramstedt's operation (pyloromyotomy)	24	14.3
Gastrectomy	22	13.1
Laparotomy ± biopsy only (for malignant obstruction)	7	4.2
Truncal vagotomy	5	3.0
Heineke-Mikulicz pyloroplasty	4	2.4
Gastric polyp excision	2	1.2

The majority of patients, 142 (77.2%) were admitted through surgical outpatient clinic and the remaining 42 (22.8%) patients were admitted through the Accident & Emergency department. Thirty-eight (20.7%) patients were, after operation, admitted in the Intensive Care Unit (ICU) before being admitted to the general surgical wards. Out of these, 30 (78.9%) were subjected to ventilatory support for a median duration of 8 days (range 1–14 days).

Treatment modalities
A total of 168 (91.3%) patients underwent surgery. Of these, gastro-jejunostomy was the most common surgical procedure performed accounting for 61.9% of cases (Table 4). Fourteen (7.6%) patients were treated successively with Histamine-2 (H2) blockers and proton pump inhibitors. The remaining two (1.2%) patients were unfit for surgery due to advanced disease. One patient, who had gastro-duodenal tuberculosis, after histological conformation of tuberculosis, was treated postoperatively with anti-tuberculous drugs with good results.

Treatment outcome
Fifty-four (32.1%) patients had 68 post-complications as shown in Table 5. Surgical site infection was the most common post-operative complication accounting for 38.2% of cases.

The overall length of hospital stay (LOS) ranged from 4 to 72 days with a median of 14 days. The median LOS for non-survivors was 7 days (range 1-14 days). Patients who developed post-operative complications stayed longer in the hospital and this was statistically significant (P = 0.002).

In this study, thirty-four patients died giving a mortality rate of 18.5%. According to multivariate logistic regression analysis, age > 60 years (OR = 2.3, 95% C.I. (1.2-6.9), p= 0.003), co-existing medical illness (OR = 8.5, 95% C.I. (2.5-18.9), p = 0.011), malignant cause (OR = 1.3, 95% CI (1.9- 8.4), p = 0.021), HIV positivity (OR = 2.9, 95% CI (1.1- 8.8), p = 0.012), low CD 4 count (<200 cells/µl) (OR = 2.0, 95% CI (1.9-10.5), p = 0.001), high ASA class (OR = 8.1, 95% CI (2.6-12.7), p = 0.014), surgical site infection (OR = 4.5, 95% CI (1.1-8.6), p = 0.022) were the main predictors of mortality.

Table 5 Distribution of patients according to post-operative complications (N= 68)

Post –operative complications	Frequency	Percentage
Surgical site infection	26	38.2
Postoperative pyrexia	10	14.7
Pneumonia	8	11.8
Postoperative vomiting	6	8.8
Afferent loop syndrome	4	5.9
Dumping	4	5.9
Diarrhea	3	4.4
Deep venous thrombosis	3	4.4
Urinary tract infection	2	2.9
Paralytic ileus	1	1.5
Peritonitis	1	1.5
Total	**68**	**100**

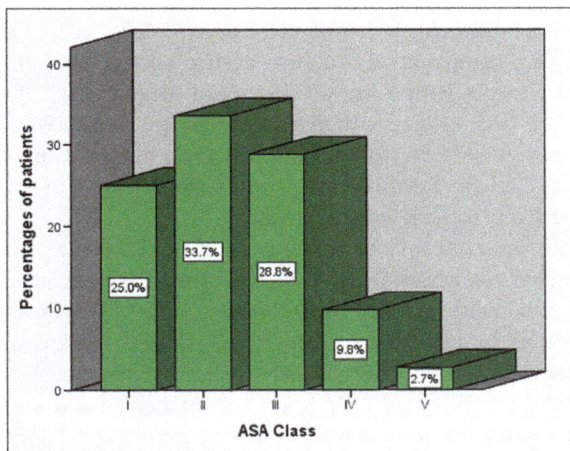

Figure 2 Distribution of patients according to ASA classification.

Follow up of patients

Out of 150 survivors, one hundred thirty-two (88.0%) patients were discharged well, twelve (8.0%) were discharged for terminal care and the remaining six (4.0%) patients were discharged against medical advice. No patient among survivors in this study had permanent disabilities (Figure 3). Of the 150 survivors, fifty-four (36.0%) patients were available for follow up at three to six months after discharge and the remaining 96 (64.0%) patients were lost to follow up.

Discussion

Gastric outlet obstruction poses diagnostic and therapeutic challenges to general surgeons practicing in resource-limited countries and contributes significantly to high morbidity and mortality [1-6]. This study was conducted in our environment to describe our own experiences in the management of this challenging disease; the problem not previously studied at our centre or any other hospital in the country. In this review, the highest age incidence of the patients at presentation was in the fourth decade of age and males were more affected. Most of the patients with benign gastric outlet obstruction in our study were in younger age group while malignant causes were in elder age group. The incidence of malignant gastric outlet obstruction in patients of older age group was also reported by others [1,7,13]. Our demographic profile is in sharp contrast to what is reported in other studies [6,9] where the majority of the patients are in the fifth and sixth decade of life. This discrepancy in age incidence may be attributed to by the large number of children in the current study. We could not establish the reasons for the male predominance.

Gastric outlet obstruction has been reported to be more prevalent in people with low socio-economic status [6]. This is reflected in our study where most of patients had either primary or no formal education and more than seventy-five percent of them were unemployed. The majority of patients in the present study came from the rural areas located a considerable distance from the study area and more than eighty percent of them had no identifiable health insurance. Similar observation was reported by others [6,13]. This observation has an implication on accessibility to health care facilities and awareness of the disease.

The majority of patients in this study had malignant gastric outlet obstruction which is in agreement with other studies reported elsewhere [1,3-5], but at variant with Kolisso [6] in Ethiopia who reported benign gastric outlet obstruction (peptic ulcer disease) as the most common cause of gastric outlet obstruction. In our study, gastric cancer was the commonest cause of malignant gastric outlet obstruction while peptic ulcer disease was the commonest benign cause. This is keeping with other studies which reported similar etiological pattern [1,13,14]. The predominant causes of gastric outlet obstruction have changed substantively with the identification of *Helicobacter pylori* and the use of proton pump inhibitors. Until the late 1970s, benign disease was responsible for the majority of cases of gastric outlet obstruction in adults, while malignancy accounted for only 10 to 39 percent of cases [2,13]. By contrast, in recent decades, 50 to 80 percent cases have been attributable to malignancy [2,13,15,16].

The clinical presentation of gastric outlet obstruction in our patients is not different from those in other studies [2-7], with non-bilious vomiting being common to all the patients. In keeping with other studies [6,16], the majority of our patients had symptoms of more than 6 months duration at the time of presentation. Late presentation in our study may be attributed to lack of accessibility to health care facilities and lack of awareness of the disease. It is worth noting that seventeen (18%) of our gastric outlet obstruction patients secondary to complicated peptic ulcer had no previous history of ulcer symptoms prior to the onset of illness. Patients with no previous diagnosis of peptic ulcer have a higher risk of developing complications such as gastric outlet obstruction than patients with a known history of ulcer disease. This may be because preventative measures are more likely to have been taken in patients with a known history of peptic ulcer disease. Furthermore, these patients are perhaps more likely to seek treatment earlier.

The presence of co-existing medical illness has been reported elsewhere to have an effect on the outcome of patients with gastric outlet obstruction [6]. This is reflected in our study where patients with co-existing medical illness had significantly high mortality rate.

The prevalence of HIV infection in the present study was 9.8%, a figure that is significantly higher than that in the general population in Tanzania (6.5%) [17]. This difference was statistically significant (P < 0.001). However,

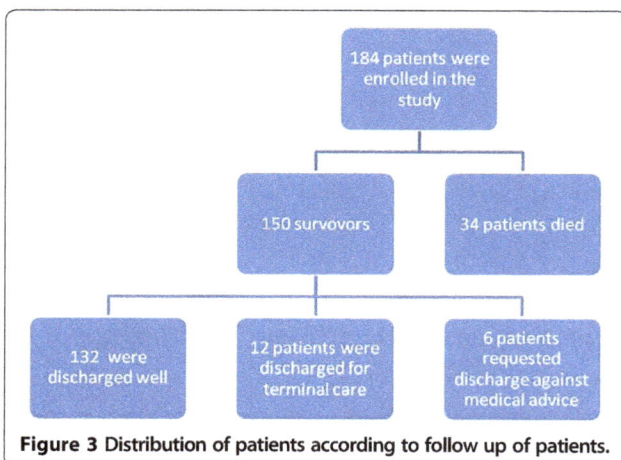

Figure 3 Distribution of patients according to follow up of patients.

failure to detect HIV infection during window period and exclusion of some patients from the study may have underestimated the prevalence of HIV infection among these patients. We could not establish the reason for the high HIV seroprevalence in our study population and we could not find any literature regarding the effect of HIV infection on the etiology and outcome of patient with gastric outlet obstruction. This calls for a need to research on this observation. In this study, HIV infection was found to be associated with poor postoperative outcome. This observation calls for routine HIV screening in patients with gastric outlet obstruction.

In agreement with other studies [1,6], the diagnosis of gastric outlet obstruction in this study was based on clinical presentation, an upper gastrointestinal barium study, and/or an inability during upper endoscopy to intubate the second portion of the duodenum (upper gastrointestinal endoscopy) and confirmed by histology and intra-operative findings. Other diagnostic investigations included abdominal ultrasound and computerized tomography (CT) scan.

The treatment of gastric outlet obstruction depends on the cause, but is usually either surgical or medical. In most patients with peptic ulcer disease, the edema will usually settle with conservative management with nasogastric suction, replacement of fluids and electrolytes and proton pump inhibitors [8]. Surgery is indicated in cases of gastric outlet obstruction in which there is significant obstruction and in cases where medical therapy has failed [8,18]. In the current study, gastro-jejunostomy was the most frequent type of surgical procedure performed. This is in line with other studies done elsewhere [19-21]. The high rate of gastro-jejunostomy in our study is attributed to the large number of patients with malignant gastric outlet obstruction. Traditionally, malignant gastric outlet obstruction has been treated surgically, usually by creating a gastro-jejunostomy. More recently, the use of endoscopically placed self-expandable metal stents (SEMS) has become a routine practice [9,10]. However, this procedure was not popular in our study due to lack of this facility in our centre.

The presence of complications has an impact on the final outcome of patients presenting with gastric outlet obstruction [18]. In our review, the postoperative complication rate was 32.1%, a figure which is higher than that reported by other authors [22,23]. In agreement with other studies [6,22,23], surgical site infection was the most common postoperative complications in the present study. High rate of surgical site infection in this study may be attributed to HIV seropositivity and low CD 4 count.

The overall median duration of hospital stay in the present study was 14 days which is higher than that reported by Kolisso [6] in Ethiopia. This can be explained by the presence of large number of patients with postoperative complications in our study. However, due to the poor socio-economic conditions in Tanzania, the duration of inpatient stay for our patients may be longer than expected. Prolonged duration of hospital stay has an impact on hospital resources as well as on increased cost of health care, loss of productivity and reduced quality of life.

The overall mortality rate in this study was 18.5% and it was significantly associated with the age > 60 years, co-existing medical illness, malignant cause, HIV positivity, low CD 4 count (<200 cells/µl), high ASA class and presence of surgical site infection. Addressing these factors responsible for high mortality in our patients is mandatory to be able to reduce mortality associated with this disease.

Self discharge by patient against medical advice is a recognized problem in our setting. Similarly, poor follow up visits after discharge from hospitals remain a cause for concern. These issues are often the results of poverty, long distance from the hospitals and ignorance and need to be addressed.

Delayed presentation and the large number of loss to follow up were the major limitations in this study. However, despite these limitations, the study has provided local data that can be utilized by health care providers to plan for preventive strategies as well as establishment of management guidelines for these patients. The challenges identified in the management of patients with gastric outlet obstruction in our environment need to be addressed, in order to deliver optimal care for these patients.

Conclusion

Gastric outlet obstruction is a common surgical problem in our setting and poses diagnostic and therapeutic challenges. It is more common among males with malignant causes being more prevalent. The benign gastric outlet obstruction is seen in young patients while malignant causes in elder age group. Gastric cancer is the commonest malignant cause of gastric outlet obstruction whereas peptic ulcer diseases the commonest benign etiology. In children, congenital pyloric stenosis is the commonest cause of gastric outlet obstruction. The majority of patients present late with poor general condition. Gastro-jejunostomy is the most common surgical procedure performed. The result of this study suggests that early recognition of the diagnosis, aggressive resuscitation and early institution of surgical management is of paramount importance if morbidity and mortality associated with gastric outlet obstruction are to be avoided.

Competing interests
The authors declare that they have no competing interests.

Authors' contributions

HJ and PLC conceived the study and participated in the literature search, writing of the manuscript and editing the article. PLC submitted the manuscript and is the corresponding author. MDM and PFR participated in study design, data analysis, manuscript writing & editing. In addition, HJ did the endoscopic examination and PFR did the histopathological examination. All the authors read and approved the final manuscript.

Acknowledgements

The authors would like to acknowledge all those who participated in the preparation of this manuscript, and those who were involved in the care of our patients.

Author details

[1]Department of Internal Medicine, Catholic University of Health and Allied Sciences- Bugando, Mwanza, Tanzania. [2]Endoscopic unit, Bugando Medical Center, Mwanza, Tanzania. [3]Department of Surgery, Muhimbili University of Health and Allied Sciences, Dar Es Salaam, Tanzania. [4]Department of Pathology, Catholic University of Health and Allied Sciences- Bugando, Mwanza, Tanzania. [5]Department of Surgery, Catholic University of Health and Allied Sciences- Bugando, Mwanza, Tanzania.

References

1. Samad A, Whanzada TW, Shoukat I: Gastric outlet obstruction: change in etiology. *Pak J Surg* 2007, **23**:29–32.
2. Johnson CD: Gastric outlet obstruction-malignant until proven otherwise. *Am J Gastroenterol* 1995, **90**:1740.
3. Tendler DA: Malignant gastric outlet obstruction: bridging another divide. *Am J Gastroenterol* 2002, **97**:4.
4. Sachdeva AK, Zaren HA, Sigel B: Surgical treatment of peptic ulcer disease. *Med Clin North Am* 1991, **75**:999–1012.
5. Sohn TA, Lillemoe KD, Cameron JL: Surgical palliation of unresectable periampullary adenocarcinoma in the 1990s. *J Am Coll Surg* 1999, **188**:658–666.
6. Kotisso R: Gastric outlet obstruction in Northwestern Ethiopia. *East Centr Afr J Surg* 2000, **5**:25–29.
7. Appasani S, Kochhar S, Nagi B, Gupta V, Kochhar R: Benign gastric outlet obstruction–spectrum and management. *Trop Gastroenterol* 2011, **32**:259–266.
8. Doherty GM, Way LW (Eds): *Current Surgical Diagnosis & Treatment*. 12th edition. New York: Mcgraw-Hill; 2006.
9. Gaidos JKJ, Draganov PV: Treatment of malignant gastric outlet obstruction with endoscopically placed self -expandable metal stents. *World J Gastroenterol* 2009, **15**:4365–4371.
10. Baron TH: Expandable metal stents for the treatment of cancerous obstruction of the gastrointestinal tract. *N Engl J Med* 2001, **344**:1681–1687.
11. Wolters U, Wolf T, Stutzer H, Schroder T: ASA classification and perioperative variables as predictors of postoperative outcome. *Brit J Anesthesia* 1996, **77**:217–222.
12. Lyamuya EF, Aboud S, Urassa WK, Sufi J, Mbwana J, Ndungulile F, Massambu C: Evaluation of rapid HIV assays and development of national rapid HIV test algorithms in Dar es salaam. *Tanzania BMC Infect Dis* 2009, **9**:19.
13. Shone DN, Nikoomanesh P, Smith-Meek MM, Bender JS: Malignancy is the most common cause of gastric outlet obstruction in the era of H2 blockers. *Am J Gastroenterol* 1995, **90**:1769–1770.
14. Misra SP, Dwivedi M, Misra V: Malignancy is the most common cause of gastric outlet obstruction even in a developing country. *Endoscopy* 1998, **30**:484–486.
15. Johnson CD, Ellis H: Gastric outlet obstruction now predicts malignancy. *Br J Surg* 1990, **77**:1023.
16. Chowdhury A, Dhali GK, Banerjee PK: Etiology of gastric outlet obstruction. *Am J Gastroenterol* 1996, **91**:1679.
17. Urassa M, Isingo R, Kumogola Y, Mwidunda P, Helelwa M, Changulucha J, Mngara J, Zaba B, Calleja T, Slaymaker E: *Effect of PMTCT availability on choice of ANC in Mwanza and Magu districts and its impact on HIV sentinel surveillanc*. Tanzania: Report of ANC surveillance Mwanza and Magu Districts; 2007.
18. Mieny CJ: *General Surgery.6th Ed*. Pretoria: Van Schaik; 2006.
19. Kikuchi S, Tsutsumi O, Kobayashi N: Does gastrojejunostomy for unresectable cancer of the gastric antrum offer satisfactory palliation? *Hepatogastroenterology* 1999, **46**:584–587.
20. Mittal A, Windsor J, Woodfield J, Casey P, Lane M: Matched study of three methods for palliation of malignant pyloroduodenal obstruction. *Br J Surg* 2004, **91**:205–209.
21. Alam TA, Baines M, Parker MC: The management of gastric outlet obstruction secondary to inoperable cancer. *Surg Endosc* 2003, **17**:320–323.
22. Dogo D, Yawe T, Gali BM: Gastric outlet obstruction in Maiduguri. *Afr J Med Sci* 1999, **28**:199–201.
23. Olaolorun DA, Oladiran IO: Gastric outlet obstruction in Ogbomoso, Nigeria. *West Afr J Med* 2001, **20**:234–237.

5

Pylorus preserving loop duodeno-enterostomy with sleeve gastrectomy - preliminary results

Jodok Matthias Grueneberger[1*], Iwona Karcz-Socha[2], Goran Marjanovic[1], Simon Kuesters[1], Krystyna Zwirska-Korczala[2], Katharina Schmidt[3] and W Konrad Karcz[3]

Abstract

Background: Bariatric operations mostly combine a restrictive gastric component with a rerouting of the intestinal passage. The pylorus can thereby be alternatively preserved or excluded. With the aim of performing a "pylorus-preserving gastric bypass", we present early results of a proximal postpyloric loop duodeno-jejunostomy associated with a sleeve gastrectomy (LSG) compared to results of a parallel, but distal LSG with a loop duodeno-ileostomy as a two-step procedure.

Methods: 16 patients underwent either a two-step LSG with a distal loop duodeno-*ileostomy* (DIOS) as revisional bariatric surgery or a combined single step operation with a proximal duodeno-*jejunostomy* (DJOS). Total small intestinal length was determined to account for inter-individual differences.

Results: Mean operative time for the second-step of the DIOS operation was 121 min and 147 min for the combined DJOS operation. The overall intestinal length was 750.8 cm (range 600-900 cm) with a bypassed limb length of 235.7 cm in DJOS patients. The mean length of the common channel in DIOS patients measured 245.6 cm. Overall excess weight loss (%EWL) of the two-step DIOS procedure came to 38.31% and 49.60%, DJOS patients experienced an %EWL of 19.75% and 46.53% at 1 and 6 months, resp. No complication related to the duodeno-enterostomy occurred.

Conclusions: Loop duodeno-enterosomies with sleeve gastrectomy can be safely performed and may open new alternatives in bariatric surgery with the possibility for inter-individual adaptation.

Background

Bariatric surgery has proven to be the most effective treatment for long-term weight loss and metabolic rebalancing in obese patients [1,2]. Most procedures combine a restrictive gastric component with a rerouting of the intestinal passage. Prominent examples are the Roux-en-Y gastric bypass (RYGB) or the biliopancreatic diversion (BPD). Gastric restriction either involves the entire stomach therefore preserving the pylorus when reconstructing the intestinal passage, or only the proximal part of the stomach is used to form a gastric pouch thus leaving a remnant stomach. Passage reconstruction then requires a gastro-enterostomy.

Preserving the pylorus when bypassing the duodenum has led to important technical changes in bariatric surgery. In order to avoid a dumping syndrome and marginal ulcers that occasionally occurred after Scopinaro´s initial BPD, Marceau et al. successfully changed the technique to perform a biliopancreatic diversion with duodenal switch (BPD/DS) with similar limb variations, using however a postpyloric reconstruction [3].

The RYGB generally is one of the best established procedures in bariatric surgery [4]. However the failure rate with weight regain due to a dilatation of the gastric pouch, gastro-jejunostomy and proximal jejunum is up to 35% [5]. Recently, bile reflux was identified as one important cause of postoperative pain [6]. Again, a postpyloric reconstruction seems tempting for this procedure.

We here present perioperative data of a proximal (similar to RYGB) and distal (similar to BPD/DS) postpyloric loop duodeno-enterostomy with sleeve gastrectomy. The distal duodeno-enterostomy, based on the

* Correspondence: jodok.grueneberger@uniklinik-freiburg.de
[1]Department of General and Visceral Surgery, University of Freiburg, Hugstetter Strasse 55, 79106 Freiburg, Germany
Full list of author information is available at the end of the article

earlier described single anastomosis duodeno-ileostomy associated to a sleeve gastrectomy (SADI-S) operation [7], was performed as revisionary bariatric operation.

Methods

Patients

From October 2011 to September 2012, 16 patients underwent loop duodeno-enterostomies for bariatric surgery. Explicit written informed consent for operation and data recording was obtained from all patients. Data recording and evaluation was approved by the ethics committee of the University of Freiburg (ref. number 321/13) and was in accordance with the Declaration of Helsinki. A proximal duodeno-jejunostomy with sleeve gastrectomy (DJOS) was conducted as an alternative to RYGB in 7 selected patients eligible for bariatric surgery with a body mass index (BMI) range from 35.7 to 47.9 kg/m^2 (median BMI 42.7 kg/m^2). In case of previous gastric banding and relevant perigastric scar tissue, instead of a sleeve gastrectomy, a gastric plicature was performed (n = 3/7) to minimize operative risk. Two-step DIOS was performed as revisionary surgery after failed RYGB due to dumping syndrome (n = 2/9) or after sleeve gastrectomy with insufficient weight loss alone (3/9) or in combination with persisting type 2 diabetes (T2DM, 4/9). All operations were performed by the same senior surgeon. In order to prevent vitamin deficiencies, besides a multivitamin, patients are prescribed Calcium (500 mg twice daily), Vitamin D3 (1000 IU daily), folic acid (5 mg daily) and iron (100 mg daily) supplementation.

Data recording included length of hospital stay, preoperative BMI, presence of medical comorbidities, intra- and postoperative complications, management of complications, total operative time, common channel length and weight loss. Total intestinal length was recorded only after February 2012. All data were entered prospectively into a custom-designed database. The patients had the same follow-up protocol at the outpatient clinic at 1, 3, 6, and 12 months after surgery, followed by an annual visit.

Operative technique

The patient is placed in the split-leg position with the operating surgeon standing between the legs. Trocar positions are similar to those used for banded sleeve gastrectomy [8].

Sleeve gastrectomy is conducted as described earlier [8]. In case of a stomach plication, we use a modified technique described by Talebpour et al. applying at least two rows of plication using a 3-0 V-Loc™ Suture (Covidien, Dublin, Ireland) [9]. The second part of the operation (second step, when performing a two-step procedure) begins with separation of the duodenum

with an endstapling device (GIA- Roticulators, Covidien, Dublin, Ireland, violet cartridge) under preservation of the right gastric artery. Before performing the duodeno-enterostomy, the length of the small bowel is determined to account for inter-individual differences. After measurement, the omega loop should be placed near the postpyloric duodenum with special attention to intestinal alignment to avoid mesenteric malrotation. The position of the duodeno-enterostomy is determined to be aboral to the Treitz ligament, 1/3 of total small bowel length for DJOS (Figure 1), and 2/3 for DIOS (Figure 2). The duodeno-enterostomy is performed as an antecolic, continuous end-to-side hand-sewn anastomosis using 3-0 V-loc™ sutures (Covidien, Dublin, Ireland, Figure 3). Diluted half-strength methylene blue dye (150-200 ml) is used for leak testing. Finally, a drain is put towards the duodenal stump. In case of a two-step procedure, the second part of the operation is conducted separately, then sparing the top left 5 mm trocar needed for sleeve gastrectomy.

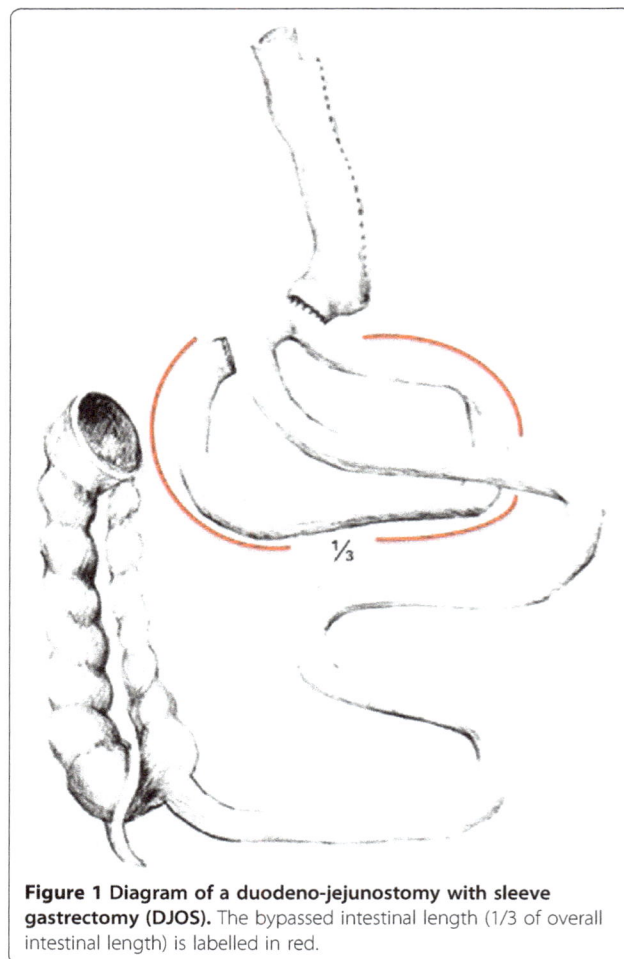

Figure 1 Diagram of a duodeno-jejunostomy with sleeve gastrectomy (DJOS). The bypassed intestinal length (1/3 of overall intestinal length) is labelled in red.

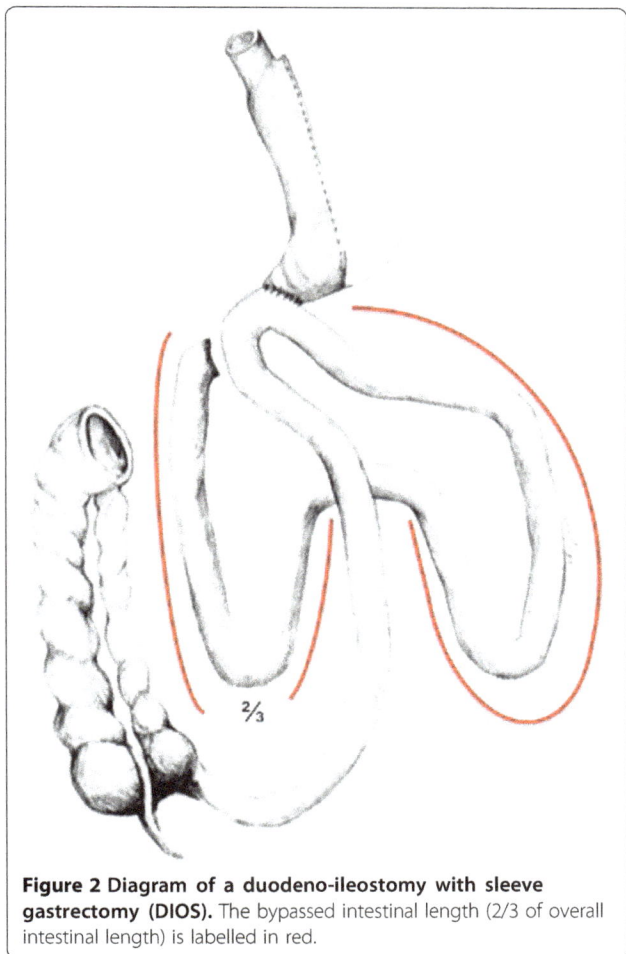

Figure 2 Diagram of a duodeno-ileostomy with sleeve gastrectomy (DIOS). The bypassed intestinal length (2/3 of overall intestinal length) is labelled in red.

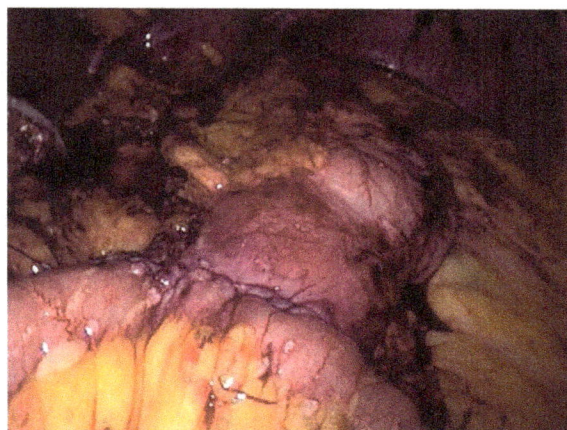

Figure 3 Final aspect of the duodeno-enterostomy.

Statistical analysis

Prism 5 for Mac OS X (GraphPad Software, Inc.) was used for all statistical analyses. Statistical significance was set at an alpha of 0.05 for all analyses.

Results

16 patients underwent laparoscopic DIOS and DJOS operations with a mean duration of 121 min and 147 min, respectively. Overall, 9 patients had undergone previous weight loss surgery, mainly gastric banding (Table 1). A complex gastric reconstruction from RYGB to a sleeve stomach due to uncontrolled dumping syndrome had been conducted earlier in 2 patients. The mean latency between the sleeve and the second step DIOS operation was 17.9 months (Table 1).

One intestinal perforation occurred upon insertion of the first trocar in a patient with previous gastric banding and subsequent adhesions to the abdominal wall. No complications specific to the duodeno-enterostomy were noted (Table 2).

Intestinal length

The overall total intestinal length was 750.8 cm (Table 2). Although there was no correlation of total intestinal length and preoperative bodyweight (linear regression p = 0.76), the total small intestinal length in DIOS patients was significantly longer than in DJOS patients (Mann-Whitney P = 0.038, Table 2).

Weight loss

The mean preoperative BMI was 40.63 kg/m^2 in DIOS and 41.60 kg/m^2 in DJOS patients (Table 1). Patients after primary DJOS operation presented with an excess weight loss (%EWL) of 19.75% and 46.53% at 1 and 6 months (Figure 4A). The overall %EWL of the combined DIOS procedure was 38.31% and 49.60% (Figure 4B). Mean weight loss through LSG alone was 31.73% (range -2.67 - 69.54). Further %EWL came to 18.73% at 1 and 33.03% at 6 months following the second step operation. In this early follow-up, 1 patient did not lose any additional weight after the second step operation despite bypassing 520 cm of small intestine and clinical signs of malabsorption. Furthermore, control CT sleeve volumetry revealed a small volume of 142 ml at 10 months postoperatively indicating sustained restriction.

Comorbidities

Prior to LSG, 88.9% of patients suffered from T2DM. At the time of the second-step DIOS operation, 44.4% had remained on anti-diabetic medication, 33.3% on insulin therapy (Table 3). 3 months after completion of the second step, only 11.1% (1 patient) still needed anti-diabetic medication. Glycated haemoglobin levels dropped from 6.8% to 5.7% in DIOS and from 8.0% to 6.9% in DJOS patients 6 months after the operation (both NS). LSG alone led to a relief of arterial hypertension in 50% of DIOS patients, with 3 patients remaining on antihypertensive drugs up to the second step operation. Only 1

Table 1 Patient characteristics

	DIOS	DJOS	Overall
Patients	9	7 (gastric plicature: n = 3)	16
Male/Female	3/6	1/6	4/12
Age	52	44	49
Body weight prior to duodeno-enterostomy	114.2 kg (85 – 145 kg)	117.4 kg (103 – 145 kg)	
BMI prior to duodeno-enterostomy	40.63 kg/m^2 (33.20 – 55.94 kg/m^2)	41.60 kg/m^2 (35.74 – 47.90 kg/m^2)	
Body weight prior to LSG	140.1 kg (105 – 175 kg)		
Gap between LSG and DIOS	17.9 months (3.65 – 41.96 months)		
%EWL before 2nd step surgery	31.73% (-2.67 – 69.54)		
Previous bariatric surgery	5 of 9 (gastric ballon 2, LGB 1, RYGB 2)	4 of 7 (LGB 4)	9 of 16

Values are expressed as means; laparoscopic gastric banding (LGB), Roux-en-Y gastric bypass (RYGB), % excess weight loss (%EWL).

patient remained on antihypertensive drugs 3 months after the DIOS operation. Interestingly, this is the same patient who also had to continue insulin treatment.

Reflux was present in the majority of patients (Table 3) with overall 87.5% of patients requiring proton-pump-inhibiting treatment. Corresponding to the shorter common channel, diarrhoea was present in 66.7% of DIOS and in 28.6% of DJOS patients. Overall, 62.5% of patients complaining of diarrhoea reported only occasional episodes. Occasional episodes of dumping were reported by only 1 patient after a DJOS operation.

Discussion

Major bariatric surgery combines a restrictive gastric component with a rearrangement of the small intestinal passage. Whenever reconnecting the stomach pouch to the intestine, the pylorus can either be preserved (BPD-DS), or excluded, as it is after common RYGB and Mini-Gastric-Bypass (MGB) [3,10]. In order to preserve the pylorus for a bypass-like procedure, we combined a LSG with an end-to-side duodenojeunostomy – DJOS.

Why should the pylorus be preserved? Historically, this debate was initiated after Watson introduced a pylorus-preserving alternative to the classic Whipple procedure in performing a pancreatic head resection [11]. This modification should prevent the patient from typical post-gastrectomy symptoms such as dumping, diarrhoea and dyspepsia [12]. A prospective randomized trial comparing the two procedures could later demonstrate an increased quality of life regarding appetite, nausea and diarrhoea resulting in a faster regain of bodyweight [13]. For bariatric surgery, Hess et al. demonstrated a reduction of marginal ulcers by 90% and no dumping syndrome when the pylorus was preserved during a BPD/DS [14].

Postpyloric anastomosis furthermore allows for loop reconstruction, whereas a "prepyloric" gastro-entero anastomosis necessitates rerouting the biliopancreatic fluids via a foot-point or a Roux-en-Y reconstruction to avoid biliary reflux. Disregarding this principle, surgeons use a loop reconstruction without rerouting biliopancreatic fluids in performing a MGB [10,15]. Although this operation enables excellent weight loss with a low complication rate, operative revision after MGB was mostly due to internal bile reflux and marginal ulcers [16]. Marginal ulcers furthermore also occur after conventional RYGB in about 13% of patients, even though a

Table 2 Perioperative data

	DIOS	DJOS	Overall
Surgical complication	0 of 9	1 of 7 (trocar perforation)	1 of 16 (6.3%)
Operative revision	0 of 9	1 of 7	1 of 16 (6.3%)
Expansion on surgery	5 of 9 (cholecystectomy 3, appendectomy 2, umbilical hernia repair 1, end-to-end jejunojejunostomy after RYGB 1)	1 of 7 (gastric band removal 1)	
Duration of surgery	120.6 min	147 min	$P = 0.112^{\psi}$
Length of small intestine	808.3 cm (range: 760 – 850 cm)	701.4 cm (range: 600 – 900 cm)	750.8 cm $P = 0.038^{\psi}$
Length of bilio-pancreatic channel	538.3 cm	235.7 cm	
Length of common channel	245.6 cm	465.7 cm	

Values are expressed as means or absolute numbers.
$^{\psi}$Mann-Whitney test DIOS vs. DJOS.

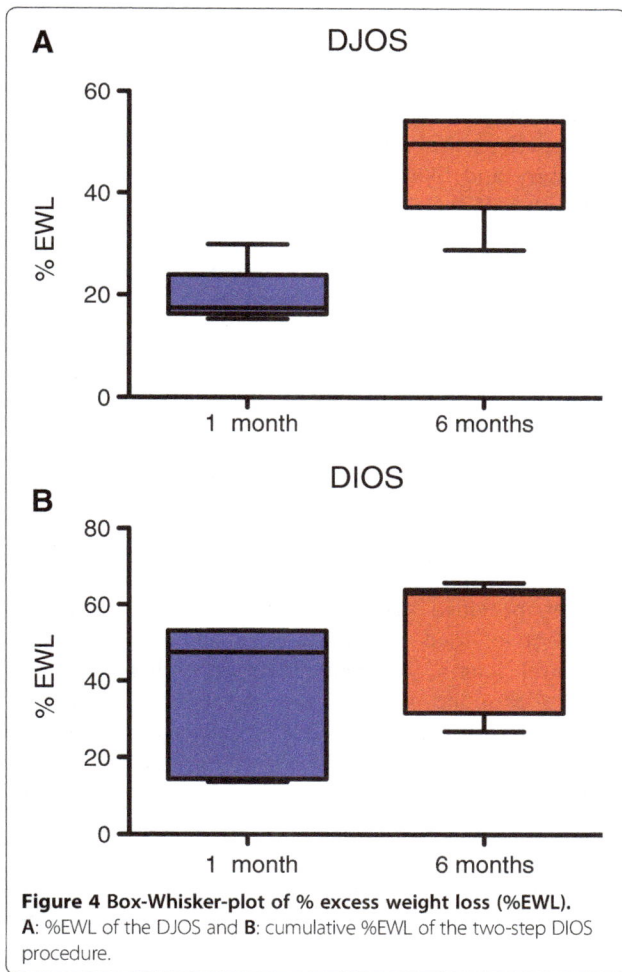

Figure 4 Box-Whisker-plot of % excess weight loss (%EWL).
A: %EWL of the DJOS and **B**: cumulative %EWL of the two-step DIOS procedure.

syndrome showed severe problems of fatigue in 12% of patients 2 years after RYGB [20]. The current analysis of postoperative bowel habits after DJOS operations revealed that only 1 patient complained of occasional dumping-related symptoms.

Surprisingly, reflux was present in 86% of patients after the DJOS operation, despite PPI treatment and grossly asymptomatic patients preoperatively. Although we cannot test for this hypothesis, we believe that reflux is a consequence of the LSG in which it is a common phenomenon [21]. However, the reflux incidence in our own isolated LSG collective is much lower and other authors report an incidence of 25-47% [21,22]. We earlier demonstrated a thoracic sleeve migration as a cause of reflux after LSG [23]. Although performing only a limited duodenal mobilisation maintaining the right gastric artery, disruption at the duodenum and pyloric mobilisation may facilitate such a migration. Long-term follow up with close attention on reflux including structured analysis such as 24-hour pH-manometry will further clarify the cause of increased reflux and show, whether these high numbers indeed prove to be an obstacle after DJOS operations.

In the current series, a gastric plicature was used in 3 patients after previous gastric banding. This constellation is a known risk factor for sleeve leak when performing a conventional LSG [24,25]. Gastric plicature has been introduced by Talebpour et al. as an alternative to LSG [9]. Weight loss through this technique alone may be inferior to conventional sleeve gastrectomy and randomized controlled trials have not been conducted to date [26]. However, in case of previous gastric banding and relevant perigastric scar tissue, a gastric plicature may pose an alternative to LSG as the stomach and surrounding scar tissue has not to be cut, especially when combined with additional bariatric options such as a rerouting of the intestine. Certainly to date, this option is relevant only for individual patient cases.

This early follow-up period of 6 months in a small and heterogeneous group does not allow for valid evaluation of weight loss capacity, yet weight loss noted after DJOS is within the range reported by others

Roux-en-Y reconstruction had been performed in these patients [17].

Furthermore, pylorus preservation leaves a physiological control mechanism of food output into the small intestine preventing a dumping syndrome [18]. Dumping syndrome is an important issue after RYGB and the overall incidence may rise up to 75.9% [19]. Recently, a detailed examination of postoperative dumping

Table 3 Morbidity

	DIOS	DJOS	
Flatulence	55.6% (all regularly)	71.4% (1 regularly, 4 occ.)	
Dumping	0%	14.3% (all occ.)	
Diarrhoea	66.7% (2 regularly, 4 occ.)	28.6% (1 regularly, 1 occ.)	
Reflux	44.4%	85.7%	$P = 0.145^{T}$
PPI treatment	100%	71.4%	

Values are expressed as fractions with subgroup differentiation in absolute number (peramphases).
^{T}Fisher´s exact test DIOS vs. DJOS.

following RYGB [27,28]. Overall %EWL of DIOS patients was considerably lower when compared to Sachez-Peraut's SADI-S collective, yet again the majority of patients had undergone pervious weight loss surgery which is known to considerably effect weight loss [7].

Weight regain is a major problem after conventional gastric bypass with up to 35% of patients experiencing an %EWL less than 60%. Causes noted are dilatation of the gastric pouch or enlargement of the gastro-jejunal anastomosis [29]. Clinically, we and others observe that patients regaining weight after RYGB have often lost their feeling of satiety and subsequently consume large meals [5]. We speculate that the DJOS operation has two distinct advantages targeting these drawbacks after conventional RYGB: 1. Anastomotic dilatation will be prevented through pyloric physiological muscle calibration and, 2. LSG is known to create an excellent feeling of satiety due to a deceleration of food transit in the longitudinal part of the sleeve stomach [30].

The major predicament in analysing limb-length variations is the fact that surgeons creating a gastric bypass commonly measure the alimentary and biliopancreatic limb but neglect the common channel length. Surgeons forming a BPD, by contrast, determine the length of the common channel and alimentary limb, and in turn neglect the length of the biliopancreatic limb. Furthermore, the total small intestinal length is highly variable and ranges between 4 to nearly 10 meters [31]. We measured a comparable range of small bowel length of 6-9 m, yet the length variation of bowel measured was large. Compared to the historical measurement of small bowel length in lean adults, the total small bowel length of obese patients was comparable to lean individuals [32].

Establishing the loop duodeno-*jejunostomy* the key issue was to determine an adequate anastomosis position. In conventional RYGB, weight loss is mainly due to calorie restriction, which is substantially caused by appetite control due to a modulation of entero-endocrine peptides, mainly located in the terminal ileum [33]. As this modulation is well known for current limb length variations in RYGB, the focus was to find an anastomosis position similar to conventional RYGB. Here, the alimentary limb ranges from 75 cm to 150 cm with a biliopancreatic limb length of approximately 30 cm [34]. Randomized controlled trials suggest that a long alimentary limb (150 cm) might be preferable for the super-obese [35,36]. However, Stefinidis et al. reviewing the "Importance of the Length of the Limbs for Gastric Bypass Patients" find no clear recommendation [34]. In MGB, the gastro-jejunostomy in usually formed at 150 cm [10]. Some authors suggest an increase in length by 10 cm for every BMI point above 40 kg/m^2 (MGB for all) [15].

To account for inter-individual differences, as outlined above, we decided to place the duodeno-jejunostomy after 1/3 of small bowel length, bypassing an average of 236 cm in performing a DJOS operation. Taking into account that the loop reconstruction combines the alimentary and biliopancreatic limb, DJOS resembles a long limb RYGB (150 cm plus 30 cm).

For the malabsorptive DIOS operation, the adequate anastomosis position had to be carefully selected in order to prevent excessive malabsorption. As there is no alimentary limb when conducting a loop reconstruction, the common channel had to be considerably longer than in classic BPD surgery. Sanchez-Pernaute et al. extensively reviewed limb length variations when initially describing the SADI-S operation, ultimately deciding to form a common channel of 200 cm [37]. As the SADI-S operation has proven to be safe and effective with no relevant malabsorption in mid-term follow up, anastomosis position for the DIOS operation should be similar [7]. Yet, provided that the overall proportional energy resorption of food consumed does not grossly depend on bowel length, it seems consistent that leaving a 200 cm common channel at a total bowel length of 500 cm causes greater possible malabsorption than the same common channel at 900 cm overall bowel length.

Based on the considerations above, we decided to place the duodeno-ileostomy after 2/3 of the small intestine, leaving a common channel of 1/3. For maximum safety, the common channel was never under 200 cm in length. The 2/3 position left a mean common channel length of 245 cm, thus approximately 20% more compared to the SADI-S operation [7].

Conclusions

Although two different metabolic principles underlie the DJOS and DIOS operation, performing loop duodeno-enterostomies with sleeve gastrectomy essentially breaks down bariatric surgery into exactly these two distinct elements, leaving the possibility for individual adaptation. The early results of this small and heterogeneous series most importantly show no mortality and no complication related to the duodeno-enterostomy. Pylorus-preserving duodeno-enterostomies with sleeve gastrectomy may open new technical alternatives in bariatric surgery. If the DJOS and DIOS operations prove to be beneficial will have to be evaluated in randomized controlled trials.

Abbreviations

BMI: Body mass index; BPD: Biliopancreatic diversion; BPD/DS: Biliopancreatic diversion with duodenal switch; CT: Computed tomograpy; DIOS: Duodeno-ileostomy with sleeve gastrectomy; DJOS: Duodeno-jejunostomy with sleeve gastrectomy; LSG: Laparsocopic sleeve gastrectomy; MGB: Mini gastric bypass; RYGB: Roux-en-Y gastric bypass; SADI-S: Single anastomosis duodeno-ileostomy associated to a sleeve gastrectomy; %EWL: Excess weight loss.

Competing interests

Jodok Matthias Grueneberger, Iwona Karcz-Socha, Goran Marjanovic, Simon Kuesters, Krystyna Zwirska-Korczala, Katharina Schmidt and W. Konrad Karcz have no conflicts of interest.

Authors' contributions

MG, GM, SK and KK participaed as surgeons for DIOS and DJOS operations, MG, KS and KK have drafted the manuscript, IK-S and KZ-K critically revised the manuscript. All authors read and approved the final manuscript.

Author details

[1]Department of General and Visceral Surgery, University of Freiburg, Hugstetter Strasse 55, 79106 Freiburg, Germany. [2]Department of Physiology, Silesian Medical University, Katowitz, Poland. [3]Department of General Surgery, University of Schleswig-Holstein, Campus Lübeck, Lübeck, Germany.

References

1. Mingrone G, Panunzi S, De Gaetano A, Guidone C, Iaconelli A, Leccesi L, Nanni G, Pomp A, Castagneto M, Ghirlanda G, Rubino F: **Bariatric surgery versus conventional medical therapy for type 2 diabetes.** *N Engl J Med* 2012, **366:**1577–1585.
2. Sjostrom L, Lindroos AK, Peltonen M, Torgerson J, Bouchard C, Carlsson B, Dahlgren S, Larsson B, Narbro K, Sjostrom CD, Sullivan M, Wedel H, Swedish Obese Subjects Study Scientific Group: **Lifestyle, diabetes, and cardiovascular risk factors 10 years after bariatric surgery.** *N Engl J Med* 2004, **351:**2683–2693.
3. Marceau P, Biron S, Bourque RA, Potvin M, Hould FS, Simard S: **Biliopancreatic Diversion with a New Type of Gastrectomy.** *Obes Surg* 1993, **3:**29–35.
4. Padwal R, Klarenbach S, Wiebe N, Birch D, Karmali S, Manns B, Hazel M, Sharma AM, Tonelli M: **Bariatric surgery: a systematic review and network meta-analysis of randomized trials.** *Obes Rev* 2011, **12:**602–621.
5. Christou NV, Look D, Maclean LD: **Weight gain after short- and long-limb gastric bypass in patients followed for longer than 10 years.** *Ann Surg* 2006, **244:**734–740.
6. Swartz DE, Mobley E, Felix EL: **Bile reflux after Roux-en-Y gastric bypass: an unrecognized cause of postoperative pain.** *Surg Obes Relat Dis* 2009, **5:**27–30.
7. Sanchez-Pernaute A, Herrera MA, Perez-Aguirre ME, Talavera P, Cabrerizo L, Matia P, Diez-Valladares L, Barabash A, Martin-Antona E, Garcia-Botella A, Garcia-Almenta EM, Torres A: **Single anastomosis duodeno-ileal bypass with sleeve gastrectomy (SADI-S). One to three-year follow-up.** *Obes Surg* 2010, **20:**1720–1726.
8. Karcz WK, Marjanovic G, Grueneberger J, Baumann T, Bukhari W, Krawczykowski D, Kuesters S: **Banded sleeve gastrectomy using the GaBP ring–surgical technique.** *Obes Facts* 2011, **4:**77–80.
9. Talebpour A, Motamedi SM, Vahidi H: **Twelve year experience of laparoscopic gastric plication in morbid obesity: development of the technique and patient outcomes.** *Ann Surg Innov Res* 2012, **6:**7.
10. Rutledge R, Walsh TR: **Continued excellent results with the mini-gastric bypass: six-year study in 2,410 patients.** *Obes Surg* 2005, **15:**1304–1308.
11. Watson K: **Carcinoma of ampulla of vater successful radical resection.** *Brit J Surg* 1944, **31:**368–373.
12. Traverso LW, Longmire WP Jr: **Preservation of the pylorus in pancreaticoduodenectomy.** *Surg Gynecol Obstet* 1978, **146:**959–962.
13. Wenger FA, Jacobi CA, Haubold K, Zieren HU, Muller JM: **[Gastrointestinal quality of life after duodenopancreatectomy in pancreatic carcinoma. Preliminary results of a prospective randomized study: pancreatoduodenectomy or pylorus-preserving pancreatoduodenectomy].** *Chirurg* 1999, **70:**1454–1459.
14. Hess DS, Hess DW: **Biliopancreatic diversion with a duodenal switch.** *Obes Surg* 1998, **8:**267–282.
15. Noun R, Skaff J, Riachi E, Daher R, Antoun NA, Nasr M: **One thousand consecutive mini-gastric bypass: short- and long-term outcome.** *Obes Surg* 2012, **22:**697–703.
16. Johnson WH, Fernanadez AZ, Farrell TM, Macdonald KG, Grant JP, McMahon RL, Pryor AD, Wolfe LG, DeMaria EJ: **Surgical revision of loop ("mini") gastric bypass procedure: multicenter review of complications and conversions to Roux-en-Y gastric bypass.** *Surg Obes Relat Dis* 2007, **3:**37–41.
17. Obeid A, Long J, Kakade M, Clements RH, Stahl R, Grams J: **Laparoscopic Roux-en-Y gastric bypass: long term clinical outcomes.** *Surg Endosc* 2012, **26:**3515–3520.
18. Shah M, Simha V, Garg A: **Review: long-term impact of bariatric surgery on body weight, comorbidities, and nutritional status.** *J Clin Endocrinol Metab* 2006, **91:**4223–4231.
19. Mallory GN, Macgregor AM, Rand CS: **The Influence of Dumping on Weight Loss After Gastric Restrictive Surgery for Morbid Obesity.** *Obes Surg* 1996, **6:**474–478.
20. Laurenius A, Olbers T, Naslund I, Karlsson J: **Dumping syndrome following gastric bypass: validation of the dumping symptom rating scale.** *Obes Surg* 2013, **23:**740–755.
21. Carter PR, LeBlanc KA, Hausmann MG, Kleinpeter KP, deBarros SN, Jones SM: **Association between gastroesophageal reflux disease and laparoscopic sleeve gastrectomy.** *Surg Obes Relat Dis* 2011, **7:**569–572.
22. Himpens J, Dobbeleir J, Peeters G: **Long-term results of laparoscopic sleeve gastrectomy for obesity.** *Ann Surg* 2010, **252:**319–324.
23. Baumann T, Grueneberger J, Pache G, Kuesters S, Marjanovic G, Kulemann B, Holzner P, Karcz-Socha I, Suesslin D, Hopt UT, Langer M, Karcz WK: **Three-dimensional stomach analysis with computed tomography after laparoscopic sleeve gastrectomy: sleeve dilation and thoracic migration.** *Surg Endosc* 2011, **25:**2323–2329.
24. Alevizos L, Linardoutsos D, Menenakos E, Stamou K, Vlachos K, Zografos G, Leandros E: **Routine abdominal drains after laparoscopic sleeve gastrectomy: a retrospective review of 353 patients.** *Obes Surg* 2011, **21:**687–691.
25. Goitein D, Feigin A, Segal-Lieberman G, Goitein O, Papa MZ, Zippel D: **Laparoscopic sleeve gastrectomy as a revisional option after gastric band failure.** *Surg Endosc* 2011, **25:**2626–2630.
26. Shen D, Ye H, Wang Y, Ji Y, Zhan X, Zhu J, Li W: **Comparison of short-term outcomes between laparoscopic greater curvature plication and laparoscopic sleeve gastrectomy.** *Surg Endosc* 2013, **27:**2768–2774.
27. Brethauer SA, Heneghan HM, Eldar S, Gatmaitan P, Huang H, Kashyap S, Gornik HL, Kirwan JP, Schauer PR: **Early effects of gastric bypass on endothelial function, inflammation, and cardiovascular risk in obese patients.** *Surg Endosc* 2011, **25:**2650–2659.
28. Lakdawala MA, Bhasker A, Mulchandani D, Goel S, Jain S: **Comparison between the results of laparoscopic sleeve gastrectomy and laparoscopic Roux-en-Y gastric bypass in the Indian population: a retrospective 1 year study.** *Obes Surg* 2010, **20:**1–6.
29. Kuesters S, Grueneberger JM, Baumann T, Daoud M, Hopt UT, Karcz WK: **Revisionary bariatric surgery: indications and outcome of 100 consecutive operations at a single center.** *Surg Endosc* 2012, **26:**1718–1723.
30. Baumann T, Kuesters S, Grueneberger J, Marjanovic G, Zimmermann L, Schaefer AO, Hopt UT, Langer M, Karcz WK: **Time-resolved MRI after ingestion of liquids reveals motility changes after laparoscopic sleeve gastrectomy–preliminary results.** *Obes Surg* 2011, **21:**95–101.
31. Savassi-Rocha AL, Diniz MT, Savassi-Rocha PR, Ferreira JT, Rodrigues de Almeida Sanches S, Diniz Mde F, Gomes de Barros H, Fonseca IK: **Influence of jejunoileal and common limb length on weight loss following Roux-en-Y gastric bypass.** *Obes Surg* 2008, **18:**1364–1368.
32. Underhill BM: **Intestinal length in man.** *Br Med J* 1955, **2:**1243–1246.
33. le Roux CW, Welbourn R, Werling M, Osborne A, Kokkinos A, Laurenius A, Lonroth H, Fandriks L, Ghatei MA, Bloom SR, Olbers T: **Gut hormones as mediators of appetite and weight loss after Roux-en-Y gastric bypass.** *Ann Surg* 2007, **246:**780–785.
34. Stefanidis D, Kuwada TS, Gersin KS: **The importance of the length of the limbs for gastric bypass patients–an evidence-based review.** *Obes Surg* 2011, **21:**119–124.
35. Brolin RE, Kenler HA, Gorman JH, Cody RP: **Long-limb gastric bypass in the superobese. A prospective randomized study.** *Ann Surg* 1992, **215:**387–395.

6

Complications and nutrient deficiencies two years after sleeve gastrectomy

Nicole Pech[1], Frank Meyer[2], Hans Lippert[2], Thomas Manger[1] and Christine Stroh[1*]

Abstract

Background: The aim of this systematic study was to investigate patient outcomes and nutritional deficiencies following sleeve gastrectomy (SG) during a median follow-up of two years.

Methods: Over a period of 56 months, all consecutive patients who underwent SG were documented in this prospective, single-center, observational study. The study endpoints included complication rates, nutritional deficiencies and percentage of excess weight loss (%EWL).

Results: From September 26, 2005 to May 28, 2009, 100 patients (female: male = 59:41) with a mean age of 43.6 years (range: 22–64) and a preoperative BMI of 52.3 kg/m^2 (range: 36–77) underwent SG. The mean operative time was 86.4 min (range: 35–275). Major complications were observed in 8.0 % of the patients. During the follow-up period, 25 patients (25.0 %) underwent a second bariatric intervention (22 DS and 3 RYGBP). Out of the total 100 patients, 48 % were supplemented with iron, 33 % with zinc, 34 % with a combination of calcium carbonate and cholecalciferol, 24 % with vitamin D, 42 % with vitamin B12 and 40 % with folic acid. The patients who received only a SG (n = 75) had %EWL of 53.6, 65.8 and 62.6 % after 6, 12 and 24 months, respectively.

Conclusions: SG is a highly effective bariatric intervention for morbidly obese patients. Nutritional deficiencies resulting from the procedure can be detected by routine nutritional screening. Results of the study show that Vitamin B12 supplementation should suggested routinely.

Keywords: Sleeve gastrectomy, Laparoscopic sleeve gastrectomy, Obesity, Metabolic surgery, Bariatric surgery, Nutritional deficiencies

Background

Obesity has developed into an epidemic. Approximately 1.7 billion people are overweight, and 312 million are obese [1,2]. In Germany in 2009, 60.1 % of male and 42.9 % of female population was overweight [3]. There are currently no conservative treatments that produce the %EWL results and stable courses observed following bariatric surgery. Obesity is associated with an increased mortality risk [4]. Obesity is also associated with increased health costs. A BMI = 35 kg/m^2 is associated with a 200 % increase in health care costs compared the normal weight range [5].

As a result of the obesity epidemic bariatric and metabolic surgeries have grown in popularity in recent years, resulting that the number of operations is rapidly increasing. Laparoscopic sleeve Gastrectomy (SG) was performed as the single step procedure for surgically induced weight loss in 2000 [6].

SG can be suggested as a first step procedure for multimorbid patients with a BMI > 50 kg/m^2, considering the high mortality rate of 6 % following biliopancreatic diversion (BPD) with DS [7,8]. In literature is the lack of studies with high evidence levels on SG reporting long term follow up data, results on reoperation rate or long term complication rate for surgical complications as well as nutrient deficiencies.

The aim of the following systematic study was to investigate nutritional deficiencies and outcomes following SG during a mean follow up period of two years.

Methods

From September 26, 2005 to May 28, 2009, 100 patients underwent SG in the Surgery Department of the SRH

* Correspondence: christine.stroh@wkg.srh.de
[1]Department of General, Abdominal and Pediatric Surgery, Municipal Hospital Gera, Strasse des Friedens 122, Gera 07548, Germany
Full list of author information is available at the end of the article

Wald-Klinikum Gera Hospital. All patients had to agree with an informed consent. Data collection and analysis was performed in compliance with the Helsinki Declaration.

After we ensured compliance with international and German guidelines all patients had to take part in an informational seminar [9]. Patient´s evaluation was performed by experienced bariatric surgeons.

Data collection took place prospectively and analyzed retrospectively. Patients were classified according to the WHO classifications of obesity (35–39.9 kg/m²; 40–49.9 kg/m²) with expansions to "super obesity" (50–59.9 kg/m²) and "super-super obesity" (= 60 kg/m²). Analyzed parameters are listed in Table 1 (Table 1). Acute and postoperative complications were evaluated.

Sleeve gastrectomy- operation technique

SG was performed in the French position in a 30° reverse Trendelenburg position. Pneumoperitoneum was established to 15 mmHg. First trocar for placing the camera was inserted 15 cm distal to the xiphoid process. Another trocar was placed on the epigastric angle for liver retraction. Two trocars were located on the right and left upper quadrants. A bougie 31–36 French was used. The dissection of the greater curve began 5–6 cm proximal to the pylorus and extended to the angle of His. Sleeve resection of the stomach was performed using an Endo GIA stapler (green) made by Covidien, Germany® using staple line reinforcement in 88 % of the patients. Staple line was not oversewn. To exclude leakage of staple line a methylene blue test was performed. The resected stomach was filled with water to determine the resected gastric volume. Histopathological analysis was performed on the specimen. In all patients for single shot antibiosis a third generation cephalosporine was given.

Postoperative follow up

All of the patients were examined throughout a 24-month follow-up period (at 3, 6, 12, 18 and 24 months postoperatively) in our clinical outpatient department.

Furthermore, short- and long-term results with regard to BMI, weight, %EWL and important laboratory parameters (iron, zinc, selenium, alkaline phosphatase, hemoglobin, MCV, albumin, vitamin B12, folic acid, calcium and parathyroid hormone levels) were registered (Table 1).

Results
Demographic data

From September 26, 2005 to May 28, 2009, 100 patients (sex ratio, females: males = 59:41 [1.4:1]) with a mean age of 43.6 years (range, 22–64) and a preoperative BMI of 52.3 kg/m² (range, 36–77) underwent SG. Operation was performed by three surgeons, operating as a team in all the 100 recorded operations. Patient´s outcome and operation time were not influenced by changing the surgeon in these team. Demographic data are shown in Table 2 (Table 2).

Surgical outcome

Operation data Of the 100 patients, 99 underwent primarily laparoscopic surgery. In 6.1 % of these patients (6 of 99), a conversion from laparoscopy to laparotomy was necessary. In one case, a primary laparotomy was performed because of an abdominal wall hernia, resection of an anus praeter, subtotal colectomy with an ileorectostomy. Subtotal colectomy was performed due to the fact of several colon operations in an outside hospital. Postoperative course of the patient was uneventful. In 4 cases, this conversion was performed because of an insufficient laparoscopic overview with high intraabdominal pressure and in 2 cases due to the fact of laparoscopically uncontrollable bleeding (Table 3).

The mean operation time was 86.4 min. The mean resected gastric volume was 995.6 ml. A 34-French calibration tube was used in 89 % of the patients (89). Staple line reinforcements were used in 88 % of the patients (88) (Table 2). Comparing leakage rate and bleeding in patients using staple line reinforcement or oversewing was no difference.

There were significant differences among the durations of the OP. When staple line reinforcements were used, the mean OP duration was 79.3 min, compared to 141.1 min without using staple line reinforcements ($p = 0.010$).

A conversion to laparotomy was significantly more necessary for patients with a BMI > 60 kg/m² compared to patients with a lower BMI ($p > 0.001$). The duration of the OP averaged 70.4 min for patients with a BMI between 35 and 39.9 kg/m², 70.2 min for patients with a BMI between 40 and 49.9 kg/m², 92.9 min for patients with a BMI between 50 and 59.9 kg/m² and 101.2 min for patients with a BMI > 60 kg/m². Patients with a BMI

Table 1 Recorded parameters

Age	OP duration
Sex	Use of staple line reinforcement
Length of hospital stay	Bougie size
Type of Operation	Resected gastric volume
Laboratory parameters	
Iron	Albumin
Zinc	Vitamin B12
Selenium	Folic acid
Alkaline phosphatase	Calcium
Hemoglobin	Parathyroid hormone

Table 2 Data from patients and operations

		BMI				Total
	[kg/m²]	35-39,9	40-49,9	50-59,9	> 60	
Sex						
Male	[%]	62.5	24.1	46.3	45.5	41.0
Female	[%]	37.5	75.9	53.7	54.5	59.0
Total	[n]	8	29	41	22	100
Mean Age Age range	[years]	44.6 33-64	44.3 22-59	43.8 22-58	41.7 25-59	43.6 22-64
Mean BMI BMI range	[kg/m²]	38.3 36.0-39.5	44.4 40.0-49.8	53.5 50.0-59.1	65.5 60.0-77.0	52.3 36.0-77.0
Operation						
Laparoscopy	[%]	100.0	96.6	95,1	81.8	93.0
Laparoscopy with conversion	[%]		3.4	2,4	18.2	6.0
Laparotomy	[%]			2,4		1.0
Mean Operative time Operative time range	[min]	70.4 41-101	70.2 44-120	92.9 35-275	101.2 45-225	86.4 35-275
Mean Resected gastric volume	[ml]	785.7 (650–900)	882.4 (600–1200)	1081.8 (500–1700)	1045.5 (700–1700)	995.6 (500–1700)
Bougie size						
31 French			3.4			1.0
32 French	[%]	12.5	3.4	7,3	9.1	7.0
34 French	[%]	75.0	93.1	87,8	90.9	89.0
36 French	[%]	12.5		4,9		3.0
Staple line reinforcement	[%]	87.5	96.6	85,4	81,8	88.0

> 50 kg/m² had significantly longer OP durations compared to patients with a BMI < 50 kg/m² (95.7 vs. 70.2; p = 0.001). The resected gastric volume was significantly higher in patients with BMI > 50 kg/m² compared to those with BMI < 50 kg/m² (1072.7 vs. 854.2; p = 0.001).

Intraoperative and early postoperative surgical complications Twenty patients (20.0 %) suffered on intraoperative or/and postoperative complications (Table 3). Postoperative complications occurred in 17 patients (17.0 %). One patient with BMI 55.5 kg/m² died (1.0 %).

Table 3 Acute and postoperative complications

Complications (20/100; 20.0 %)			
Cause of acute complications / conversions		**Postoperative complications**	
	[n]		[n]
Insufficient intraabdominal view	4	Leakage	3
Insufficient intraabdominal view Bleeding	2	Abscess	5
		Severe sepsis	2
		Perforation of duodenum	1
		Pleural effusion	2
		Pneumonia	3
		Thrombosis	1
		Wound infection	6
		Death	1

At the tenth postoperative day patient complained of left upper abdominal pain. The CT scan showed an insufficient suture with a subcardial abscess. A CT-guided puncture ensued. Patient's cardiac situation worsened and ARDS developed. Acute complications were observed significantly more frequently in patients with BMI > 60 kg/m² (p < 0.001). The major complication rate was 8 % (Table 3).

Mortality rate Mortality rate after 24 month of total follow up is 2 %. Above mentioned patient died during hospital stay 73 days after operation, due to SIRS and ARDS. Second patient died several months after SG in fact of his cardiac situation without any relation to operation.

Follow up data Follow up rate was 80 % (80/100). All of these patients were clinical examined with a laboratory test 24 months after SG, so mean follow up time is 24 months.

The mean preoperative BMI of all of the patients examined was 52.3 kg/m². At the end of the follow up, there was a significant reduction in BMI to 35.4 kg/m² (p < 0.0005). The greatest weight loss occurred within the first 12 postoperative months (52.3 kg/m² to 36.3 kg/m²). Afterwards we observed a weight loss from 36.3 kg/m² to 35.4 kg/m² for all of the patients.

The %EWL in the BMI categories between 35 and 39.9 kg/m² and 40 and 49.9 kg/m² was 47.4 % and 47.5 %, respectively, after 3 months. The greatest %EWL in these categories was achieved after 12 (72.6 %) and 24 (74.2 %) months. Patient´s with a BMI between 35 and 39.9 kg/m² showed a slight tendency toward increased weight after this time. Patient´s with a BMI between 40 and 49.9 kg/m², 50 and 59.9 kg/m² and over 60 kg/m² showed continuous weight loss throughout the entire 24-month follow-up period (Table 4). On average, there was a tendency toward increased weight after 18 months. The most significant weight loss was achieved within the first postoperative year ($p < 0.0005$). Regarding the percentage overweight loss, the highest %EWL of 67.1 % occurred after 18 months, and after 24 months, there was a further %EWL of 62.6 %. The highest %EWL of 83.3 % was observed in patients with a BMI between 35 and 39.9 kg/m² after 12 and 18 months (Table 4).

Revisional procedures after SG Over the total observation period of 24 months, a second operation to induce weight loss was required in 25.0 % (25) of the patients to develop further weight loss or amelioration on comorbidities. Three patients underwent RYGBP and 22 patients DS.

Nutrient deficiencies, laboratory parameters and supplementation
In patients after SG as a single step procedure a postoperative routine supplementation was not performed. Supplementation was suggested according laboratory examination performed every 6 months in case of deficiencies.

Iron Iron supplementation was performed in 48 patients (48.0 %). Seven of these patients developed microcytic anemia, which required the initiation of iron supplementation. In 23 of these 48 patients, iron supplementation

was performed as prophylaxis after RYGBP or DS. The other 25 patients (25.0 %) 21 of them female were supplemented after SG. Further we examined iron supplementation in fertile woman. Women had a mean age of 42.8 years (25–59). Thirteen of these 21 women recorded a reduced iron value, and the other 8 women were supplemented with a combination of folic acid and iron.

Zinc The highest average value for zinc of 14.70 µmol/L was determined preoperatively (reference range: 10–23 µmol/L). There were no significant differences among the average values in the follow-up period. In total, 33 patients underwent zinc supplementation, and 5 of these complained of hair loss. Nineteen patients were supplemented after RYGBP or DS. Fourteen patients (14.0 %) were supplemented following SG due to zinc deficiency. For supplementation patients were given 15 mg Zink daily.

Selenium The highest average value for selenium of 81.60 µg/L (reference range: 50–120 µg/L) was determined preoperatively. After 3 months, a significant decrease to 61.13 µg/L ($p < 0.0005$) occurred. No other significant differences were observed over the course of the follow-up. Due to selenium deficiency in laboratory eight patients after SG were treated with selenium supplementation using 100 µg twice a day. Among the 75 patients who did not undergo a second operation, there was a gradual increase in the concentration of selenium (OP: 81.5 µg/L; 3rd month: 62.1 µg/L; 6th month: 63.0 µg/L; 12th month: 66.9 µg/L; 18th month: 66.8 µg/L; 24th month: 69.7 µg/L). The increase in selenium from 3 months after the operation achieved a significant level after 12 months ($p = 0.043$).

Calcium and parathyroid hormone In 62 of the 100 patients, PTH levels were preoperatively determined, and 22.6 % of the patients (14) had hyperparathyroidism. The average PTH levels (reference range: 10.0–69.0 ng/L) for patients with BMIs over 60 kg/m² were 83.15 ng/L preoperatively, 73.30 ng/L after 6 months and 61.55 ng/L after 18 months (Table 5; 6). Thirty-four patients (34.0 %) were supplemented with calcium carbonate and cholecalciferol, including 15 patients

Table 4 Weight progression (BMI in kg/m²) of patients without a second operation during the follow-up period (n = 75) and %EWL of patients without a second operation during the follow-up period

months BMI	OP	3	6	12	18	24
35-39.9 kg/m²	38.2	31.0	30.2	27.4	27.5	28.4
40-49.9 kg/m²	44.2	35.0	31.1	29.4	30.0	29.9
50-59.9 kg/m²	53.2	44.0	39.5	37.6	36.9	38.2
≥60 kg/m²	65.6	52.5	48.1	44.0	42.3	43.7
Total	51,0	40.8	38.4	34.4	34.4	35.6
%EWL						
35-39,9 kg/m²		53.4	62.5	83.3	83.3	76.3
40-49,9 kg/m²		48.6	67.4	76.4	75.0	74.5
50-59,9 kg/m²		33.6	48.5	54.7	57.3	52.8
≥60 kg/m²		30.3	42.6	52.5	58.6	53.8
Total		40.7	53.6	65.8	67.1	62.6

Table 5 Postoperative course of calcium (mmol/l)

Timeline [months] BMI [kg/m²]	OP	3	6	12	18	24
35 - 39,9	2,36	2,36	2,37	2,40	2,40	2,44
40 - 49,9	2,38	2,37	2,40	2,35	2,38	2,36
50 - 59,9	2,37	2,35	2,38	2,34	2,35	2,30
≥ 60	2,33	2,44	2,40	2,34	2,35	2,33
Total	2,36	2,37	2,39	2,35	2,36	2,34

Table 6 Postoperative course of parathormone (ng/l)

Timeline [months] BMI [kg/m^2]	OP	3	6	12	18	24
35 - 39,9	44,93	45,45	41,98	42,04	44,70	39,90
40 - 49,9	57,34	65,65	51,73	54,23	56,01	54,94
50 - 59,9	48,98	46,93	53,29	55,95	55,79	56,28
≥ 60	83,15	108,82	73,30	60,41	61,55	64,81
Total	59,55	66,67	56,72	55,13	56,44	56,52

supplemented after RYGBP or DS. For calcium supplementation patients were supplemented with 500 mg calcium with 10 mg cholecalciferol four times daily. Twenty-four patients (24.0 %) were treated with separate or additional vitamin D supplementation due to high levels of PTH, including 9 patients treated preventively after a second operation.

Under supplementation, a rising concentration of PTH appeared 3 months after the operation. After 6 months, a significant decrease in the concentration of PTH was identified ($p = 0.045$). Course of PTH levels is shown in table 6 (Table 6).

Albumin SG did not significantly affect the patients' albumin levels (reference range: 34.0-48.0 g/L) during the follow-up period.

Vitamin B12 Overall, forty-two patients (42.0 %) received vitamin B12 supplementation. For vitamin B12 supplementation 1000 µg Vitamin B12 monthly was ordinated. 24 patients with SG as a standalone procedure (24.0 %) were supplemented within the first postoperative year and 18 patients after RYGBP or DS. (Table 7). Under supplementation, the vitamin B12 levels achieved stable average values (reference range: 175–810 pmol/L) during the entire follow-up period.

The 75 patients after SG as a standalone procedure demonstrated stable and not significantly different vitamin B12 concentrations (OP: 285.6 pmol/L; 3rd month:

288.1 pmol/L; 6th month: 269.0 pmol/L; 12th month: 253.8 pmol/L; 18th month: 254.2 pmol/L; 24th month: 265.2 pmol/L) (Table 7).

Folic acid Regarding folic acid (reference range: 10.40-42.40 nmol/L), there was a significant decrease 3 months after the operation from 18.87 nmol/L to 15.29 nmol/L ($p < 0.0005$). 19 patients were supplemented. After RYGBP or DS 21 patient were given a supplementation according national and international guidelines. After the third month following the operation, an increasing concentration of folic acid was observed with a maximum average of 20.96 nmol/L after 24 months. Supplementation was performed with a combination of folic acid 0.5 mg and iron 40 mg daily.

Discussion

SG is an effective operative method for inducing weight loss. SG can be performed as the first step of a two-stage procedure for high-risk patients to reduce the perioperative risks of DS or RYGBP.

Literature shows the benefits of LSG compared to laparoscopic gastric banding (LAGB) and laparoscopic RYGBP. Advantages of SG are non-resection of the pylorus, which prevents dumping syndrome; no intestinal anastomoses, no risk of developing an internal hernia and nearly regular intestinal absorption [10]. Complication rate of SG procedure is still high, especially short term complications as leakage and staple line insufficiency influences the complication rate. In literature an increasing long term complication rate is reported due to stenosis, gastroesophageal reflux and re-operation rate due insufficient weight loss, regain of weight or insufficient amelioration of comorbidities [11]. Evidence based data on nutrient deficiencies, especially vitamin B12 and iron, after SG is not available.

SG, however, reduces perioperative risks of morbidly obese patients with BMI > 60 kg/m^2 as a first step procedure [12]. The reported initial weight loss after SG

Table 7 Necessity of vitamin B12 supplementation during the follow-up period

	BMI									
	35-39.9 kg/m^2		40-49.9 kg/m^2		50-59,9 kg/m^2		≥ 60 kg/m^2		Total	
Vitamin B12	[n]	[%]	[n]	%	[n]	[%]	[n]	[%]	[n]	[%]
After OP	0	0.0	0	0.0	0	0.0	1	4.5	1	1.0
After 3 months	1	12.5	4	13.8	5	12.2	2	9.1	12	12.0
After 6 months	0	0.0	2	6.9	4	9.8	2	9.1	8	8.0
After 12 months	0	0.0	1	3.4	0	0.0	2	9.1	3	3.0
After 24 months	0	0.0	0	0.0	0	0.0	0	0.0	0	0.0
After 2nd OP	1	12.5	2	6.9	10	24.4	5	22.7	18	18.0
Total	2	25.0	9	31.0	19	46.3	12	54.5	42	42.0

spans a wide range, between 33 and 83 % [13,14]. In a prospective study of 100 patients, Johnston et al. presented a %EWL of 60 % after 5 years [15]. That study group achieved a %EWL of 60.3 % after 12 months and 63.8 % after 24 months.

Over a 24-month period, the entire patient population experienced continuous weight loss. The weight loss remained constant (BMI 35.4 kg/m^2) in clinical examinations through the 24th months. SG as a single step operation is suitable for patients with BMIs < 50 kg/m^2. Only 8.1 % of these patients (3/37) required a second intervention to induce further weight loss within the follow-up period (vs. 34.9 % with BMI of 50 kg/m^2). After 24 months, patients with a BMI between 35 to 39.9 kg/m^2 achieved the highest %EWL. Therefore, there was no correlation between the resected volume of the stomach and the %EWL. Only one patient (12.5 %) needed to undergo a second operation for further weight loss.

After 18 months, patients who only underwent SG demonstrated increased mean weights, which may have been due to sleeve dilatation. This possibility was considered by Gluck et al., who presented %EWLs of 67.9 % after 1 year, 62.4 % after 2 years and 62.2 % after 3 years for patients after SG with preoperative BMIs between 35 and 43 kg/m^2 [16].

There is not always sufficient weight loss after SG; insufficient changes in food patterns or potential recidivism to old food patterns may cause a sleeve dilatation. One option for treatment may be a re-sleeve operation. There are inadequate data to properly appraise this option, and further studies must clarify the utility of this procedure in comparison to RYGBP or DS as a second operation.

In addition because of the moderate rate of major complications of 8.0 % (8/100), SG can be recommended as a first-step operation before malabsorptive interventions. Regarding postoperative complications, there were no significant differences among the BMI categories. However, patients with BMI > 60 kg/m^2 required a change to laparotomy significantly more often because of an insufficient intraabdominal view. Preoperative implantation of a gastric balloon to reduce morbidity for patients with BMI > 60 kg/m^2 still needs to be addressed. Especially in patients with BMI above 60 kg/m^2 general complication rate is increasing, due to the fact of an increased pulmonary complication risk, longer operation time and a higher risk for renal complications especially rhabdomyolysis [17].

In this study, there was a 30-day mortality of 0.0 %, a hospitalization mortality of 1.0 %, and a one-year mortality of 2.0 %. There were 2 patients who did not benefit from SG. One patient with a preoperative BMI of 50.5 kg/m^2 first lost weight after SG, but his weight eventually increased to a higher level than before SG

(59.7 kg/m^2 by the end of the follow-up). An insufficient change in food patterns and intake of high-calorie foods appeared to be the cause. The other patient, with a preoperative BMI of 55.5 kg/m^2, died after a prolonged course with various complications on day 73 after SG. One other multimorbid patient with a preoperative BMI of 68.0 kg/m^2 died 10 months postoperatively. A causal relationship with SG was excluded after consultation with the family doctor.

The definitive success rate for SG in this study was 98.0 %, with a mortality of 1.0 % and a non-responder rate of 1.0 %. Twenty-five percent of the patients in this study required a second operation via a two-stage procedure for further weight loss.

Nutritional deficits after LSG are rarely evaluated. In postoperative course there is no suggestion for vitamin supplementation. Evidence based data on necessity of supplementation after SG does not exist in literature. After evaluating nutritional deficiencies, there is no need for supplementation after SG, although preoperative existing deficits should be supplemented. Laboratory parameters should be monitored regularly to detect early nutritional deficiencies and to initiate appropriate therapies.

Vitamin B12 levels were in the lower third of the reference range during supplementation. Therefore, it is likely that without supplementation, vitamin B12 deficiencies would have occurred. Therefore, a general vitamin B12 supplementation is advisable to avoid pernicious anemia and to prevent neuropathic pain.

Patients with deficiencies in albumin, vitamin D or calcium have a higher risk of developing osteoporosis; therefore, it is recommended that appropriate supplementations be initiated, even if the concentrations of these parameters are only slightly decreased. PTH levels should be determined to diagnose secondary hyperparathyroidism.

Based on to parameters, iron supplementation should be initiated similar to the supplementation of folic acid. Moreover, supplementation of zinc should be based on symptoms (hair loss, immune deficiency, dry skin). Medication of zinc and calcium should be suggested to intake at different times, because zinc reduces calcium absorption. Supplementation of selenium is not generally necessary because postoperative deficiencies normalize on their own without supplementation, and an adequate, varied food intake seems to be sufficient. Regular determination of laboratory parameters should be performed 6 months after the operation and semiannually thereafter; if the patient's weight stabilizes, laboratory parameters should be determined once a year.

Conclusions

Our results following SG and those reported in the literature are promising. Adequate long-term results are still unavailable because long-term studies (> 6 years)

are rarely performed. The effectiveness and safety of SG are encouraging.

The operative treatment is not comparable among studies because of a lack of standardization [9]. Also, the 3rd International Consensus Statement on Sleeve Gastrectomy could not recommend which part of the antrum should be left and to what degree the antrum should be minimized to achieve a long-term volume reduction in the sleeve [8]. Evidence-based data are unavailable concerning the size of the bougie or whether the use of staple line reinforcement could reduce the rates of leakage [18].

Our data suggest:

SG is an effective intervention for weight loss. For patients with a BMI of 35–49.9 kg/m^2, a single-step procedure is suitable. For patients with a BMI > 50 kg/m^2, SG is suitable as a first-step procedure for reducing perioperative risks for DS [8; 17].

for patients with BMI > 60 kg/m^2, preoperative implantation of a gastric balloon should be discussed with the aim to reduce morbidity and mortality.

Supplementation of vitamin B12 is indicated and should generally be initiated after SG.

Supplementation of iron and folic acid should depend on laboratory parameters for both genders.

A deficiency in albumin was not reproducible in our patients.

Supplementation of zinc should be based on symptoms. Substitution of selenium is not necessary.

Competing interests

The undersigned authors attest that we have no commercial associations (e.g., equity ownership or interest, consultancy, patent and licensing agreements, or institutional and corporate associations) that might present a conflict of interest in relation to the submitted manuscript. (N. Pech on behalf of the co-authors).

Author details

[1]Department of General, Abdominal and Pediatric Surgery, Municipal Hospital Gera, Strasse des Friedens 122, Gera 07548, Germany. [2]Department of General, Abdominal and Vascular Surgery, University Hospital, Magdeburg, Germany.

Authors' contribution

All authors read and approved the final manuscript.

References

1. James PT, Rigby N, Leach R: **The obesity epidemic, metabolic syndrome and future prevention strategies.** *Eur J Cardiovasc Prev Rehabil* 2004, **11**(1):3–8.
2. Deitel M: **Overweight and obesity worldwide now estimated to involve 1.7 billion people.** *Obes Surg* 2003, **13**(3):329–330.
3. : *Statistisches-Bundesamt. 2010. Mikrozensus. 2009 Wiesbaden: Statistisches Bundesamt. Federal Statistical Office. 2010 Microcensus. 2009 Wiesbaden: Federal Statistical Office.*
4. Katzmarzyk PT, Craig CL, Bouchard C: **Original article underweight, overweight and obesity: relationships with mortality in the 13-year follow-up of the Canada Fitness Survey.** *J Clin Epidemiol* 2001, **54**(9):916–920.
5. von Lengerke T, Reitmeir P, John J: **Direct medical costs of obesity: a Bottom-up comparison of over- vs. normalweight adults of KORA- study region.** *Health service* 2006, **2006**(02):110–115.
6. Gagner M, Rogula T: **Laparoscopic reoperative sleeve gastrectomy for poor weight loss after biliopancreatic diversion with duodenal switch.** *Obes Surg* 2003, **13**(4):649–654.
7. Felberbauer FX, Langer FB, Shakeri-Leidenmuhler S, Bohdjalian A, Prager G: **What means and to which end we perform obesity surgery?** *J nutri med* 2010, **12**(2):19.
8. Deitel M, Gagner M, Erickson AL, Crosby RD: **Third International Summit: Current status of sleeve gastrectomy.** *Surg Obes Relat Dis* 2011 Nov-Dec, **7**(6):749–59. Epub 2011 Aug 10.
9. Runkel N, Colombo-Benkmann M, Hüttl TP, Tigges H, Mann O, Flade-Kuthe R, Shang E, Susewind M, Wolff S, Wunder R, Wirth A, Winckler K, Weimann A, de Zwaan M, Sauerland S: **Evidence-based German guidelines for surgery for obesity.** *Int J Colorectal Dis* 2011, **26**(4):397–404. Epub 2011 Feb 12.
10. Cottam D, Qureshi FG, Mattar SG, Sharma S, Holover S, Bonanomi G, Ramanathan R, Schauer P: **Laparoscopic sleeve gastrectomy as an initial weight-loss procedure for high-risk patients with morbid obesity.** *Surg Endosc* 2006, **20**(6):859–863.
11. Himpens J, Dobbeleir J, Peeters G: **Long-term results of laparoscopic sleeve gastrectomy for obesity.** *Ann Surg* 2010, **252**(2):319–24.
12. Buchwald H, Avidor Y, Braunwald E, Jensen MD, Pories W, Fahrbach K, Schoelles K: **Bariatric surgery: a systematic review and meta-analysis.** *JAMA* 2004, **292**(14):1724–37. Review. Erratum in: JAMA. 2005 Apr 13;293(14):1728.
13. Aggarwal S, Kini SU, Herron DM: **Laparoscopic sleeve gastrectomy for morbid obesity: a review.** *Surg Obes Relat Dis* 2007, **3**(2):189–194.
14. Hüttl TP, Obeidat FW, Parhofer KG, Zugel N, Huttl PE, Jauch KW, Lang RA: **Operative techniques and outcomes in metabolic surgery: sleeve gastrectomy.** *Zentralbl Chir* 2009, **134**(1):24–31.
15. Johnston D, Dachtler J, Sue-Ling HM, King RF, Martin G: **The Magenstrasse and Mill operation for morbid obesity.** *Obes Surg* 2003, **13**(1):10–16.
16. Gluck B, Movitz B, Jansma S, Gluck J, Laskowski K: **Laparoscopic Sleeve Gastrectomy is a Safe and Effective Bariatric Procedure for the Lower BMI (35.0–43.0 kg/m(2)) Population.** *Obes Surg* 2011 Aug, **21**(8):1168–71.
17. Gagner M, Boza C: **Laparoscopic duodenal switch for morbid obesity.** *Expert Rev Med Devices* 2006, **3**(1):105–12. Review.
18. Stroh C, Birk D, Flade-Kuthe R, Frenken M, Herbig B, Höhne S, Köhler H, Lange V, Ludwig K, Matkowitz R, Meyer G, Pick P, Horbach T, Krause S, Schäfer L, Schlensak M, Shang E, Sonnenberg T, Susewind M, Voigt H, Weiner R, Wolff S, Wolf AM, Schmidt U, Lippert H, Manger T, Bariatric Surgery Working Group: **Results of sleeve gastrectomy-data from a nationwide survey on bariatric surgery in Germany.** *Obes Surg* 2009, **19**(5):632–40. Epub 2009 Jan 29.

7

Trends and results in treatment of gastric cancer over last two decades at single East European centre: a cohort study

Antanas Mickevicius[1*], Povilas Ignatavicius[1,2], Rytis Markelis[1], Audrius Parseliunas[1], Dainora Butkute[3], Mindaugas Kiudelis[1], Zilvinas Endzinas[1], Almantas Maleckas[1] and Zilvinas Dambrauskas[1,2]

Abstract

Background: A steady decline in gastric cancer mortality rate over the last few decades is observed in Western Europe. However it is still not clear if this trend applies to Eastern Europe where high incidence rate of gastric cancer is observed.

Methods: This was a retrospective non-randomized, single center, cohort study. During the study period 557 consecutive patients diagnosed with gastric cancer in which curative operation was performed met the inclusion criteria. The study population was divided into two groups according to two equal time periods: 01-01-1994 – 31-12-2000 (Group I – 273 patients) and 01-01-2001 – 31-12-2007 (Group II – 284 patients). Primary (five-year survival rate) and secondary (postoperative complications, 30-day mortality rate and length of hospital stay) endpoints were evaluated and compared.

Results: Rate of postoperative complications was similar between the groups, except for Grade III (Clavien-Dindo grading system for the classification of surgical complications) complications that were observed at significantly lower rates in Group II (26 (9.5%) vs. 11 (3.9%), p = 0.02). Length of hospital stay was significantly (p = 0.001) shorter (22.6 ± 28.9 vs. 16.2 ± 17.01 days) and 30-day mortality was significantly (p = 0.02) lower (15 (5.5%) vs. 4 (1.4%)) in Group II. Similar rates of gastric cancer related mortality were observed in both groups (92.3% vs. 90.7%). However survival analysis revealed significantly (p = 0.02) better overall 5-year survival rate in Group II (35.6%, 101 of 284) than in Group I (23.4%, 64 of 273). There was no difference in 5-year survival rate when comparing different TNM stages.

Conclusions: Gastric cancer treatment results remain poor despite decreasing early postoperative mortality rates, shortening hospital stay and improved overall survival over the time. Prognosis of treatment of gastric cancer depends mainly on the stage of the disease. Absence of screening programs and lack of clinical symptoms in early stages of gastric cancer lead to circumstances when most of the patients presenting with advanced stage of the disease can expect a median survival of less than 30 months even after surgery with curative intent.

Keywords: Gastric cancer, Complications, Survival, Mortality

Background

Although a steady decline in gastric cancer mortality rates over the last few decades is observed, gastric cancer still remains the fourth most common cancer and is the second leading cause of cancer death worldwide with poor survival rates [1]. While incidence rates of gastric cancer in North America, Africa, South and West Asia are declining, rates in North-East Asia, Eastern part of South America and Eastern Europe stay high [1-3]. Surgery remains the major and potentially curative treatment method for resectable gastric cancer. Considering the location and size of the tumor as well as invasion to the adjacent organs, routinely standard radical total or subtotal gastrectomy with lymphadenectomy or multiorgan resections are performed [4-6]. The overall 5-year survival rate of patients with advanced resectable gastric cancer differs between different countries and different centres, but in general it ranges from 10% to 30% [5,7,8].

* Correspondence: a_mickevicius@yahoo.com
[1]Department of Surgery, Lithuanian University of Health Sciences, Eiveniu Str. 2, Kaunas LT-50009, Lithuania
Full list of author information is available at the end of the article

Previous studies have shown that age, lymph node and liver metastasis, disease stage and tumour size are important predictive factors for survival in patients with resectable gastric cancer [9-11]. However it is not certainly clear if these predictive factors are the same in all regions and why incidence rates of gastric cancer are still high in the region of Eastern Europe.

The aim of this single centre study was to compare the clinical course and outcomes, such as postoperative complications, the length of hospital stay and mortality rate, over two distinctive time periods.

Methods

This was a retrospective non-randomized, single center, cohort study. Data collection was performed at the Department of Surgery, Lithuanian University of Health Sciences using specially developed and maintained database from 01-01-1994 to 31-12-2007. During this period 708 patients underwent radical gastrectomy. Five hundred fifty seven consecutive patients were included in the study according to the following inclusion criteria: (1) histologically proven gastric adenocarcinoma; (2) diagnosis based on the UICC TNM staging classification; (3) curative D1 or D2 gastrectomy performed; (4) available complete medical record; (5) postoperative follow-up. Patients with proven distant metastatic disease and in whom only palliative surgery was performed, were excluded from the study. The study population was divided in two groups according to two equal time periods: 01-01-1994 – 31-12-2000 (Group I – 273 patients) and 01-01-2001 – 31-12-2007 (Group II – 284 patients). During the first time period patients diagnosed

with gastric cancer were treated according to the guidelines of that time. Standardized protocol was introduced in the year 2001: preoperative evaluation and care (preoperative computed tomography (CT) staging, prophylactic antibiotics), surgical treatment and postoperative care (prophylaxis of thromboembolic disorders; early mobilisation; on day 2 after surgery patients were allowed to drink clear liquids; on postoperative day 3 the soft diet was allowed; drain's placement was at the discretion of the surgeon). The Kaunas Regional Biomedical Research Ethics Committee approved the study (protocol no. BE-2-10) and allowed the use of publicly unavailable database. All patients provided written informed consent. The primary outcome was measured as the five-year survival rate. The gastric cancer- related survival, rates of postoperative complications, the length of hospital stay and 30-day mortality rate were considered as secondary outcomes. The outcomes were studied to evaluate the progress in gastric cancer treatment results over time.

Surgical procedure

All the surgical procedures were based on the intention to cure. The extent of the surgical procedure was planned based on pre-operative and intra-operative findings, physical condition of the patient. Considering the location of the tumor, routinely standard total (adenocarcinoma involving the proximal third of the stomach) or subtotal (adenocarcinoma of the distal and middle thirds of the stomach) gastrectomy with D1 or D2 lymphadenectomy and a Roux-en-Y reconstruction was performed. Surgical procedures and the definition of

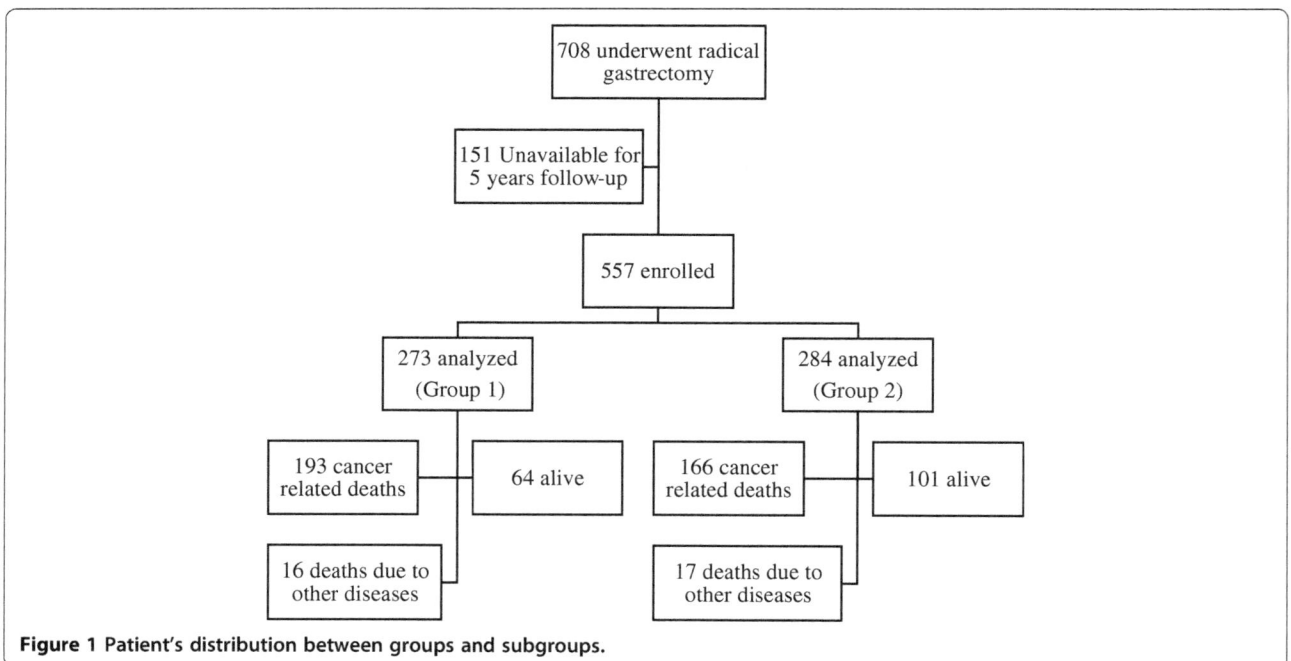

Figure 1 Patient's distribution between groups and subgroups.

Trends and results in treatment of gastric cancer over last two decades at single East...

43

lymphadenectomy referred to the Japanese Classification of Gastric Carcinoma [12]. Combined multiorgan resections were performed in cases of advanced tumors involving the pancreas, colon or spleen. Surgery was considered as a curative when there was no macroscopically residual tumor after surgery and resection margins were histologically clear (R0).

Postoperative course

Postoperative complications were classified according Clavien-Dindo grading system for the classification of surgical complications (Grade I - V) [13].

Different mainly fluorouracil (5-FU) based adjuvant chemotherapy regiments were inconsistently used postoperatively in the period from 1994 to 2000. Whereas patients during the period from 2001 to 2007 as a standard received a combined 5-FU and leucovorin adjuvant chemotherapy or concurrent chemoradion treatment (5-FU and leucovorin with 45 Gy radiation dose) in more advanced cancer cases.

Statistical analysis

Statistical analysis was performed using SPSS 14.0 for Windows *(SPSS Inc., Chicago, USA)*. The data are presented as mean ± Standard deviation or median and range. The cumulative survival was determined by the Kaplan-Meier method, and univariate comparisons between the groups were performed using the log-rank test. The independent prognostic factors were examined by Cox regression analysis. For comparison between groups, the Mann–Whitney test or Student's t test were employed where appropriate. $P < 0.05$ was considered statistically significant.

Results

Seven hundred and eight patients with proven gastric adenocarcinoma underwent a subtotal or total gastrectomy

Table 1 Patients' characteristics

Parameter	Group I	Group II	P value
Gender			
Male	155 (56.8%)	164 (57.7%)	0.944
Female	118 (43.2%)	120 (42.3%)	0.938
Age	63.2 ± 12.7	64.3 ± 12.1	0.331
≤ 65	135 (49.5%)	134 (47.2%)	0.767
> 65	138 (50.5%)	150 (52.8%)	0.772
Procedure			
Total gastrectomy	80 (29.3%)	52 (18.3%)	0.019
Subtotal gastrectomy	193 (70.7%)	232 (81.7%)	0.273
D1 lymphadenectomy	7 (2.6%)	5 (1.8%)	0.572
D2 lymphadenectomy	266 (97.4%)	279 (98.2%)	0.952
Total	273	284	

Table 2 Staging of the disease

Parameter	Group I	Group II	P value
Pathological stage			
T1	21 (7.7%)	39 (13.7%)	0.042
T2	42 (15.4%)	101 (35.6%)	0.0001
T3	118 (43.2%)	116 (40.8%)	0.775
T4	92 (33.7%)	28 (9.9%)	0.0001
N stage			
N0	86 (31.5%)	91 (32.0%)	0.931
N1	68 (24.9%)	87 (30.6%)	0.276
N2	92 (33.7%)	73 (25.7%)	0.133
N3	27 (9.9%)	33 (11.6%)	0.589
TNM Stage			
IA	18 (6.6%)	30 (10.6%)	0.135
IB	30 (11.0%)	47 (16.5%)	0.114
IIA	43 (15.8%)	61 (21.5%)	0.165
IIB	51 (18.7%)	47 (16.5%)	0.586
IIIA	58 (21.2%)	65 (22.9%)	0.765
IIIB	51 (18.7%)	24 (8.5%)	0.002
IIIC	22 (8.1%)	10 (3.5%)	0.044

and D1 or D2 lymphadenectomy with curative intent between 1994 and 2007. One hundred fifty one patients were unavailable for 5 years follow-up. The most frequent detected reason of the unavailability was moving abroad. Data from 557 patients which were followed-up postoperatively was analysed. The distribution of patients between groups and subgroups is shown in Figure 1. There were no significant differences between the groups in gender and age. The number of elderly (>65 years) patients was also similar (50.5% vs. 52.8%). Total gastrectomy was statistically significantly more often performed in Group I (29.3%) than in Group II (18.3%). D2 lymphadenectomy was more often performed than D1 lymphadenectomy in both groups (Table 1). Gastric cancer in early stages (IA - IIA)

Table 3 Postoperative course and outcomes

Parameter	Group I	Group II	P value
Hospital stay (days)	22.61 ± 28.96	16.20 ± 17.01	0.001
Complications*	55 (20.1%)	42 (14.8%)	0.187
I	13 (4.7%)	15 (5.4%)	0.848
II	8 (2.9%)	6 (2.1%)	0.598
III	26 (9.5%)	11 (3.9%)	0.017
IV	4 (1.5%)	5 (1.7%)	1.000
V	4 (1.5%)	5 (1.7%)	1.000
30-day mortality	15 (5.5%)	4 (1.4%)	0.017

*- According to Clavien-Dindo grading system for the classification of surgical complications.

Table 4 Postoperative survival analysis

Parameter	Group I	Group II	P value
Overall survival (months)	48.40+/−65,966	43.78+/− 39.736	0.319
1-year survival rate	137 (50.2%)	203 (71.5%)	0.013
2-years survival rate	110 (40.3%)	150 (52.8%)	0.083
5-year survival rate	64 (23.4%)	101 (35.6%)	0.021
IA	11 (61.1%)	25 (83.3%)	0.644
IB	22 (73.3%)	33 (70.2%)	1.000
IIA	17 (39.5%)	23 (37.7%)	1.000
IIB	7 (13.7%)	13 (27.7%)	0.221
IIIA	7 (12.1%)	5 (7.7%)	0.552
IIIB	0	2 (8.3%)	0.111
IIIC	0	0	-
Deaths	209 (76.6%)	183 (64.4%)	0.210
Gastric cancer related	193 (92.3%)	166 (90.7%)	0.942
Other causes	16 (7.7%)	17 (9.3%)	0.717

was more frequently diagnosed in Group II than in Group I and in late stages (IIB - IIIC) more frequently in Group I. Statistically significant difference was found only when comparing stages IIIB-IIIC. Significantly more patients were diagnosed with lower stage of the primary tumor

(T stage) in Group II (13.7% vs 7.7% in T1 stage (P = 0.04) and 35.6% vs 15.4% in T2 stage (P = 0.0001)). On the contrary in Group I more patients were diagnosed in T4 stage (33.7% vs 9.9%, P = 0.0001) (Table 2).

When analyzing postoperative course of the disease shorter hospital stay (16.20 ± 17.01 vs. 22.61 ± 28.96 days, P = 0.001) and lower 30-day mortality rate (1.4% vs 5.5%, P = 0.0173) was identified in Group II. During postoperative period in 6 patients (2.2%) of Group I and in 7 patients (2.5%) of Group II anastomotic leakage was identified. However grade of postoperative complications was similar between both groups. Only Grade III (Complications requiring surgical, endoscopic or radiological intervention) complications were statistically significant more often identified in Group I (9.5% vs 3.9%, P = 0.017) (Table 3).

The survival analysis revealed higher median overall survival (months) in Group I (48.40 ± 65.966 vs. 43.78 ± 39.736). However Group I patients are observed for a longer time period and long-term survivors among them could influence this outcome. In contrary when analysing 1-year and 5-year survival rates, significantly higher survival is observed in Group II (71.5% vs. 50.2% and 35.6% vs. 23.4%). Patients with more advanced T stage and involved lymphnodes had worse 5-year survival prognosis as compared with patients with les advanced

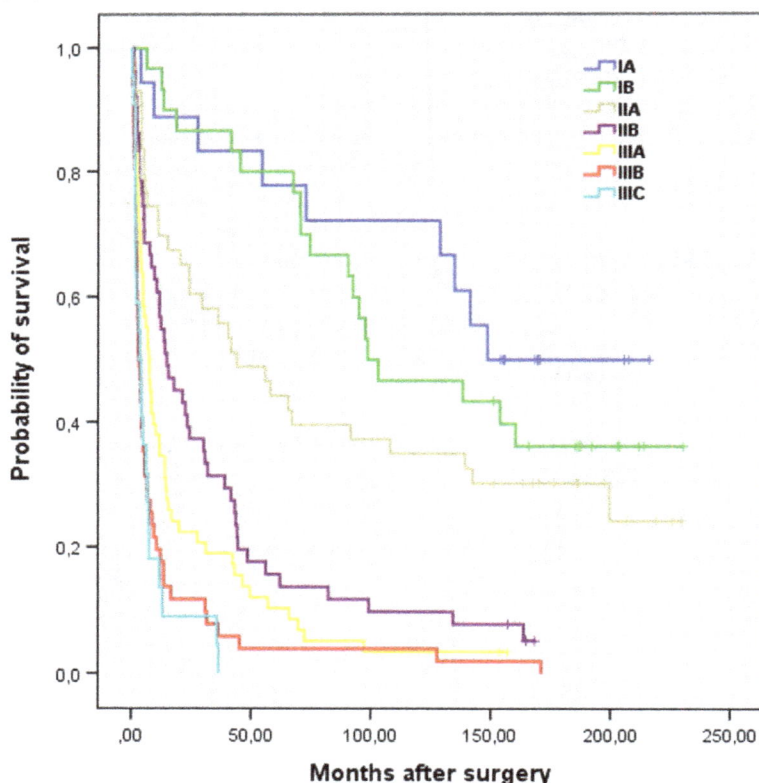

Figure 2 Overall survival (in months) after surgery according to TNM stage (Group I).

T stage and no lymphnodes involvement. However statistically significant difference was found only when analyzing lymphnodes involvement (p < 0.05).

In both groups the reasons of death were similar; the majority of patients died of gastric cancer (92.3% vs. 90.7%). There was no difference in 5-year survival rate when comparing different TNM stages between both groups (Table 4). However in early stages (IA - IIA) survival rate was higher comparing with advanced stages (IIB - IIIC) (Figures 2 and 3).

Discussions

The incidence of gastric cancer in Eastern Europe remains high following Eastern Asia and South America. The highest gastric cancer incidence rate in European Union (EU) is reported in Lithuania [14]. In this single-institutional study we present case series from large university hospital in Lithuania raising a question: is there a significant progress in terms of treatment success and survival among patients diagnosed with gastric cancer and treated with curative surgery over time? To clarify changes, positive or negative tendencies the two groups on background of time of surgery were created.

Most of demographic data, clinicopathologic characteristics in our study are comparable to the groups presented

from other European countries. Regrettably, gastric cancer remains often diagnosed in advanced stages in Lithuania, leading to poor prognosis. Late diagnosis of gastric cancer is a well-known problem among patients from Western countries. Hundahl et al. [7] from United States (US) report 65% of gastric cancers presenting at an advanced stage (T3-T4) with a nearly 85% of tumours accompanied with lymph node affection at the time of surgery. The data are very close to ours (T3-T4 - 63.6%; N+ 68.2%). However higher gastric cancer incidence rate in Lithuania leads to even more actual problem.

The interesting difference identified between our data and studies done in Western Europe - a lack of growing incidence of upper-third gastric cancer. In contrary, we even had more distal and middle third tumours and higher proportion of patients underwent subtotal gastrectomy in Group II. Although we have not analysed this factor in our study, high prevalence of Helicobacter pylori infection in Lithuania (78.5% in the year 1999 and 69.7% in the year 2005) could be related to the high incidence of gastric cancer [15].

The overall incidence of directly surgery-related postoperative complications in our study (anastomosis or duodenal stump leakage) <3% is comparable to majority of published data [16-18]. The rate and grade of postoperative

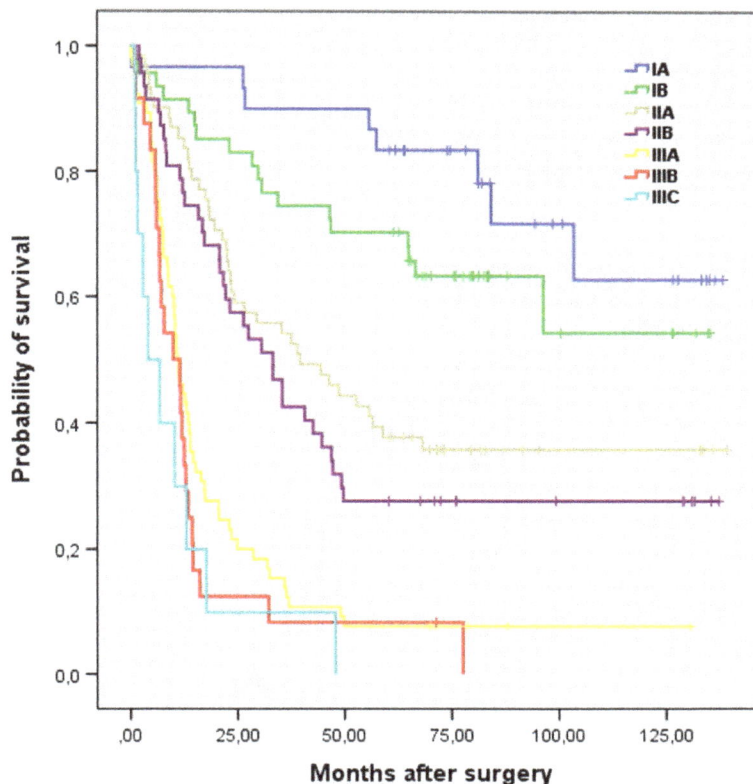

Figure 3 Overall survival (in months) after surgery according to TNM stage (Group II).

complications (except Grade III complications) in our study was similar in both groups; however 30-day mortality rate and in-hospital stay decreased significantly in Group II. These results should be considered as a consequence of more detailed preoperative patients' selection, standardised surgery technique, and improved perioperative care over time.

The overall 5-year survival rate was slightly higher in Group II, however remaining below 40% in entire cohort. The higher survival rate possibly caused by a higher rate of early detection (standardized protocol of diagnosis) of gastric cancer (more T1, T2 tumours, less IIIB, IIIC stages in Group II), perioperative care improvement over time and possibilities of palliation procedures in cases of recurrent disease. The most common cause of treatment failure in our study was peritoneal recurrence and spread of the disease. Similar data are presented by other authors [19,20]. Observed 5-year survival rate in early stages (IA 61.1% vs. 83.3% and IB 73.3% vs. 70.2%) of gastric cancer is lower than in Eastern countries, but is similar to the data presented by the Western European countries from the similar time period [21,22].

Regarding the surgical technique and extent of lymph node dissection, it became highly standardised over last 15 years. The patients in our study mainly underwent gastrectomy with a Roux-en-Y reconstruction and D2 lymphadenectomy (97.4% vs. 98.2%). There has been controversy regarding the extent of lymph node dissection around the European centres in last decade, pointing on higher postoperative morbidity after D2 dissection, however most experts suggest that extended lymphadenectomy could be performed with acceptable morbidity and mortality rate by specialized surgeons in large-volume centres [23-25].

Conclusions

Despite some positive changes in early postoperative mortality rate, hospital stay and overall survival over the time, gastric cancer treatment results remain poor. Prognosis of treatment of gastric cancer depends mainly on the stage of the disease. Absence of screening programs and lack of clinical symptoms in early stages of gastric cancer lead to circumstances when most of the patients presenting with advanced stage of the disease can expect a median survival of less than 30 months even after curative intent surgery. The most efficient way to reach more significant progress in gastric cancer treatment should concentrate mostly on earlier diagnosis, when survival results after radical surgery are far more promising.

Competing interests
The authors declare that they have no competing interests.

Authors' contributions
AM, PI, RM, AP, DB, MK, ZE collected, analysed and interpreted the data. AM, AM, ZD drafted the study concept and design, supervised the study,

analysed and interpreted the data. AM, PI, ZD drafted the manuscript. All authors read and approved the final manuscript.

Author details
[1]Department of Surgery, Lithuanian University of Health Sciences, Eiveniu Str. 2, Kaunas LT-50009, Lithuania. [2]Laboratory of Surgical Gastroenterology, Institute for Digestive System Research, Lithuanian University of Health Sciences, Eivenių str. 2, Kaunas LT-50009, Lithuania. [3]Department of Oncology, Lithuanian University of Health Sciences, Eivenių str. 2, Kaunas LT-50009, Lithuania.

References
1. Parkin DM, Bray F, Ferlay J, Pisani P: Global cancer statistics, 2002. CA Cancer J Clin 2005, 55(2):74–108.
2. Yamaoka Y, Kato M, Asaka M: Geographic differences in gastric cancer incidence can be explained by differences between Helicobacter pylori strains. Intern Med 2008, 47(12):1077–1083.
3. Smailyte G, Kurtinaitis J: Cancer mortality differences among urban and rural residents in Lithuania. BMC Public Health 2008, 8:56.
4. Fukuda N, Sugiyama Y, Wada J: Prognostic factors of T4 gastric cancer patients undergoing potentially curative resection. WJG 2011, 17(9):1180–1184.
5. Dikken JL, van de Velde CJ, Coit DG, Shah MA, Verheij M, Cats A: Treatment of resectable gastric cancer. Ther Adv Gastroenterol 2012, 5(1):49–69.
6. Lee JH, Kim KM, Cheong JH, Noh SH: Current management and future strategies of gastric cancer. Yonsei Med J 2012, 53(2):248–257.
7. Hundahl SA, Phillips JL, Menck HR: The National Cancer Data Base Report on poor survival of U.S. gastric carcinoma patients treated with gastrectomy: Fifth Edition American Joint Committee on Cancer staging, proximal disease, and the "different disease" hypothesis. Cancer 2000, 88(4):921–932.
8. Cenitagoya GF, Bergh CK, Klinger-Roitman J: A prospective study of gastric cancer. 'Real' 5-year survival rates and mortality rates in a country with high incidence. Digestive surgery 1998, 15(4):317–322.
9. Shiraishi N, Sato K, Yasuda K, Inomata M, Kitano S: Multivariate prognostic study on large gastric cancer. J Surg Oncol 2007, 96(1):14–18.
10. Seo SH, Hur H, An CW, Yi X, Kim JY, Han SU, Cho YK: Operative risk factors in gastric cancer surgery for elderly patients. J Gastric Cancer 2011, 11(2):116–121.
11. Smith JK, McPhee JT, Hill JS, Whalen GF, Sullivan ME, Litwin DE, Anderson FA, Tseng JF: National outcomes after gastric resection for neoplasm. Arch Surg 2007, 142(4):387–393.
12. Japanese Gastric Cancer A: Japanese classification of gastric carcinoma: 3rd English edition. Gastric Cancer 2011, 14(2):101–112.
13. Clavien PA, Barkun J, de Oliveira ML, Vauthey JN, Dindo D, Schulick RD, de Santibanes E, Pekolj J, Slankamenac K, Bassi C, Graf R, Vonlanthen R, Padbury R, Cameron JL, Makuuchi M: The Clavien-Dindo classification of surgical complications: five-year experience. Ann Surg 2009, 250(2):187–196.
14. Levi F, Lucchini F, Negri E, La Vecchia C: Trends in mortality from major cancers in the European Union, including acceding countries, in 2004. Cancer 2004, 101(12):2843–2850.
15. Jonaitis L, Ivanauskas A, Janciauskas D, Funka K, Sudraba A, Tolmanis I, Krams A, Stirna D, Vanags A, Kupcinskas L, Leja M, Lin JT: Precancerous gastric conditions in high Helicobacter pylori prevalence areas: comparison between Eastern European (Lithuanian, Latvian) and Asian (Taiwanese) patients. Medicina 2007, 43(8):623–629.
16. Gockel I, Pietzka S, Gonner U, Hommel G, Junginger T: Subtotal or total gastrectomy for gastric cancer: impact of the surgical procedure on morbidity and prognosis–analysis of a 10-year experience. Langenbecks Arch Surg 2005, 390(2):148–155.
17. Oh SJ, Choi WB, Song J, Hyung WJ, Choi SH, Noh SH, Yonsei Gastric Cancer C: Complications requiring reoperation after gastrectomy for gastric cancer: 17 years experience in a single institute. J Gastrointest Surg 2009, 13(2):239–245.
18. Otsuji E, Fujiyama J, Takagi T, Ito T, Kuriu Y, Toma A, Okamoto K, Hagiwara A, Yamagishi H: Results of total gastrectomy with extended lymphadenectomy for gastric cancer in elderly patients. J Surg Oncol 2005, 91(4):232–236.

19. Yoo CH, Noh SH, Shin DW, Choi SH, Min JS: Recurrence following curative resection for gastric carcinoma. *Br J Surg* 2000, **87**(2):236–242.

20. Moriguchi S, Maehara Y, Korenaga D, Sugimachi K, Nose Y: **Risk factors which predict pattern of recurrence after curative surgery for patients with advanced gastric cancer.** *Surg Oncol* 1992, 1(5):341–346.

21. Lamb P, Sivashanmugam T, White M, Irving M, Wayman J, Raimes S: **Gastric cancer surgery–a balance of risk and radicality.** *Ann R Coll Surg Engl* 2008, **90**(3):235–242.

22. Bonenkamp JJ, Hermans J, Sasako M, van de Velde CJ, Welvaart K, Songun I, Meyer S, Plukker JT, Van Elk P, Obertop H, Gouma DJ, Van Lanschot JJ, Taat CW, De Graaf PW, Von Meyenfeldt MF, Tilanus H, Dutch Gastric Cancer Group: **Extended lymph-node dissection for gastric cancer.** *N Engl J Med* 1999, **340**(12):908–914.

23. Hartgrink HH, van de Velde CJ, Putter H, Bonenkamp JJ, Klein Kranenbarg E, Songun I, Welvaart K, van Krieken JH, Meijer S, Plukker JT, Van Elk PJ, Obertop H, Gouma DJ, Van Lanschot JJ, Taat CW, De Graaf PW, Von Meyenfeldt MF, Tilanus H, Sasako M: **Extended lymph node dissection for gastric cancer: who may benefit? Final results of the randomized Dutch gastric cancer group trial.** *J Clin Oncol* 2004, **22**(11):2069–2077.

24. Cuschieri A, Weeden S, Fielding J, Bancewicz J, Craven J, Joypaul V, Sydes M, Fayers P: **Patient survival after D1 and D2 resections for gastric cancer: long-term results of the MRC randomized surgical trial. Surg Co-operative Group.** *Br J Cancer* 1999, **79**(9–10):1522–1530.

25. Songun I, Putter H, Kranenbarg EM, Sasako M, van de Velde CJ: **Surgical treatment of gastric cancer: 15-year follow-up results of the randomised nationwide Dutch D1D2 trial.** *Lancet Oncol* 2010, **11**(5):439–449.

8

Impact of neoadjuvant chemotherapy with PELF-protocoll versus surgery alone in the treatment of advanced gastric carcinoma

Catharina Ruf[1], Oliver Thomusch[1], Matthias Goos[1], Frank Makowiec[1], Gerald Illerhaus[2] and Guenther Ruf[1*]

Abstract

Background: In a retrospective study we analyzed the impact of neoadjuvant chemotherapy (CTx) with the PELF - protocol (Cisplatin, Epirubicin, Leukovorin, 5-Fluoruracil) on mortality, recurrence and prognosis of patients with advanced gastric carcinoma, UICC stages Ib-III.

Methods: 64 patients were included. 26 patients received neoadjuvant CTx followed by surgical resection, 38 received surgical resection only. Tumor staging was performed by endoscopy, endosonography, computed tomography and laparoscopy. Patients staged Ib – III received two cycles of CTx according to the PELF-protocol. Adjuvant chemotherapy was not performed at all.

Results: Complete (CR) or partial response (PR) was seen in 20 patients (77%), 19% showing CR and 58% PR. No benefit was observed in 6 patients (23%). Two of these 6 patients displayed tumor progression during CTx. Major toxicity was defined as grade 3 to 4 neutropenia or gastrointestinal side effects. One patient died under CTx because of neutropenia and was excluded from the overall patient collective. The curative resection rate was 77% after CTx and 74% after surgery only. The perioperative morbidity rate after CTx was 39% versus 66% after resection only. Recurrence rate after CTx was 38% and 61% after surgery alone; we detected an effective reduction of locoregional recurrence (12% vs. 26%). The overall survival was 38% after CTx and 42% after resection only. The 5-year survival rates were 45% in responders, 20% in non - responders and 42% in only resected patients. A subgroup analysis indicates that responders with stage III tumors may benefit with respect to their 5-year survival in comparable patients without neoadjuvant CTx. As to be expected, non-responders with stage III tumors did not benefit with respect to their survival. The 5-year-survival was approximated using a Kaplan-Meier curve and compared using a log-rank test.

Conclusion: In patients with advanced gastric carcinoma, neoadjuvant CTx with the PELF- protocol significantly reduces the recurrence rate, especially locoregionally, compared to surgery alone. In our study, there was no overall survival benefit after a 5-year follow-up period. Alone a subgroup of patients with stage III tumors appear to benefit significantly in the long term from neoadjuvant CTx.

Keywords: Neoadjuvant chemotherapy, PELF, Advanced gastric cancer

* Correspondence: guenther.ruf@uniklinik-freiburg.de
[1]Department of Surgery, University of Freiburg, Universitätsklinikum, Hugstetterstr. 55, D-79106 Freiburg, Germany
Full list of author information is available at the end of the article

Background

Gastric carcinoma is the second most common GI-cancer with a poor overall prognosis [1]. Surgical resection is the only curative treatment option in afflicted patients. Detrimentally, the overall resection rate is as low as 33%, and in less than 60% of these patients R0-resection is possible [2,3]. At the time of diagnosis, half of patients suffer from advanced tumor disease making curative resection uncertain at best [1,2]. The probability of lymph node metastasis rapidly increases with the depth of infiltration. Already patients with stage Ib tumors have a high likelihood of lymph node metastases and therefore have a high recurrence rate of up to 69%, even following curative surgery [1,2,4]. Locoregional recurrence is most common (87%), but peritoneal and liver metastasis occur as well (13%) [5,6]. These data dramatically illustrate the importance of detecting gastric carcinoma at earlier stages.

The current survival rate across all tumor stages ranges between 40% and 50% and is still achieved primarily by curative surgical resection [7]. Only patients with Ia-tumors have a reasonably good prognosis with a 5-year survival rate of 83%. The survival rates of patients with more advanced tumors quickly decreases to 69% in patients with Ib tumors, 43% in stage II, 28% in stage III and 8.7% in stage IV patients [8-15].

Perioperative chemotherapy was thought to improve this dire prognosis, especially in patients with advanced tumor stages (UICC Ib-III) by down-staging the tumor and increasing the rate of curative resection [1,2,16]. Intraoperative radiation or adjuvant radio-/chemotherapy with various regimens do in fact successfully reduce locoregional recurrence, but fail to improve the long-term outcome [5,11-15].

Neoadjuvant chemotherapy (CTx) on the other hand is believed to reduce intraoperative tumor cell dissemination as well as occult micrometastases. Strategically, it is hoped that this may increase the curative resection rate and reduce locoregional recurrence, thus improving the prognosis of advanced gastric carcinoma [2,7,17].

Methods

From January 2000 to December 2006, we treated a total of 124 patients with gastric carcinoma. All patients with an early tumor stage (UICC Ia), distant metastases (liver or peritoneum), oesophageal tumor localization, concomitant active malignant disease or poor liver and kidney functions and patients who denied CTx were excluded from our study. 64 patients with stage Ib – III gastric carcinoma were included. They received either a combined modality treatment with neoadjuvant CTx and surgery or surgical resection only. All patients chose chemotherapy after informed consent. All data were assessed retrospectively.

Staging was performed using the AJCC/UICC classification by means of endoscopy, endoscopic sonography, computed tomography and laparoscopy. The standard surgical procedure consisted of total gastrectomy and entailed D-2 lymphadenectomy. Subtotal gastrectomy and D2-lymphadenectomy were restricted to early stages of intestinal-type cancers of the distal third of the stomach. The resection margins were examined by frozen sections intraoperatively. Neoadjuvant CTx was administered according to the PELF-protocol in two cycles at 0 and 6 weeks: Cisplatin 40 mg/m^2, Epirubicin 35 mg/m^2, Leucovorin 500 mg/m^2 and 5-Fluoruracil 500 mg/m^2. Chemotherapy was terminated in cases of gastrointestinal and grade 2 to 4 hematologic toxicities. Subsequent to CTx, a second CT-scan, endoscopy and endoscopic sonography were performed to restage the tumor. Objective response was evaluated by histological examination and classified as "complete", "partial" or "no response". Histological regression was graded as "little", "moderate" or "strong". Both groups were compared with respect to age, sex, symptoms, diagnosis, tumor localization (proximal/distal), histology (Lauren type and WHO classification), grading (low, medium, high), extent of surgery (total/subtotal gastrectomy), and resection status (R0/R1). Endpoint criteria were complications during therapy, tumor recurrence and survival. Furthermore, responders and non-responders were compared with regard to completion of CTx, distribution of tumor stages, resection status and long-term survival (5-year follow-up). The 5-year-survival was approximated using a Kaplan-Meier curve and compared using a log-rank test. Clinical follow-up spanned the time from initial diagnosis of gastric cancer until the last registered visit in the clinical records of our 'Comprehensive Cancer Care Center Freiburg' or the day of death. All cases of postoperative death, including patients who died of other causes, were included in the survival analysis.

All statistical calculations were performed using SPSS 15 (SPSS Inc., Chicago) software. Statistical analysis was performed using X test, t test, and Fisher's exact test. Results were considered statistically significant at $P < 0.05$.

Results

One Patient, who died under neoadjuvant chemotherapy, was excluded. In total, 64 patients with advanced gastric carcinoma staged UICC Ib-III were included in the study. 26 of these received preoperative CTx followed by surgical resection. The other 38 patients received resection only. Patient characteristics were well balanced in both groups (Table 1). Median age was 67.86 years. There were 21 women and 43 men. Stage Ib was diagnosed in 12 patients (19%), stage II in 20 (31%) and stage III in 32 (50%). The tumor was located in the proximal stomach in 46 patients. Most frequently, an poorly differentiated (G3) intestinal Lauren type (36/64) tumor was found. All 64 patients underwent surgical Resection. 56 patients received total gastrectomy with D2-lymphadenectomy, 8

Table 1 Patients characteristics (n = 64)

	Neoadjuvant CTx (n = 26/64)	Surgery n (n = 38/64)
Age		
Median (years)	64.5	73
(range)	(38–76)	(43–91)
Sex		
Males	20	23
Females	6	15
Tumor localization		
Proximal	20	26
Distal	6	12
Surgical procedure		
Total gastrectomy	25	31
Subtotal gastrectomy	1	7
D2-lymphadenectomy	26	38
Resection		
Curative (R0)	20	28
Palliative (R1)	6	10
UICC stage, pretherapeutic		
Ib	2	10
II	7	13
III	17	15
WHO classification		
Adenocarcinoma	20	31
Signet-cell carcinoma	6	7
Grading		
G 1-2	6	21
G 3	20	17
Lauren-classification		
Intestinal	15	21
Diffuse	11	17

Table 2 Comparison of tumor stage distribution before and after chemotherapy (downstaging) and resection only

UICC	Neoadjuvant CTx (n = 26/64)		Surgery (n = 38/64)	
	Before CTx	Postoperative	Preoperative	Postoperative
Ib	2	10	10	16
II	7	7	13	9
III	17	3	15	7
IV	0	6	0	6

regressiongrade 2; the examination of the resected tissue of the remaining patients showed complete necrosis. (Regression grade was examined by JRSGC). The histological response was particularly significant among patients staged UICC III. Table 2 illustrates pre- versus postoperative tumor staging in both groups. The curative resection rate after neoadjuvant CTx was 77% (n = 20/26) and was accomplished in 17 responders and 3 non-responders. R1-resection was diagnosed in 6 cases (3 responders and 3 non-responders).

Postoperative complications developed in 35 of 64 patients. The complication rate was 39% in the group with chemotherapy (n = 10/26) and 66% after surgical resection only (n = 25/38). Common complications like pneumonia (7/64), pulmonary embolism (2/64) and urinary infection (1/64) occurred more frequently in the group without neodjuvant CTx. Complication like deep vein thrombosis appeared in both groups with the same frequency (2/64). Between the two groups, there was no difference with respect to the surgical complication rate, which arose in 8 of 26 patients subsequent to CTx and 15 of 38 patients after resection only. Anastomotic leakage occurred in 12% after CTx and 11% after resection only. Also intestinal obstruction (3/64), delayed nourishment (5/64) and wound infection (8/64) weren't more frequent in the group with CTx (Table 3).

Overall recurrence rate was 52% (n = 33/64). CTx reduced the overall recurrence rate and was 39% in the neoadjuvant group versus 63% in the only surgery group

patients received subtotal gastrectomy in cases of early tumor stages and intestinal-type tumors with distal localization. The overall curative resection rate (R0) was 75% (n = 48/64). Thus by definition, 16 patients received not curative resection (R1).

Preoperative CTx was administered in 26 and completed in 18 patients. In 8 cases, CTx was aborted due to gastrointestinal toxicity, i.e. nausea, vomiting and diarrhea (n = 3/26), hematologic toxicity, i.e. neutropenia (n = 2/26), complete early tumor regression in one case and tumor progression in 2 further patients. We observed a histological response rate of 77% (n = 20/26), 5 patients showing complete and 15 patients displaying partial response. No histological benefit was detected in 6 patients (23%). In respect of the regression grade 75% showed submucosal subtotal cicatrisation, which complies with

Table 3 Complications

	Neoadjuvant CTx (n = 26/64)	Surgery (n = 38/64)
Anastomotic leakage	3	4
Delayed nourishment	0	5
Intestinal obstruction	2	1
Wound infection	3	5
Pneumonia	1	6
Urinary infection	0	1
Lung embolism	0	2
Deep vein thrombosis	1	1

Table 4 Localization of recurrence

	Neoadjuvant CTx (n = 26/64)	Surgery (n = 38/64)
Local	3	10
Peritoneal	3	4
Lymph node metastases	0	5
Distant metastases	4	5

(Table 4). Especially locoregional recurrence was reduced after chemotherapy and occurred in 12% versus 26% after resection only. Lymph node metastases merely occurred in only resected patients. However, peritoneal recurrence or distant metastases couldn't be prevented by CTx.

The overall survival was not improved by CTx (Figure 1). The 5-year survival rate was 38% after CTx versus 42% after surgery only. Not even a subgroup analysis comparing responders with only resected patients showed a benefit of CTx. The 5-year survival rate of responders was 44% versus the above mentioned 42% after surgery only. Non-responders to CTx had a worse survival rate of 20% (Figure 2).

A subgroup analysis of patients with preoperative stage III tumors showed a significantly improved survival in responders to chemotherapy compared to patients without response (p = 0.002) (Figure 3).

Discussion

The poor prognosis of gastric carcinoma has remained unchanged for the past 2 decades with a 5-year-survival rate ranging between 40% and 50%. Surgery is the only curative treatment option for locally advanced disease. Furthermore, most patients are initially diagnosed at advanced tumor stages. Despite curative resection (R0), the overall recurrence rate is 69%. Locoregional relapse

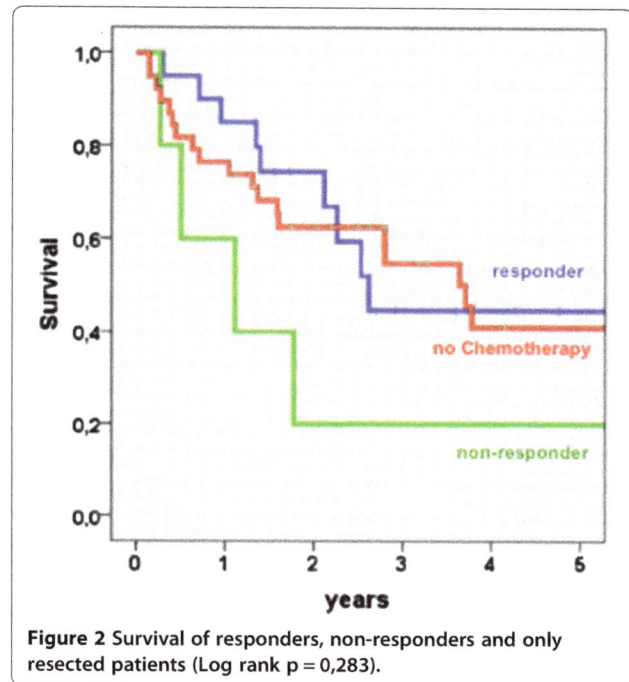

Figure 2 Survival of responders, non-responders and only resected patients (Log rank p = 0,283).

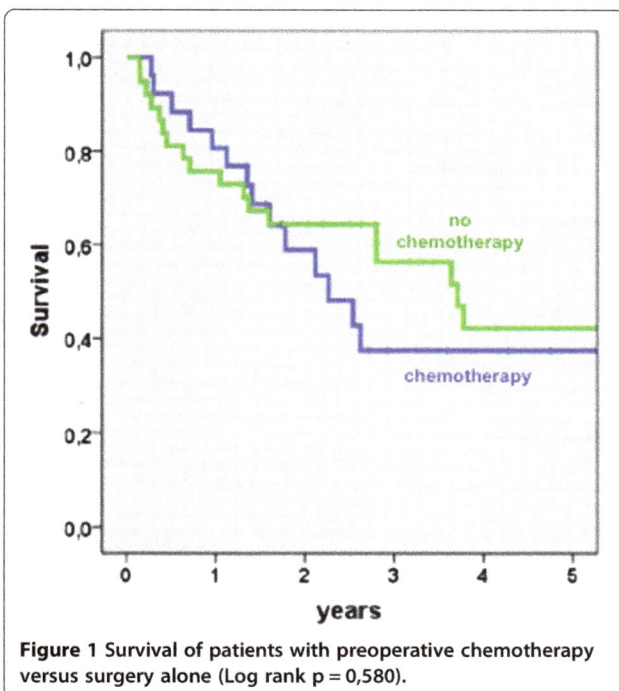

Figure 1 Survival of patients with preoperative chemotherapy versus surgery alone (Log rank p = 0,580).

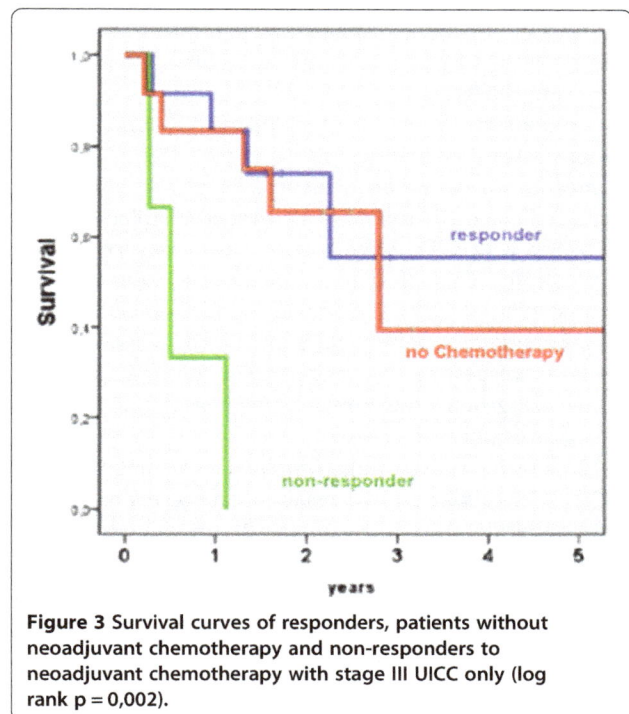

Figure 3 Survival curves of responders, patients without neoadjuvant chemotherapy and non-responders to neoadjuvant chemotherapy with stage III UICC only (log rank p = 0,002).

(87%) as well as lymphatic and peritoneal metastasis have a high likelihood [1,4,6]. Radiation and chemotherapy aim at controlling local tumor spread and eliminating disseminated tumor cells to prolong survival [18]. Intraoperative radiation succeeded in reducing locoregional relapse, but failed in improving overall survival [5]. The palliative implementation of PELF-CTx had a significant impact on the median survival [19]. Therefore, we investigated the influence of this protocol in the neoadjuvant setting on morbidity and mortality, tumor recurrence and prognosis.

Regarding size, our study ranges in the lower third of current literature [1,2,5,20]. With respect to age (median 69 years), lack of specific symptomatology in early tumor stages and typical symptoms in advanced stages of gastric cancer, diagnosis/staging and tumor localization, our study population compares well with similar trials [1,2,5,20]. Furthermore, our inclusion criteria are very similar to comparable studies [1,2,20]. In our study, patients with UICC stages Ib-III, diagnosed by imaging, were included. In comparable trials, only patients with stage IV and M + or only stages IIIa/b and IV were included [1,7,20].

Preoperative CTx aims at devitalizing and downsizing tumor tissue to increase the chance of curative resection [6]. In 20 patients (77%), there was an objective histological response. This is considerably more than in other studies where histological response was observed in 17% to 50% of cases [1,2,20-22]. An exceptional response was observed in cases of UICC stage III tumors (Table 2). In these patients a clear down-staging was recognizable [2,6,20]. Following CTx, the curative resection rate was 77%, thus exceeding reported R0-resection rates of around 60% [2,20]. However, compared to the result in patients who received surgical resection only (74%), we found no significant difference.

A comparison of pre- and postoperative tumor staging demonstrates a surprisingly low accuracy of implemented diagnostics. In the group without CTx, only 7 cases of 15 diagnosed stage III tumors were verified histologically. In the group with CTx, only 3 of 17 cases were confirmed histologically. This effect may however be explained by a down-staging of CTx. The similar high R0-resection rates in both study groups may be indicative of diagnostic imprecision, suggesting that more earlier tumor stages were in the CTx group. Unfortunately, explaining this in retrospect proves unfeasible.

Preoperative CTx is hoped to reduce recurrence rates (69%) by making curative resection more probable and by eliminating micrometastases [2]. In our study, the relapse rate was 38% after CTx versus 63% following surgery. Other studies report recurrence rates of 60% to 70% following CTx [5,20]. Especially local recurrence seems to be reduced after preoperative chemotherapy. 26% after surgery only and 12% of patients with CTx developed locoregional recurrence. These results are comparable with the local relapse after intraoperative radiation (10%) [5]. Recurrence in lymph nodes was only seen in patients without CTx and is explainable by the observed response especially of lymphatic micrometastases [20,22]. Nevertheless, recurrence in the peritoneum, 12% after CTx and 20% after surgery, and liver metastases couldn't be prevented and were comparable with other trials [23].

First and foremost, neoadjuvant CTx aims prolonging overall survival [6]. Unfortunately, our results show that the overall survival is not improved under these conditions. The 5-year survival rate with chemotherapy was 38% versus 42% without. A comparable trial failed to show a benefit of chemotherapy as well [2,20]. Current trials hypothesize that an objective histological response is an important prognostic factor [2,6]. However, in our study responders had no better long-term outcome than patients without CTx (45% versus 42%) (Figure 2) [2,6,20]. The only exception to our observation was seen in a subgroup analysis of responders with stage III tumors. In this subgroup, the 5-year survival rate was 46% after CTx versus 31% after resection only (Figure 3).

Conclusion

We regard advanced gastric cancer as a systemic disease. Meaningful prognostic criteria are intraperitoneal and local recurrence. Neoadjuvant CTx succeeds in reducing local relapse, but does not appear to impact the overall survival. Despite this lack of benefit as seen across all tumor stages, a subgroup of patients with stage III tumors seems to benefit significantly from neoadjuvant CTx. However, it remains challenging to select these patients due to the low accuracy of current diagnostics. In summary, additional therapeutic modalities, such as antibody treatment in combination with current standards of treatment will be necessary to improve the prognosis of advanced gastric cancer.

Abbreviations
CTx: Chemotherapy; PELF: Cisplatin, Epirubicin, Leukovorin, 5-Fluoruracil; UICC: Union internationale contre le cancer; CR: Complete response; PR: Partial response; AJCC: American joint committee on cancer; JRSGC: Japanese research society for gastric cancer 1995.

Competing interests
The authors declare that they have no competing interests.

Authors' contributions
RC was responsible for the data gathering and analysis of the data and also did the literature research. TO and RG did the surgery and RG also created the study design. GM and IG took care of the patients during chemotherapy and ensured the right application according to the PELF-protocol. MF performed the statistic analysis. All authors read and approved the final manuscript.

Author details
[1]Department of Surgery, University of Freiburg, Universitätsklinikum, Hugstetterstr. 55, D-79106 Freiburg, Germany. [2]Department of Oncology, University of Freiburg, Freiburg, Germany.

References

1. Macdonald JS, Fleming TR, Peterson RF, Berenberg JL, McClure S, Chapman RA, Eyre HJ, Solanki D, Cruz AB Jr, Gagliano R, et al: Adjuvant chemotherapy with 5-FU, adriamycin and mitomycin-C (FAM) versus surgery alone for patients with locally advanced gastric adenocarinoma: a Southwest Oncology Group study. *Ann Surg Oncol* 1995, 2(6):488–494.

2. Gallardo-Rincón D, Oñate-Ocaña LF, Calderillo-Ruiz G: Neoadjuvant chemotherapy with P-ELF (cisplatin, etoposide, leucovorin, 5-fluorouracil) followed by radical resection in patients with initially unresectable gastric adenocarcinoma: a phase II study. *Ann Surg Oncol* 1999, 7(1):45–50.

3. Nitti D, Wils J, Dos Santos JG, Fountzilas G, Conte PF, Tres A, Coombes RC, Crivellari D, Marchet A, Sanchez E, Bliss JM, Homewood J, Couvreur ML, Hall E, Baron B, Woods E, Emson M, Van Cutsem E, Lise M, EORTC GI Group, ICCG: Randomized phase III trials of adjuvant FAMTX or FEMTX compared with surgery alone in resected gastric cancer. A combined analysis of ther EORTC GI Group and the ICCG. *Ann Oncol* 2006, 17:262–269.

4. Lake JC, Lopez PP: Gastric cancer: diagnosis and treatment options. *Am Fam Physician* 2004, 69(5):1133–1140.

5. Drognitz O, Henne K, Weissenberger C, Bruggmoser G, Göbel H, Hopt UT, Frommhold H, Ruf G: Long-term results after intraoperative radiation therapy for gastric cancer. *Int J Radiat Oncol Biol Phys* 2007, 70(3):715–721.

6. Fink U, Stein HJ, Siewert JR: Multimodal therapy of tumors of the uppergastrointestinal tract. *Chirurg* 1998, 69(4):349–359.

7. Lim L, Michael M, Mann GB, Leong T: Adjuvant therapy in gastric cancer. *J Clin Oncol* 2005, 23(25):6220–6232.

8. Maley CC, Glaipeau PC, Li X, Sanchez CA, Paulson TG, Blount PL, Reid BJ: The Combination of genetic instability and clonal expansion predicts progression to eosophageal adenocarinoma. *Cancer Res* 2004, 64(20):7629–7633.

9. Okuda M, Miyashiro E, Nakazawa T: Helicobacter pylori infection in childhood. *J Gastroenterol* 2004, 39(8):809–810.

10. Tatsuguchi A, Miyake K, Gudis K, Futagami S, Tsukui T, Wada K, Kishida T, Fukuda Y, Sugisaki Y, Sakamoto C: Effect of Helicobacter pylori infection on ghrelin expression in human gastric mucosa. *Am J Gastroenterol* 2004, 99(11):2121–2127.

11. Crabtree JE, Court M, Aboshkiwa MA, Jeremy AH, Dixon MF, Robinson PA: Gastric mucosal cytokine and epithelial response to Helicobacter pylori infection in Mongolian gerbils. *J Pathol* 2004, 202(2):197–207.

12. Nardone G, Rocco A, Vaira D, Staibano S, Budillon A, Tatangelo F, Sciulli MG, Perna F, Salvatore G, Di Benedetto M, De Rosa G, Patrignani P: Expression of COX-2, mPGE-synthase1, MDR-1 (P-gp), and Bcl-xL: a molecular pathway of H pylori-related gastric carcinogenesis. *J Pathol* 2004, 202(3):305–312.

13. Lee KA, Ki CS, Kim HJ, Sohn KM, Kim JW, Kang WK, Rhee JC, Song SY, Sohn TS: Novel interleukin 1beta polymorphism increased the risk of gastric cancer in a Korean population. *J Gastroenterol* 2004, 39(5):429–433.

14. Glas J, Török HP, Schneider A, Brünnler G, Kopp R, Albert ED, Stolte M, Folwaczny C: Allele 2 of the interleukin-1 receptor antagonist gene is associated with early gastric cancer. *J Clin Oncol* 2004, 22(23):4746–4752.

15. Matsuhisa T, Matsukura N, Yamada N: Topography of chronic active gastritis in Helicobacter pylori-positive Asian populations: age-, gender-, and endoscopic diagnosis-matched study. *J Gastroenterol* 2004, 39(4):324–328.

16. Ychou M, Boige V, Pignon JP, Conroy T, Bouche O, Lebreton G, Ducortieux M, Bedenne L, Fabre JM, Saint-Aubert B, Genere J, Lasser P: Rogier Perioperative chemotherapy compared with surgery alone for resectable gastroesophageal adenocarcinoma: an FNCLCC and FFCD multicenter phase III trial. *J Clin Oncol* 2011, 29:1715–1721.

17. Li W, Quin J, Sun Y-H, Liu TS: Neoadjuvant chemotherapy for advanced gastric cancer: a meta-analysis. *World J Gastroenterol* 2010, 16:5621–5628.

18. Hallissey MT, Dunn JA, Ward LC, Allum WH: The second British stomach cancer group trial of adjuvant radiotherapy or chemotherapy in resectable gastric cancer: five-year follow-up. *Lancet* 1994, 343(8909):1309–1312.

19. Cascinu S, Graziano F, Barni S, Labianca R, Comella G, Casaretti R, Frontini L, Catalano V, Baldelli AM, Catalano G: A phase II study of sequential chemotherapy with docetaxel after the weekly PELF regimen in advanced gastric cancer. A report from the Italian group for the study of digestive tract cancer. *Br J Cancer* 2001, 84(4):470–474.

20. Nakajima T, Ota K, Ishihara S, Oyama S, Nishi M, Ohashi Y, Yanagisawa A: Combined intensive chemotherapy and radical surgery for incurable gastric cancer. *Ann Surg Oncol* 1997, 4(3):203–208.

21. Gold JS, Jaques DP, Bentrem DJ, Shah MA, Tang LH, Brennan MF, Coit DG: Outcome of patients with known metastatic gastric cancer undergoing resection with therapeutic intent. *Ann Surg Oncol* 2006, 14(2):365–372.

22. Cunningham D, Allum WH, Stenning SP, Thompson JN, Van de Velde CJ, Nicolson M, Scarffe JH, Lofts FJ, Falk SJ, Iveson TJ, Smith DB, Langley RE, Verma M, Weeden S, Chua YJ, MAGIC Trial Participants: Perioperative chemotherapy versus surgery alone for resectable gastroesophageal cancer. *N Engl J Med* 2006, 355(1):11–20.

23. Mori T, Fujiwara Y, Sugita Y, Azama T, Ishii T, Taniguchi K, Yamazaki K, Takiguchi S, Yasuda T, Yano M, Monden M: Application of molecular diagnosis for detection of peritoneal micrometastasis and evaluation of preoperative chemotherapy in advanced gastric carcinoma. *Ann Surg Oncol* 2003, 11(1):14–20.

9

Robotic transthoracic esophagectomy

Shailesh Puntambekar[1*], Rahul Kenawadekar[1,2], Sanjay Kumar[1], Saurabh Joshi[1], Geetanjali Agarwal[1], Sunil Reddy[1] and Jainul Mallik[1]

Abstract

Background: We have initially published our experience with the robotic transthoracic esophagectomy in 32 patients from a single institute. The present paper is the extension of our experience with robotic system and to best of our knowledge this represents the largest series of robotic transthoracic esophagectomy worldwide. The objective of this study was to investigate the feasibility of the robotic transthoracic esophagectomy for esophageal cancer in a series of patients from a single institute.

Methods: A retrospective review of medical records was conducted for 83 esophageal cancer patients who underwent robotic esophagectomy at our institute from December 2009 to December 2012. All patients underwent a thorough clinical examination and pre-operative investigations. All patients underwent robotic esophageal mobilization. En-bloc dissection with lymphadenectomy was performed in all cases with preservation of Azygous vein. Relevant data were gathered from medical records.

Results: The study population comprised of 50 men and 33 women with mean age of 59.18 years. The mean operative time was 204.94 mins (range 180 to 300). The mean blood loss was 86.75 ml (range 50 to 200). The mean number of lymph node yield was 18. 36 (range 13 to 24). None of the patient required conversion. The mean ICU stay and hospital stay was 1 day (range 1 to 3) and 10.37 days (range 10 to 13), respectively. A total of 16 (19.28%) complication were reported in these patents. Commonly reported complication included dysphagia, pleural effusion and anastomotic leak. No treatment related mortality was observed. After a median follow-up period of 10 months, 66 patients (79.52%) survived with disease free stage.

Conclusions: We found robot-assisted thoracoscopic esophagectomy feasible in cases of esophageal cancer. The procedure allowed precise en-bloc dissection with lymphadenectomy in mediastinum with reduced operative time, blood loss and complications.

Background

The GLOBOCAN 2008 cancer fact sheet described esophageal cancer as the eighth most common cancer worldwide. There were 482,300 new cases of esophageal cancer with 406,800 estimated deaths worldwide in year 2008 [1]. For esophageal cancer, esophagectomy remains the cornerstone of the treatment with curative intent [2]. However, surgical resection of the esophageal cancer is a challenging dissection compared to other gastrointestinal cancers mainly due to anatomical difficulties. Additionally, surgeries for esophageal cancer are frequently associated with high rates of cardiopulmonary morbidity and mortality [3,4]. Minimally invasive esophagectomy

(MIE) is being used increasingly with aim to reduce the surgical trauma and thereby reducing morbidity and mortality [4-6]. The available literature data shows other advantages of MIE including decrease in operative time, blood loss, post-operative complications and hospital stay with comparable oncological clearance [4-6]. However, steep learning curve associated with MIE has been a challenge [7,8].

Robotic surgery has generated considerable excitement and interest in various oncological surgeries including esophageal surgery. Robot-assisted surgery can accelerate the learning curve of MIE with the help of magnified three-dimensional view, improved articulation of instruments with seven degree of freedom, improved dexterity and enhanced ergonomics [8-11]. Robotic assisted surgery can help the surgeon in precise dissection of the structures in the mediastinum which otherwise would

* Correspondence: shase63@gmail.com
[1]Galaxy Care Laparoscopy Institute, Opposite Garware College, 25-A, Ayurvedic Rasashala Premises, Karve Road, Pune, Maharashtra 411004, India
Full list of author information is available at the end of the article

have been challenging via conventional MIE. However, in spite of various advantages of robotic esophagectomy, it still remains in the early phase of acceptance.

We have initially published our experience with the robotic transthoracic esophagectomy in 32 patients from a single institute [11]. The present paper is the extension of our experience with robotic system and to best of our knowledge this represents the largest series of robotic transthoracic esophagectomy worldwide.

Methods

Patients

We retrospectively reviewed the medical records of 83 esophageal cancer patients who underwent robotic assisted esophagectomy at Galaxy Care Laparoscopy institute from December 2009 to December 2012. The review was conducted on the basis of prospectively recorded data from a computerized database. Care Hospitals Institutional review board and ethics committee approved the study. Each patient gave consent for conversion to either thoracoscopic or open surgery just in case of complications. Each patient's consent was also taken for use of video footage of their surgery for academic and research purposes (including specific written consent from the patient whose edited operative video is accompanying this manuscript). All patients underwent a thorough clinical examination and pre-operative investigations including routine hematogram, biochemical investigations, pulmonary function tests, chest radiograph, ECG, 2D Echo, contrast enhanced CT scan of thorax and abdomen, upper GI endoscopy with biopsy and barium swallow with stomach plates. Endoscopic ultrasound staging was done to identify the stage of the tumor.

Patients with histologically proven squamous cell carcinoma, adenocarcinoma or dysplasia as well as other resectable forms of tumors were the candidate for the surgery. The operability criteria were clearly defined as per NCCN guidelines. American Society of Anesthesiologists (ASA) class I to III was regarded appropriate for the procedure. Patients with cervical esophageal cancer were not considered suitable for the procedure.

All the patients underwent robotic esophageal mobilization. The entire thoracic esophagus along with paraesophageal, subcarinal, paratracheal and bronchial lymph nodes were removed en-bloc. Azygos vein was preserved in all cases. The resected specimen was examined by an experienced pathologist. Pre-operative investigations, clinical data, operative details, pathological details and post-operative data were gathered from medical records.

Operative technique

The patient was placed in the prone position on an operative sandbag. The robotic cart was situated to the left side of the patient. The operative trocars for the robot (one 12- mm port for the camera and two 8-mm ports for the arms) were placed (Figure 1). The first port was inserted 1 finger-breadth below and posterior to inferior angle of scapula in the 5th or 6th intercostal space. Two 8-mm trocars were positioned under direct thoracoscopic vision in a vertical line at a distance of 5 cm and in triangulation with the camera port in the third and eighth intercostal spaces, respectively. One 10-mm port for the assistant was placed between the left working port and the camera port. This was used for suction and clip application. Pneumoinsufflation was created at a pressure of 7 mm Hg. (Additional file 1).

With the patient in a prone position, the esophagus falls anteriorly out of its normal position, which creates natural tension and simplifies dissection. We used Maryland bipolar forceps in left arm and hot shears (scissors with monopolar current) in right arm of the robot. The procedure began with the incision of the visceral pleura between the esophagus and the lung just inferior to the azygos vein. This helped in keeping the esophagus attached to the pleura on the aortic side. More than 3 fourths of the circumference of the esophagus was mobilized in this way from the cranial to the caudal direction. The plane of dissection was outside the vagus. The posterior large direct aortic branches were then clipped, and the small branches were cauterized with bipolar forceps. This completed the mobilization of the esophagus all around. The caudal limit of the dissection was the hiatus. The same dissection was continued in the supra-azygos region. The vagal fibers going to the bronchus were preserved. The azygos vein was preserved. Complete mobilization of the esophagus was achieved. The specimen also included the lower and middle mediastinal, subcarinal, and right paratracheal nodes. The thoracic duct was identified and clipped in all cases.

Stomach mobilization

Stomach mobilization was done laparoscopically. All the nodes along the left gastric, paraesophageal, splenic and along the hepatic artery were removed. The stomach was mobilized on the right gastro epiploic and right gastric artery. The stomach tube was prepared extracorporially by taking 5 cm incision in the midline.

Cervical incision

Left supraclavicular 3 cm incision was taken. The two heads of the sternomastoid were separated and the esophagus was pulled up to the wound. The esophagus was cut and the NG tube was attached to the distal end. The specimen was removed abdominally. The stomach tube was attached to the NG tube and was pulled to the neck and hand sewn esophageogastric

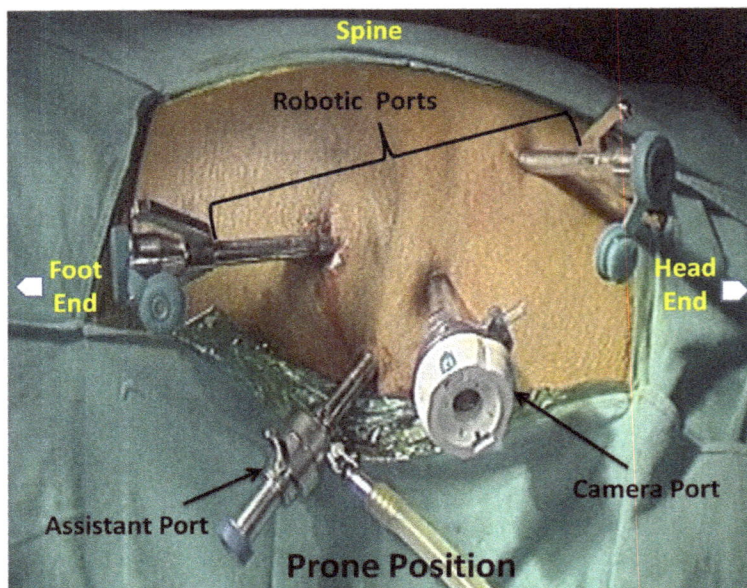

Figure 1 Patient and port positioning.

anastamoses was done. Feeding jejunostomy was done in all the patients.

Post-operative course

The patients were kept in ICU for minimum one day after which shifted to respective ward. The continuous monitoring of vital parameters was done further for next 48 hrs and then every day for the next 4 days. The chest radiograph and hematogram was done every day for 2 days and then were repeated only when the patient had respiratory signs, fever, or any other complaints. Patients were made ambulatory after 24 hrs and jejunostomy tube feeding was started after 48 hrs of surgery. The leak test was performed on the 7th day of the surgery and oral feeding was started accordingly.

The patients with nodal involvement were subjected to chemotherapy or radiotherapy or both depending on number of node positivity and histology of tumor. The patients were followed 3 monthly for clinical checkup, chest radiograph and ultrasonography for the period of one year and than six monthly for a period of two years. If any suspicion was raised PET scan was advised.

Results

The study population consisted of 83 patients, 50 men (60.24%) and 33 women (39.76%). The mean age at surgery was 59.18 years (range, 30 to 87 years). Most commonly involved site (50 cases, 60.24%) was lower third of the esophagus. The predominant histology (67 cases, 80.72%) was squamous cell carcinoma. A total of 21.69% of patients presented at least one comorbid condition, with

hypertension and diabetes observed as most common comorbidities. Information on patient demographics is presented in Table 1.

The mean operative time was 204.94 minutes (range 180 to 300). The size of the tumor did not significantly affect operative times. The mean blood loss was 86.75 ml (range 50 to 200). The mean number of lymph node yield was 18. 36 (range 13 to 24). Only two patients showed positive circumferential margin. None of the patient required conversion to thoracoscopic or open surgery. The mean ICU stay was 1 day (range 1 to 3) and the mean hospital stay was 10.37 days (range 10 to 13). Table 2 represents operative and post-operative outcomes.

Postoperative morbidity occurred in 16 cases (19.28%). A total 19 of incidents were reported in these cases. Dysphagia was the most commonly observed event (6 cases, 7.23%) followed by pleural effusion (3 cases, 3.61%). Anastomotic leak was reported in 3 cases and chyle leak was observed in one patient. There were only two incidences of recurrent palsy. One patient developed port site metastasis which was treated with excision. No treatment related mortality was observed. At the end of the study period, 66 patients (79.52%) were alive in disease free stage at the median follow-up period of 10 months. One patient was lost to follow up. Figure 2 shows the Kaplan Meier survival analysis.

Discussion

To the best of our knowledge, this is the largest study on robotic transthoracic esophagectomy till date which

Table 1 Clinico-demographic characteristics of the patients with esophageal cancer

Variable	N (%)
Gender	
Male	50 (60.24)
Female	33 (39.76)
Age distribution	
21 – 30	1 (1.20)
31 – 40	5 (6.02)
41 – 50	15 (18.07)
51 – 60	22 (26.51)
61 – 70	28 (33.73)
71 – 80	9 (10.84)
81 – 90	3 (3.61)
Histology	
Squamous cell carcinoma	67 (80.72)
Adenocarcinoma	12 (14.46)
Dysplasia	2 (2.41)
Gastrointestinal stromal tumor	1 (1.20)
Lymphoma	1 (1.20)
Site of cancer	
Middle third	50 (60.24)
Lower third	20 (24.10)
Gastroesophageal junction	13 (15.66)
TNM stage of tumor	
High-grade dysplasia	2 (2.41)
I	8 (9.64)
II	64 (77.11)
III	9 (10.84)
ASA grading	
I	2 (2.41)
II	60 (72.29)
III	19 (22.89)
IV	2 (2.41)
Preoperative morbidity	
Diabetes mellitus	11 (13.25)
Bronchial asthma	3 (3.61)
Hypertension	15 (18.07)
Stroke	1 (1.20)
Ischemic heart disease	2 (2.41)
Hemiplagia	1 (1.20)

Table 2 Operative outcomes following the robotic transthoracic esophagectomy

Variable	Mean (range) or no. (%)
Total operative time (mins)	204.94 (180–300)
Docking time (mins)	9.06 (5–30)
Undocking time (mins)	5 (2–10)
Time for esophageal mobilization (mins)	104.08 (80–170)
Estimated blood loss (ml)	86.75 (50–200)
Lymphnode yield (no.)	18.36 (13–24)
ICU stay (days)	1 (1–3)
Hospital stay (days)	10.37 (10–13)
Nil by mouth (days)	9.40 (8–12)
Conversion (no.)	Nil
Margin positivity (no.)	2 (2.41)
Adjuvant chemotherapy (no.)	15 (18.07)
Complications (no.)	
Dysphagia for solids	6 (7.23)
Pleural effusion	3 (3.61)
Aspiration pneumonia	1 (1.20)
Recurrent palsy	2 (2.41)
Anastomotic leak	3 (3.61)
Chyle leak	1 (1.20)
Port site metastasis	1 (1.20)
Surgical site infection	1 (1.20)
Sepsis	1 (1.20)

represents the comprehensive experience from our institute. As the available data in the literature on this advancement is scarce, we feel that the present study perhaps will provide a better idea on the 'real world' scenario.

Esophagectomy for esophageal carcinoma is a technically challenging procedure associated with relatively high mortality and morbidity [7,12-14]. To reduce the morbidity as a result of surgical trauma from open procedures, minimal invasive procedures were introduced in the recent past. There are published reports that favored the use of MIE due to advantages of shorter operative time; reduced blood loss and shorter hospital stay [7,12,15-17]. Nevertheless, the conventional MIE methods are limited by the technical difficulties. Mainly, the use of long instruments with limited degree of freedom and two-dimensional view can become hindrance for optimal dissection [18,19].

The more recent introduction of robotic systems in surgical oncology has answered the limitations of MIE. Compared to the traditional minimally invasive procedures, robotic-assisted surgery offers several potential advantages. The improved visualization with the magnified three-dimensional view is of particular benefit that allows a precise and atraumatic dissection of the periesophageal tissue along the vital structures, such as pulmonary vein, trachea, thoracic duct, aorta and vagus nerve [9,20]. More importantly, the magnified view of

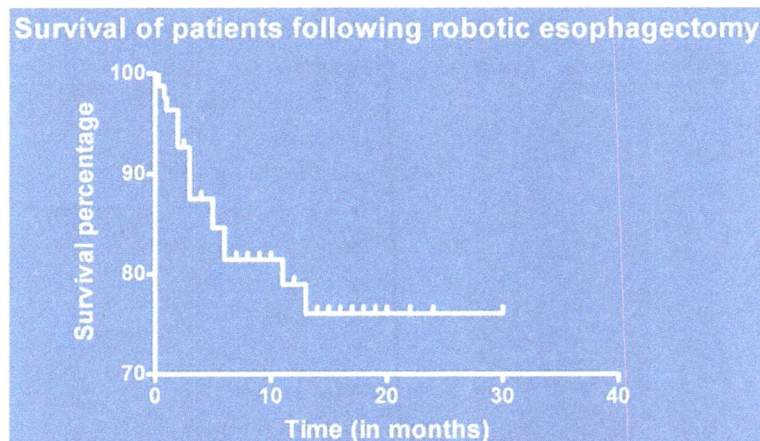

Figure 2 Disease free survival following robotic transthoracic esophagectomy (Kaplan Meier Plot).

the surgical field can assist in a more extensive dissection of the lymph nodes. The lymphatic spread of esophageal cancer is generally irregular due to submucosal lymphatic drainage system. The radical resection of esophagus with surrounding lymph nodes offers the best possible cure. With the use of robotic arms, we were able to achieve the mean lymph node yield of 18.36 (range 13 to 24). A study from van Hillegersberg R et al. harvested a median of 20 lymph nodes (range, 9–30) through robot-assisted thoracoscopic esophagectomy [9]. Cerfolio et al. reported median number of 20 through the same approach [21]. Galvani et al. achieved mean lymph nodes yield of 12 (range 7 to 27) using robot-assisted transhiatal esophagectomy [22]. The same approach was utilized by Dunn et al., who harvested a median of 20 lymph nodes (range, 3–38) [23]. Sarkaria et al. reported median number of 20 lymph nodes (range, 10–49) using combined thoracoscopic and laparoscopic robotic-assisted approach [24]. We believe that the transthoracoscopic approach offers an outstanding access to the mediastinum and thereby allows an extended lymphadenectomy. When performing the procedure through the transhiatal approach, these potential metastatic lymph nodes might be leftover in situ [25]. In fact, the R0 resection was achieved in 97.59% of our study population. Few other case series using the similar approach showed R0 resection rate varying from 76% to 100% [21,26,27].

The advantages of robotic surgery are more valuable when operating in the confined area, as in the esophageal surgery. The dexterity and articulated instruments permit seven degrees of motion including in/out; rotation; pitch at wrist; yaw at wrist; pitch at fulcrum; yaw at fulcrum and grip strength [20]. The improved tremor free motion stability can add to fine movements and facilitate a precise dissection and suturing in a confined

operating space. As a result, we enjoyed atraumatic dissection during the mediastinal dissection of the esophagus and surrounding lymph nodes. Additionally, we did not encounter any iatrogenic trauma during the procedure and achieved advantages in operative time and blood loss.

In comparison to previously reported studies, our study showed reduced total operating time. The total operating time of the procedure in our series was 204.94 mins. The first performed robotic-assisted esophagectomy in 2003 reported total operative time of 246 mins [28]. Subsequent case series by van Hillgers et al. reported total operative time of 450 (range 370–550) min and thoracoscopic time of 180 (range 120–240) mins from experience in 21 patients [9]. Boone et al. reported median operative time of 450 mins in a series of 47 patients [27]. Some of the transhiatal approached had reported total operative time of 267.71 mins [22] and 311 mins [23]. In the report from Sarkaria et al. the median total operative time was 556 min (range 395–807) [24]. The relatively low total operative time in our series was a result of increased experience in robotic surgery, a well focused operating team as well as nursing staff's familiarity with the procedures and equipments. We were able to reduce the docking time from 30 mins in initial days to 5 mins in the most recent case. This significant decrease represents the learning curve of the surgeon and team. The estimated blood loss was 86.75 ml in our study. Other publications have reported blood loss ranging from 40–625 ml using similar approach [9,21,27]. Papers focused on the transhiatal approach reported blood loss of 54 ml [22] and 97.2 ml [23]. None of our patient required blood transfusion. This is of clinical significance as various studies have indicated that esophageal cancer patients with major blood loss receiving blood transfusions have a worse prognosis [29,30].

The mean ICU stay and hospital stay in our study was 1.2 days and 8 days, respectively. Other studies have reported ICU stay ranging from 1.8 day to 4 days [9,22,27] and hospital stay ranging from 8.7 days to 18 days [9,22-24,27]. Weksler B et al. compared the robotic esophagectomy with the traditional MIE and found no significant differences in operative time, blood loss, number of resected lymph nodes, length of ICU/hospital stay and postoperative complications [31].

In our study, we did not encounter any in-hospital mortality. Approximately, 80% of the patient population was alive at the median follow up of 10 months. There were no treatment related deaths. Two patients had recurrence of the cancer, one of which died while other was disease free following the further treatment. The complication rate was low in our study with reported complications in only 19.28% of the study population. In general, the transthoracic approach is more aggressive than the transhiatal approach and is more likely to cause cardiopulmonary complications, anastomotic and chylous leaks, vocal cord paralysis, and wound infection [32]. However, a study by Satoh et al. has showed significantly reduced incidence of recurrent nerve palsy by robotic thoracoscopic esophagectomy in comparison to conventional thoracoscopic esophagectomy [33]. Although, we encountered only two cases with recurrent nerve palsy, we advocate extreme caution during the en-bloc resection as there are chances of damaging recurrent nerve and its small branches that are located in the fatty tissue of the superior mediastinum. In our series, the post-operating complications reduced markedly in due course, with reported 3 cases anastomotic leak from first 32 cases in our previous publication [11] and no further incidences from last 51 cases. Similarly, there were no further cases of chyle leak from our last 51 cases.

A prospective randomized clinical trial is underway for comparing robot-assisted thoraco-laparoscopic esophagectomy with the open transthoracic esophagectomy [34]. We are really hopeful that the trial will furnish the similar results to our study for robotic esophagectomy. If the trial hypothesis is proved, robot esophagectomy can be considered as treatment option related with a lower postoperative complications, lower blood loss and shorter hospital stay with at least similar oncologic outcomes and better postoperative quality of life [34].

The major drawback of the robotic system is the lack of haptic sensations. This limitation is mainly significant in procedures where touch is an important component. However, the recent surgical innovations are focused on the development of systems that transmits the haptic feedback to surgeon [35]. As the surgeon works alone at a console, learning procedures and training to others can be sometimes challenging [20]. Finally, the cost of the equipments could be additional limitation. However, robot- assisted surgery has already confirmed cost savings from minimal blood loss, morbidity and reduced hospital stay [8].

Conclusion

We found robot-assisted thoracoscopic esophagectomy acceptable for treatment of esophageal cancer. The procedure allowed precise en-bloc dissection with lymphadenectomy in mediastinum. The advantages of robotic system helped us to minimize operative time, blood loss and complications. We are optimistic that future randomized trials will establish this procedure as standard of care for esophageal cancer.

Competing interests
The authors declare that they have no competing interests.

Authors' contributions
Dr.SP*- conception, study design, Sole operating surgeon on robotic console and corresponding author. Dr.RK- study design, data collection, interpretation and analysis. Dr.SK- data collection, interpretation and analysis. Dr.SJ- data collection, interpretation and analysis. Dr.GA- data collection, interpretation and analysis. Dr.SR- data collection, interpretation and analysis. Dr.JM- data collection, interpretation and analysis. *Dr SP gave final approval for the final version to be published. All authors read and approved the final manuscript.

Acknowledgements
1. Dr Seema Puntambekar for Proof reading of the manuscript.
2. Mr Neelesh Sonawane for Video editing and voice over and background music.

Author details
¹Galaxy Care Laparoscopy Institute, Opposite Garware College, 25-A, Ayurvedic Rasashala Premises, Karve Road, Pune, Maharashtra 411004, India. ²Department of Surgery, JNMC, KLE University, Belgaum, India.

References
1. Jemal A, Bray F, Center MM, Ferlay J, Ward E, Forman D. Global cancer statistics. CA Cancer J Clin. 2011;61(2):69–90.
2. Mariette C, Piessen G, Triboulet JP. Therapeutic strategies in oesophageal carcinoma: role of surgery and other modalities. Lancet Oncol. 2007;8(6):545–53.
3. Law S, Wong J. Use of minimally invasive oesophagectomy for cancer of the oesophagus. Lancet Oncol. 2002;3(4):215–22.
4. Kim T, Hochwald SN, Sarosi GA, Caban AM, Rossidis G, Ben-David K. Review of minimally invasive esophagectomy and current controversies. Gastroenterol Res Pract. 2012;2012:683213.
5. Nafteux P, Moons J, Coosemans W, Decaluwé H, Decker G, De Leyn P, et al. Minimally invasive oesophagectomy: a valuable alternative to open oesophagectomy for the treatment of early oesophageal and gastro-oesophageal junction carcinoma. Eur J Cardiothorac Surg. 2011;40(6):1455–63. discussion 63–4.
6. Verhage RJ, Hazebroek EJ, Boone J, Van Hillegersberg R. Minimally invasive surgery compared to open procedures in esophagectomy for cancer: a systematic review of the literature. Minerva Chir. 2009;64(2):135–46.
7. Law S. Minimally invasive techniques for oesophageal cancer surgery. Best Pract Res Clin Gastroenterol. 2006;20(5):925–40.

8. Finley DS, Nguyen NT. Surgical robotics. Curr Surg. 2005;62(2):262–72.

9. van Hillegersberg R, Boone J, Draaisma WA, Broeders IA, Giezeman MJ, Borel Rinkes IH. First experience with robot-assisted thoracoscopic esophagolymphadenectomy for esophageal cancer. Surg Endosc. 2006;20(9):1435–9.

10. Kernstine KH. The first series of completely robotic esophagectomies with three-field lymphadenectomy: initial experience. Surg Endosc. 2008;22(9):2102.

11. Puntambekar SP, Rayate N, Joshi S, Agarwal G. Robotic transthoracic esophagectomy in the prone position: experience with 32 patients with esophageal cancer. J Thorac Cardiovasc Surg. 2011;142(5):1283–4.

12. Law S. Is minimally invasive preferable to open oesophagectomy? Lancet. 2012;379(9829):1856–8.

13. Hoppo T, Jobe BA, Hunter JG. Minimally invasive esophagectomy: the evolution and technique of minimally invasive surgery for esophageal cancer. World J Surg. 2011;35(7):1454–63.

14. Levy RM, Wizorek J, Shende M, Luketich JD. Laparoscopic and thoracoscopic esophagectomy. Adv Surg. 2010;44:101–16.

15. Nguyen NT, Follette DM, Wolfe BM, Schneider PD, Roberts P, Goodnight Jr JE. Comparison of minimally invasive esophagectomy with transthoracic and transhiatal esophagectomy. Arch Surg. 2000;135(8):920–5.

16. Luketich JD, Nguyen NT, Weigel T, Ferson P, Keenan R, Schauer P. Minimally invasive approach to esophagectomy. JSLS. 1998;2(3):243–7.

17. Luketich JD, Schauer PR, Christie NA, Weigel TL, Raja S, Fernando HC, et al. Minimally invasive esophagectomy. Ann Thorac Surg. 2000;70(3):906–11. discussion 11–2.

18. Germain A, Bresler L. Robotic-assisted surgical procedures in visceral and digestive surgery. J Visc Surg. 2011;148(5 Suppl):e40–6.

19. Ruurda JP, van Vroonhoven TJ, Broeders IA. Robot-assisted surgical systems: a new era in laparoscopic surgery. Ann R Coll Surg Engl. 2002;84(4):223–6.

20. Watson TJ. Robotic esophagectomy: is it an advance and what is the future? Ann Thorac Surg. 2008;85(2):S757–9.

21. Cerfolio RJ, Bryant AS, Hawn MT. Technical aspects and early results of robotic esophagectomy with chest anastomosis. J Thorac Cardiovasc Surg. 2013;145(1):90–6.

22. Galvani CA, Gorodner MV, Moser F, Jacobsen G, Chretien C, Espat NJ, et al. Robotically assisted laparoscopic transhiatal esophagectomy. Surg Endosc. 2008;22(1):188–95.

23. Dunn DH, Johnson EM, Morphew JA, Dilworth HP, Krueger JL, Banerji N. Robot-assisted transhiatal esophagectomy: a 3-year single-center experience. Dis Esophagus. 2013;26(2):159–66.

24. Sarkaria IS, Rizk NP, Finley DJ, Bains MS, Adusumilli PS, Huang J, et al. Combined thoracoscopic and laparoscopic robotic-assisted minimally invasive esophagectomy using a four-arm platform: experience, technique and cautions during early procedure development. Eur J Cardiothorac Surg. 2013;43(5):e107–15.

25. Boone J, Borel Rinkes IH, van Hillegersberg R. Transhiatal robot-assisted esophagectomy. Surg Endosc. 2008;22(4):1139–40.

26. Kim DJ, Hyung WJ, Lee CY, Lee JG, Haam SJ, Park IK, et al. Thoracoscopic esophagectomy for esophageal cancer: feasibility and safety of robotic assistance in the prone position. J Thorac Cardiovasc Surg. 2010;139(1):53–9. 1.

27. Boone J, Schipper ME, Moojen WA, Borel Rinkes IH, Cromheecke GJ, van Hillegersberg R. Robot-assisted thoracoscopic oesophagectomy for cancer. Br J Surg. 2009;96(8):878–86.

28. Horgan S, Berger RA, Elli EF, Espat NJ. Robotic-assisted minimally invasive transhiatal esophagectomy. Am Surg. 2003;69(7):624–6.

29. Tachibana M, Hishikawa Y, Abe S, Yoshimura H, Monden N, Dhar DK, et al. Prognostic factors in node-negative squamous cell carcinoma of the thoracic esophagus. Int J Surg Investig. 2000;1(5):389–95.

30. Dresner SM, Lamb PJ, Shenfine J, Hayes N, Griffin SM. Prognostic significance of peri-operative blood transfusion following radical resection for oesophageal carcinoma. Eur J Surg Oncol. 2000;26(5):492–7.

31. Weksler B, Sharma P, Moudgill N, Chojnacki KA, Rosato EL. Robot-assisted minimally invasive esophagectomy is equivalent to thoracoscopic minimally invasive esophagectomy. Dis Esophagus. 2012;25(5):403–9.

32. Sweed MR, Edmonson D, Cohen SJ. Tumors of the esophagus, gastroesophageal junction, and stomach. Semin Oncol Nurs. 2009;25(1):61–75.

33. Satoh S, Suda K, Kawamura Y, Yoshimura F, Taniguchi K, Uyama I. [Robotic surgery for gastroenterological malignancies]. Gan To Kagaku Ryoho. 2012;39(7):1030–4.

34. van der Sluis PC, Ruurda JP, van der Horst S, Roy JJ V, Marc GH B, Margriet JD P, et al. Robot-assisted minimally invasive thoraco-laparoscopic esophagectomy versus open transthoracic esophagectomy for resectable esophageal cancer, a randomized controlled trial (ROBOT trial). Trials. 2012;13:230.

35. Taylor GW, Barrie J, Hood A, Culmer P, Neville A, Jayne DG. Surgical innovations: Addressing the technology gaps in minimally invasive surgery. Trends in Anaesthesia and Critical Care. 2013;3(2):56–61.

10

Which criteria should be used to define type 2 diabetes remission after bariatric surgery?

Ana M Ramos-Levi[1], Lucio Cabrerizo[1], Pilar Matía[1], Andrés Sánchez-Pernaute[2], Antonio J Torres[2] and Miguel A Rubio[1*]

Abstract

Background: Comparison of diabetes remission rates after bariatric surgery using two different models of criteria.

Methods: Retrospective analysis of data from 110 patients with type 2 diabetes and morbid obesity who underwent bariatric surgery, preoperatively and at 18-month follow-up. Comparison of two models of remission: 1) 2009 consensus statement criteria; 2) simple criteria using ADA's HbA1c diabetes diagnostic cut-off values.

Results: Patients' mean ± SD preoperative characteristics were: age 53.3 ± 9.5 years, BMI 43.6 ± 5.5 kg/m^2, HbA1c 7.9 ± 1.8%, duration of diabetes 7.6 ± 7.5 years. 44.5% of patients with previous insulin therapy. With 2009 consensus statement criteria: complete, partial and no remission in 50%, 12.7% and 37.3%, respectively; with HbA1c criteria: 50%, 15% and 34.5% in the analogous categories (p = 0.673).

Conclusions: We suggest a simpler approach to evaluate diabetes remission after bariatric surgery, following the rationale of the definition of diabetes itself.

Keywords: Diabetes, Diabetes remission, Bariatric surgery, Remission criteria, Morbid obesity

Background

Buse et al. [1] proposed in 2009 a consensus definition of diabetes remission. These clear, although strict, criteria prompt the need to reconsider diabetes remission rates after bariatric surgery.

The objective of this study is to compare diabetes remission rates using Buse's consensus group criteria with those obtained with a simpler definition based on the American Diabetes Association's (ADA) glycosylated hemoglobin (HbA1c) cut-off levels used to diagnose diabetes [2], after bariatric surgery.

Methods

Data were retrospectively analyzed from a cohort of 539 patients who underwent bariatric surgery with a pre-operative diagnosis of diabetes and morbid obesity (body mass index [BMI] > 35 kg/m^2) in a single center. Information was obtained from medical records, preoperatively, and at 18 months after surgery. Duration of diabetes,

* Correspondence: marubioh@gmail.com
[1]Department of Endocrinology and Nutrition, Hospital Clínico San Carlos, Instituto de Investigación Sanitaria San Carlos (IdISSC), Facultad de Medicina, Complutense University, Madrid, Spain
Full list of author information is available at the end of the article

previous hypoglycemic treatment, age, weight, height, BMI, fasting glucose (FG) and HbA1c were recorded. All patients signed a written informed consent prior to surgery in which it was specified that clinical and analytical data collected before the bariatric procedure and during follow up could be potentially used in an anonymous way for investigation and publication. This study was approved by the Ethics Committee of the Hospital Clinico San Carlos and was in compliance with the Helsinki Declaration.

Two criteria were used to define diabetes remission: 1) 2009 consensus statement (model 1): complete remission if "normal" measures of glucose metabolism were achieved (HbA1c < 6% and FG < 100 mg/dl [< 5.6 mmol/l]; partial remission if HbA1c < 6.5% and FG 100–125 mg/dl (5.6-6.9 mmol/l), in both cases in the absence of pharmacologic therapy or ongoing procedures, for a duration of at least one year [1]. 2) "HbA1c criteria", based on HbA1c levels used to define diabetes in current ADA guidelines [2] (model 2): remission if HbA1c < 5.7%, improvement if HbA1c 5.7 - 6.5%, in both cases without hypoglycemic treatment and a duration of at least one year, and no remission if these criteria were not met.

Measurement of HbA1c was carried out in blood samples collected with EDTA 3 K, by using high performance liquid chromatography (HPLC) (Tosoh G8®). This method is monthly evaluated by the Program of External Guarantee of Quality of the Spanish Society of Clinical Chemistry, and is in compliance with ADA recommendations [2], which specify that the diagnostic test should be performed using a method that is certified by the National Glycohemoglobin Standardization Program (NGSP).

Three types of bariatric surgery were performed: laparoscopic Roux-en-Y gastric bypass, biliopancreatic diversion and sleeve gastrectomy. Eligibility for each of them varied according to the patients' previous diabetes medical history and comorbidities.

Preoperative features were compared with the 18-month follow-up ones using t test for paired samples and Wilcoxon's test. The number of patients in each remission category 18 months after surgery using both criteria was compared using Chi-square test. Preoperative characteristics were evaluated in their association with rates of the three remission categories with Kruskal Wallis and Chi square tests.

Results

We obtained data from 110 patients with type 2 diabetes (61.8% women). Mean ± SD preoperative characteristics were: age 53 ± 10 years, BMI 43.6 ± 5.5 kg/m^2, FG 165.2 ± 58.5 mg/dL and HbA1c 7.9 ±1.8%. Mean duration of diabetes was 7.6 ±7.5 years and 44.5% of patients were on insulin therapy prior to surgery.

At 18-months follow-up, mean ± SD BMI, FG and HbA1c were 29.0 ± 5.0 kg/m^2, 100.2 ± 23.9 mg/dL and 5.4 ± 0.7%, respectively, all being significantly different from their corresponding preoperative values (p < 0.001 in all cases).

Eighteen months after bariatric surgery, according to model 1, 50% obtained complete remission, 12.7% partial remission, and 37.3% no remission. With model 2, rates in the analogous categories were 50%, 15% and 34.5%, respectively (Table 1). No significant differences were found whichever the criteria used (p = 0.673). Age and preoperative BMI did not influence the rate of remission. Percentage of body weight loss (% WL) and percentage of excess body weight loss (% EWL) were greater in the complete remission group (p < 0.05). Mean duration of diabetes was significantly different across the three remission categories (p = 0.001), being greater in the non-remission group (p < 0.05). Previous insulin treatment was more frequent in the non-remission group (p = 0.000).

Discussion

This study revealed that using simpler criteria based on ADA's diabetes diagnostic HbA1c cut-off values [2] (model 2) results in remission rates comparable to those obtained with the criteria proposed by the 2009 consensus group [1] (model 1). We consider that model 2 criteria were more straightforward and of easy application, as they are based on only one biochemical parameter (the HbA1c level), in the absence of hypoglycemic treatment.

The use of Buse et al's criteria has proved to achieve lower remission rates after bariatric procedures [3],

Table 1 Patients' characteristics according to each remission category

Variable		TOTAL	2009 Consensus group criteria (Model 1)				ADA's HbA1c criteria (Model 2)			
			Complete	Partial	No remission	p	<5.7%	5.7-6.5%	>6.5% and/or treatment	p
No of patients		110	55 (50.0)	14 (12.7)	41 (37.3)		55 (50.0)	17 (15.5)	38 (34.5)	
Age (years)		53.3 ± 9.5	51.5 ± 9.8	55.6 ± 8.0	54.9 ± 9.4	0.230	52.1 ± 9.7	52.8 ± 8.4	55.2 ± 9.7	0.299
Preop - BMI (kg/m^2)		43.6 ± 5.5	44.3 ± 5.2	43.7 ± 4.8	42.8 ± 6.0	0.514	44.1 ± 4.9	43.6 ± 6.2	43.0 ± 6.0	0.595
18 m - BMI (kg/m^2)		29.0 ± 5.0	28.1 ± 4.5	31.8 ± 4.9	29.2 ± 5.4	0.049	28.3 ± 4.3	30.9 ± 6.0	29.3 ± 5.4	0.193
Preop – FG (mg/dl)		165.2 ± 58.5	156.0 ± 55.3	137.8 ± 26.6	186.9 ± 64.3	0.004	153.9 ± 55.1	142.0 ± 29.5	191.8 ± 64.4	0.001
18 m – FG (mg/dl)		100.2 ± 23.9	86.7 ± 7.5	104.6 ± 6.9	118.6 ± 30.4	0.000	87.7 ± 8.9	101.5 ± 12.4	119.8 ± 30.8	0.000
Preop - HbA1c (%)		7.9 ± 1.8	7.5 ± 1.5	7.0 ± 0.8	8.6 ± 1.9	0.002	7.3 ± 1.3	7.7 ± 1.8	8.7 ± 1.9	0.000
18 m - HbA1c (%)		5.4 ± 0.7	5.0 ± 0.6	5.5 ± 0.5	6.1 ± 0.6	0.000	4.9 ± 0.5	5.8 ± 0.1	6.1 ± 0.7	0.000
%WL		33.1 ± 9.4	36.1 ± 7.9	27.1 ± 7.2	31.0 ± 10.4	0.001	35.6 ± 8.1	29.4 ± 8.3	31.0 ± 10.5	0.014
%EWL		70.7 ± 21.0	75.9 ± 17.7	57.0 ± 15.3	68.6 ± 24.4	0.007	74.9 ± 17.7	63.3 ± 22.5	68.0 ± 23.7	0.070
Duration of diabetes (years)		7.6 ± 7.5	5.1 ± 4.0	4.4 ± 4.8	11.9 ± 9.9	0.001	5.3 ± 4.3	4.6 ± 3.5	12.6 ± 10.0	0.000
Previous treatment with insulin	No	61 (55.5)	39 (70.9)	10 (71.4)	12 (29..3)	0.000	37 (67.3)	14 (82.4)	10 (26.3)	0.000
	Yes	49 (44.5)	16 (29.1)	4 (28.6)	29 (70.7)		18 (32.7)	3 (17.6)	28 (73.7)	

Values show mean ± SD or number of patients and percentages (%).
"Preop" = preoperative; "18 m" = 18-month; "BMI" = body mass index; "FG" = fasting glucose; "HbA1c" = glycosylated hemoglobin; "%WL" = percentage body weight loss at 18 months; "%EWL" = percentage excess body weight loss at 18 months.

highlighting the importance of the definition to be able to compare the outcomes of studies. Buchwald et al. [4], in 3,188 patients with type 2 diabetes, reported a 56.7-95.1% resolution rate, depending on the bariatric procedure used, and defining remission as being off diabetes medications with normal FG (< 100 mg/dl [< 5.6 mmol/l]) or HbA1c < 6%. The elevated remission rates remarked in this meta-analysis and in other following studies [5,6] have generated controversial and confounding expectations regarding true remission rates for patients with type 2 diabetes after bariatric surgery. In our series, at 18-month follow-up, complete remission was achieved in 50% of patients, in agreement with rates previously communicated [3,7,8]. Therefore, the need for uniform inclusion criteria to define type 2 diabetes complete or partial remission after bariatric surgery becomes evident and, for this reason, this issue should be addressed by scientific societies and a consensus should be reached in specific position statements.

It has recently been outlined [9,10] that diabetes duration, use of insulin, the bariatric procedure performed and, presumably, preoperative BMI, all contribute to the wide variability of remission rates reported. In the present study, regardless of the model used, longer duration of diabetes and previous treatment with insulin, were found to be associated with a lower rate of remission, a finding which is consistent with most published analyses [9,11-13]. Knowledge of these previous factors may be useful to determine how much improvement can be potentially expected after a specific bariatric procedure. For instance, in our series, in accordance to what has recently been observed [8,10,14], remission rates in patients previously on insulin therapy were around 30%, whilst rates raised up to 70% in those patients receiving only oral medication. Similarly, and also agreeing with previous works [8,9], we observed an inverse relation between diabetes duration and resolution. Thus, in future studies, differences in remission rates should be specified according to previous hypoglycemic treatments and/or diabetes duration.

Conclusions

In conclusion, we propose simpler criteria for diabetes remission after bariatric surgery based on the ADA's definition of diabetes. These may be of a more practical and affordable clinical application, as well as realistic regarding what outcomes to expect.

Abbreviations

ADA: American Diabetes Association; BMI: Body mass index (kg/m^2); FG: Fasting glucose (mg/dl); HbA1c: Glycosylated hemoglobin (%); SD: Standard deviation; %WL: percentage of body weight loss; %EWL: percentage of excess body weight loss.

Competing interests

The authors declare no conflict of interest.

Authors' contributions

AMR researched, analyzed and interpreted data, and wrote the manuscript. LC and PM researched data and contributed to the discussion. AS and AT researched data and performed all bariatric procedures. MAR contributed to study conception and design, data analysis and interpretation, and reviewed and edited the manuscript. All authors gave final approval of the version to be published. All authors read and approved the final manuscript.

Acknowledgments

This study was granted by Fundación Mutua Madrileña de Investigación Biomédica AP 89592011.

Author details

^{1}Department of Endocrinology and Nutrition, Hospital Clínico San Carlos, Instituto de Investigación Sanitaria San Carlos (IdISSC), Facultad de Medicina, Complutense University, Madrid, Spain. ^{2}Department of Surgery, Hospital Clínico San Carlos, Instituto de Investigación Sanitaria San Carlos (IdISSC), Facultad de Medicina, Complutense University, Madrid, Spain.

References

1. Buse JB, Caprio S, Cefalu WT, et al: How do we define cure of diabetes? Diabetes Care 2009, 32:2133–5.
2. American Diabetes Association: Standards of Medical Care in Diabetes 2012. Diabetes Care 2012, 35:S11–S63.
3. Pournaras DJ, Aasheim ET, Søvik TT, et al: Effect of the definition of type II diabetes remission in the evaluation of bariatric surgery for metabolic disorders. Br J Surg 2012, 99:100–3.
4. Buchwald H, Estok R, Fahrbach K, et al: Weight and type 2 diabetes after bariatric surgery: systematic review and meta-analysis. Am J Med 2009, 122:248–256. e5.
5. Dixon JB, le Roux CW, Rubino F, Zimmet P: Bariatric Surgery for type 2 diabetes. Lancet 2012, 16(379):2300–2311.
6. Mingrone G, Panunzi S, De Gaetano A, et al: Bariatric surgery versus conventional medical therapy for type 2 diabetes. N Engl J Med 2012, 366:1577–1585.
7. Schauer P, Kashyap SR, Wolski K, et al: Bariatric surgery versus intensive medical therapy in obese patients with diabetes. N Engl J Med 2012, 366:1567–1576.
8. Blackstone R, Bunt JC, Cortés MC, Sugerman HJ: Type 2 diabetes after gastric bypass: remission in five models using HbA1c, fasting blood glucose, and medication status. Surg Obes Relat Dis 2012; 8:548-55.
9. Schernthaner G, Brix JM, Kopp HP, Schernthaner GH: Cure of type 2 diabetes by metabolic surgery? A critical analysis of the evidence in 2010. Diabetes Care 2011, 34(Suppl 2):S355–360.
10. Kashyap SR, Schauer P: Clinical considerations for the management of residual diabetes following bariatric surgery. Diabetes Obes Metab 2012, 14:733–779.
11. Schauer PR, Burguera B, Ikramuddin S, et al: Effect of laparoscopic Roux-en-Y gastric bypass on type 2 diabetes mellitus. Ann Surg 2003, 238:467–485.
12. Dixon JB, O'Brien PR, Playfair J, et al: Adjustable gastric banding and conventional therapy for type 2 diabetes: a randomized controlled trial. JAMA 2008, 299:316–323.
13. Vetter ML, Cardillo S, Rickels MR, Iqbal N: Narrative review: effect of bariatric surgery on type 2 diabetes mellitus. Ann Intern Med 2009, 150:94–103.
14. Hamza N, Abbas MH, Darwish A, Shafeek Z, New J, Ammori BJ: Predictors of remission of type 2 diabetes mellitus after laparoscopic gastric banding and bypass. Surg Obes Relat Dis 2011, 7:691–6.

11

The quality of life after a total gastrectomy with extended lymphadenectomy and omega type oesophagojejunostomy for gastric adenocarcinoma without distant metastases

Gintare Jakstaite[1], Narimantas Evaldas Samalavicius[1*], Giedre Smailyte[1] and Raimundas Lunevicius[2]

Abstract

Background: To evaluate the quality of life (QOL) in relation to age, sex, clinical stage, postoperative complication, and adjuvant chemotherapy in patients who underwent curative total gastrectomy with D2 lymphadenectomy and Omega type esophagojejunostomy for gastric adenocarcinoma.

Methods: 69 patients were included. Lithuanian version of the European Organization for Research and Treatment of Cancer Quality of Life Questionnaire Cancer 30 was sent to all of them from six months to two years after gastric surgery for self-completion. 34 questionnaires were filled and were used as material for further analysis. Influence of age ($\geq$ 65 vs < 65), sex, clinical stage (I–II vs III), surgical complication, and adjuvant chemotherapy was assessed on QOL in this retrospective cross-sectional case series study.

Results: The global health status was better in the group of patients aged over 65 (63.0 points vs 46.4, P = 0.0509). The functional scales were higher in the same group of patients. Significant difference was only observed on the social scale in favour of elders (P = 0.0039). Sex, clinical stage, surgical complications, and postoperative chemotherapy had no significant influence on any aspect of QOL.

Conclusion: The global QOL and the social functioning was better in patients aged 65 years and over, compared to patients under the age of 65 in the period of 6 to 18 months after a total gastrectomy with D2 lymphadenectomy and Omega esophagojejunostomy.

Keywords: Gastric cancer, Total gastrectomy, Extended lymphadenectomy, Omega esophagojejunostomy, Quality of life

Background

Improving cancer therapy leads to increasing survival rates. In addition to this, there is more attention being placed on the quality of life (QOL) which is mostly dependent on cancer diagnosis and complex treatment [1]. Thorough assessment on the QOL of patients is especially important when surgery is applied as a main option of treatment, as the operated patients often suffer from various functional and psychological symptoms for a considerably longer time than the average amount of months following the surgery. These symptoms and other aspects of health which necessitate for changes of lifestyle, have to be analysed by investigating the QOL.

QOL is a multidimensional construct which represents comfort and well-being of the patients, secondary to the disease and treatment [2]. Research has shown that patients want information not only about the treatment outcomes but also about the influence of treatment on their lifestyle [3]. This is the reason why the information about the QOL should become a part of fully informed consent taking procedure before surgical treatment [4]. On the other hand, when physicians consider QOL as one of the points of prognosis after particular surgical

* Correspondence: narimantsam@takas.lt
[1]Clinic of Oncosurgery of Oncology Institute, Clinic of Internal Diseases, Family Medicine and Oncology of Medical Faculty, Vilnius University, 1 Santariskiu Street, Vilnius LT-08660, Lithuania
Full list of author information is available at the end of the article

procedure, they often rely solely on their personal professional experience because there is not much formal data about QOL except for few locations of cancer, for instance, breast or prostate [5]. The rationale for this research was the fact that little attention, if any, has been focused on QOL after extended curative surgery for gastric cancer with particular type of gastrointestinal continuity reconstruction. The aim of this retrospective cross-sectional study was, therefore, to evaluate the QOL in relation to age, sex, clinical stage, postoperative complication, and adjuvant chemotherapy in patients who underwent curative total gastrectomy with D2 lymphadenectomy and Omega type esophagojejunostomy for gastric adenocarcinoma without distant metastases.

Methods

The curative R0 total gastrectomy for middle or/and proximal gastric adenocarcinoma with reconstruction of digestive tract by means of an esophagojejunostomy with a jejunal loop and Braun's side-to-side enteroanastomosis was performed on 87 patients in the Institute of Oncology of the Vilnius University, Lithuania, from January 2008 to July 2009. All specimens were evaluated histologically. Gastric adenocarcinoma was staged according to 7th edition of TNM classification of malignant tumours [6]. An extended lymphadenectomy D2 was based on principles described and developed by Japanese gastric cancer association [7]. 69 patients, who were without distant metastasis or proven recurrence 6 to 18 months after surgery, were included into the retrospective cross-sectional study. None of these patients received neoadjuvant treatment prior to surgery.

The Lithuanian version of the European Organisation for Research and Treatment of Cancer Quality of Life Questionnaire Cancer 30 (EORTC QLQ-C30) was used to assess the QOL of gastric cancer patients and sent to them for self-completion in January 2010. 36 patients (52.2%) had responded. 34 questionnaires were filled thoroughly and they were used as material for further investigation.

The main characteristics of those patients are shown in the Table 1. The influence of age ($\geq$ 65 years vs. < 65), sex, clinical stage (I–II vs III), surgical complication (yes vs. no), and adjuvant chemotherapy (yes vs. no) was assessed on QOL. All data are expressed as mean ± using standard deviation. Quality of life scores were compared between groups using the Mann–Whitney U-test. Differences with a P value of 0.05 were considered to be statistically significant. Microsoft Office XP Excel 2007 Worksheets were used for accumulation and analysis of data.

Results

The age of patients had an obvious tendency to influence the global health status (Figure 1A). It was better in the group of patients aged 65 years and over (63.0 points

Table 1 Characteristics of 34 patients who filled the EORTC QLQ-C30

Characteristics	Value/patients	Per cent
Age Median	64	–
Range	42-84	–
SD	10.91	–
$\geq$ 65	18	52.9
< 65	16	47.1
Sex		
Male	20	58.8
Female	14	41.2
Stage of gastric cancer		
I	5	14.7
II	12	35.3
III	17	50.0
Histology		
Well-differentiated adenocarcinoma	1	3.0
Moderately differentiated adenocarcinoma	8	23.4
Poorly-differentiated adenocarcinoma	25	73.6
Postoperative complication		
Yes	7	20.6
No	27	79.4
Adjuvant chemotherapy		
Yes	16	47.1
No	18	52.9

vs 46.4 points, P = 0.0509). The functional scales were also higher in the group of patients aged 65 and over. The significant difference was only observed on the social scale and the global outcome showed in favour of elders (82.4 vs. 53.2, P = 0.0039). Symptoms, especially pain (44.8 vs. 25.0) and insomnia (47.9 vs 29.6), were more common in patients under age 65. However, the differences between these groups were not significant (Figure 1B).

Analysis of the influence of sex on the global health status (54.2 vs. 56.5) and functional scales have shown no differences between male and female (Figure 2A). Although symptoms like nausea and vomiting, insomnia, constipation were more often complained by woman (24.5 vs. 8.8, 45.1 vs 31.4, 27.5 vs. 9.8, respectively), a statistical significant difference was not found (Figure 2B).

The global health status (63.7 vs. 44.6) and functional scales were higher in patients with I and II clinical stages for gastric adenocarcinoma (Figure 3A). On the other hand, these patients expressed more symptoms such as fatigue, nausea and vomiting, pain, dyspnoea, loss of

A. The functional scales and global health status

B. Symptoms' scales

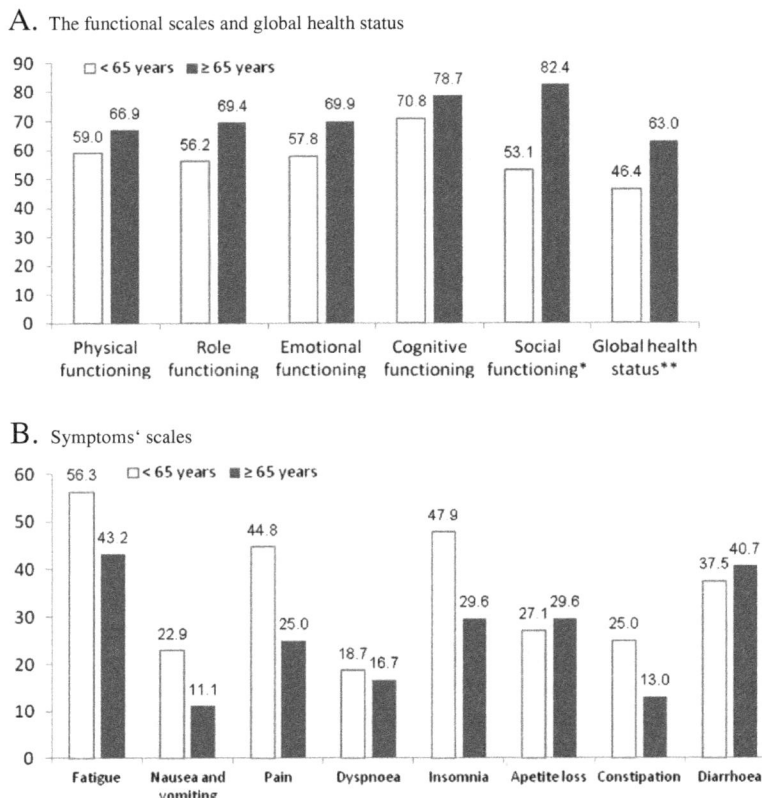

Figure 1 **Impact of age on the quality of life at time of total gastrectomy with extended lymphadenectomy and Omega type esophagojejunostomy (* P = 0.0039, ** P = 0.0509, Mann–Whitney *U* test).**

appetite, and diarrhoea (Figure 3B). Nevertheless, differences between groups were not statistical significant.

Neither statistical significant differences between groups nor obvious trends, an analysis of surgical complications and adjuvant chemotherapy on QOL were revealed.

Discussion

The studies on the QOL of gastric cancer patients mostly feature the direct interview and evaluation of patients' symptoms or performance status by physician [5], although the evaluation of QOL is more valuable when it is expressed by the patients themselves [8]. Also, any study on QOL should cover as many aspects of life as possible. Kaptein et al. wrote a review on all QOL studies of patients with gastric cancer which showed that all the studies included physiological aspects but none of them included social functioning [5]. As the biopsychosocial model of medicine is increasingly becoming significantly important, the wider spectrum QOL research is becoming increasingly valuable [5,9].

The EORTC QLQ-C30 is an extensively tested questionnaire on cancer patients which can be used to evaluate the QOL of cancer patients in any country.

Furthermore, it is a combination of adequate psychometric characteristics which give an opportunity of comparing between patients with different categories of cancer [10]. The same questionnaire was used in the studies which analysed QOL of cancer patients who followed radical surgical procedures as well [10-13]. The EORTC QLQ-C30 consists of 30 items which ask how the patient would rate his or her health and all the aspects associated with it during the last week [14]. Every item belongs to a different scale or it is a single-item measure. There are five functional scales, three symptom scales, a global health status, and six single-items in the questionnaire. All of the scales and single-item measures have been transformed linearly, ranging from 0 to 100. The data was evaluated by the guidelines of the EORTC [10,11]. It is important to note that higher scores for the functional scales and the global health status reflect better quality of life, while high scores for the symptom scales represent problems which influence the QOL negatively.

Total curative gastrectomy consists of two phases: the removal of the stomach with a limited or extended lymphadenectomy and the reconstruction of the gastrointestinal tract. Nowadays, the most popular method of

A. The functional scales and global health status

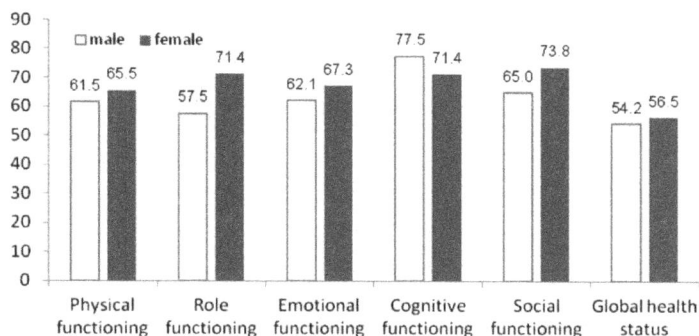

B. Symptoms' scales

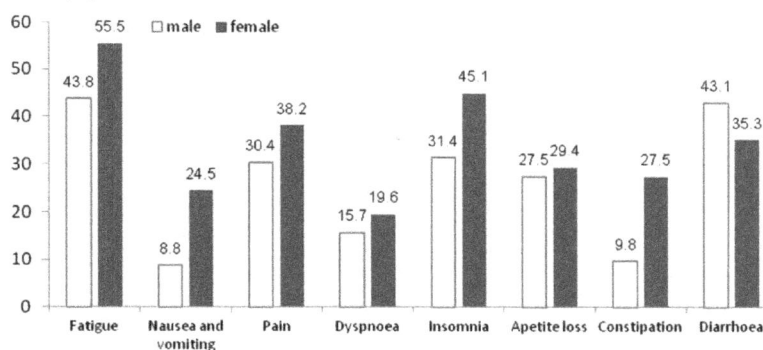

Figure 2 Influence of sex on the quality of life at time of total gastrectomy with extended lymphadenectomy and Omega type esophagojejunostomy (no significant differences).

restoration of continuity of the gastrointestinal tract is Roux-en-Y one [8]. This might be the reason why so little information on outcomes of other reconstructions as well as Omega technique can be found. The importance of knowledge on postoperative QOL as it may be an important factor in clinical decision-making, including considering surgery or not in a subgroup of patients with limited life expectancy was emphasized [15].

Several studies analysed a relation between QOL and clinical, demographic, and social parameters as it was done in this study [14,16-20]. Analysis of global health care status of our patients has shown, surprisingly, that the elder patients scored a better QOL in comparison to those younger, and is especially noticeable in social functioning. It is not simple to explain this finding of the study as other similar studies which pointed out a different trend – younger patients had better QOL after gastric surgery than older [19,20]. In our view, the fact that the global QOL and the social functioning was better in Lithuanian patients aged 65 years and over may be related with a less demanding, and, therefore, slightly more positive outlook to disease burden and surrounding environment. Nevertheless, one should be cautious in interpreting key finding of this study because of nature of

this study. On the other hand, de Liaño et al. also indicated that older patients' global health status was better, however, he also found that older patients had more clinical symptoms which is a contrasts to our study [14].

Physicians often link the advanced stage of cancer with the poorer quality of life. Although the scales of the earlier-stage cases were a little bit higher, this study as well as Huang et al. study [18] had not shown any significant differences between early and advanced cancer stages when at least 6 month had passed after surgical treatment. On the other hand, Matsushita et al. found that patients in the later stage of gastric cancer had a significantly worse quality of life [17]. Furthermore, there is no single opinion about the influence of postoperative complications following total gastrectomy on QOL. In addition to our study, de Liano et al. stated that QOL had no relation with postoperative complications. However, Matsushita et al. concluded that it negatively influences the physical functioning of gastrectomized patients after 6 months [14,17]. We have to note that women had higher scores almost in all functional and symptom's scales dimensions. Nevertheless, there were no statistically significant differences. Again, data are controversial regarding gender role on QOL [14,19,21].

A. The functional scales and global health status

B. Symptoms' scale

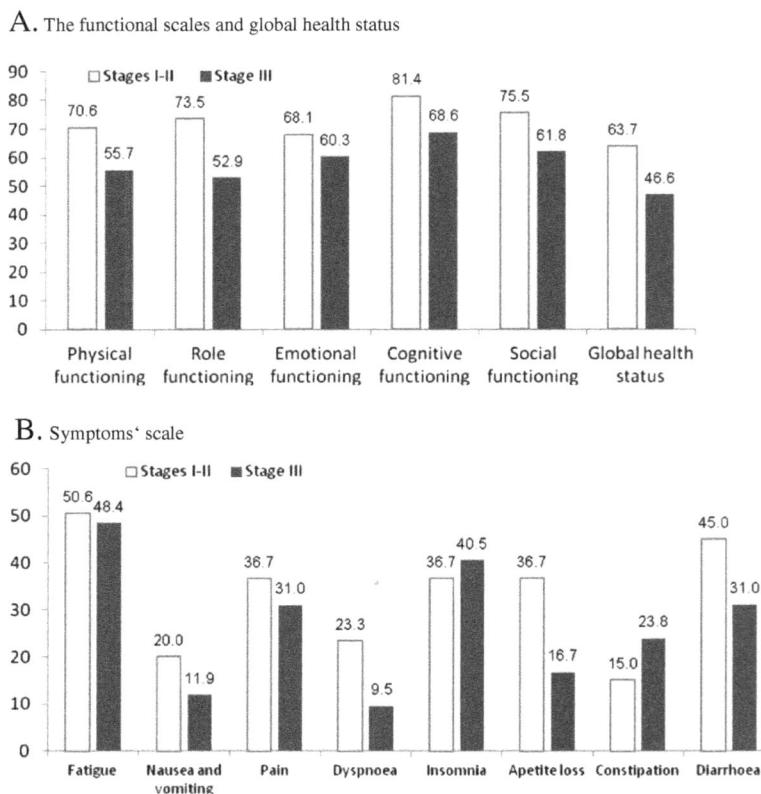

Figure 3 Impact of clinical stage of the gastric cancer on the quality of life at time of total gastrectomy with extended lymphadenectomy and Omega type esophagojejunostomy (no significant differences).

They are few limitations of this study. It is a retrospective study whereby there were a small number of patients responders involved; it undoubtedly caused a bias view. There was no control group. In addition to this, as the QOL is a subjective feature, it is influenced by not only diagnosis or treatment, but by the character and psychological state of the patients as well [17].

Conclusions

Data of the study show that the global QOL and the social functioning was better in patients aged 65 years and over, compared to patients under age 65 in the period of 6 to 18 months after a total gastrectomy with extended lymphadenectomy and Omega esophagojejunostomy for gastric adenocarcinoma without distant metastases and recurrence. In our view, this study delineated a question for further research related to type of curative surgery for elderly and survivorship. It, as a retrospective cross-sectional study of QOL after total gastrectomy with Omega reconstruction of gastrointestinal tract, can provide background for design of both retrospective case–control and prospective randomised clinical studies. Meanwhile, results of previous and current studies that include QOL in patients with gastric cancer should be

applied in preoperative as well as postoperative clinical care, which aims at improving the QOL of these patients after the total gastrectomy with particular method of gastrointestinal reconstruction.

Competing interests
The authors declare that they have no competing interests.

Author details
[1]Clinic of Oncosurgery of Oncology Institute, Clinic of Internal Diseases, Family Medicine and Oncology of Medical Faculty, Vilnius University, 1 Santariskiu Street, Vilnius LT-08660, Lithuania. [2]Liver, Renal & Surgery Department, King's College Hospital NHS Foundation Trust, King's Health Partners Academic Health Sciences Centre, Denmark Hill, London SE5 9RS, UK.

Authors' contribution
NES and RL equally participated in the design of the study, critical revision, and definitive drafting. GJ carried out the accumulation of the data, literature review, and provisional drafting. GS carried out the statistical analysis of data. All authors read and approved the final manuscript.

References
1.   Schipper H, Clinch J, Powell V: **Definitions and conceptual issues**. In *Quality of Life Assessments in Clinical Trials*. Edited by Spilker B. New York: Raven; 1990:11–24.

The quality of life after a total gastrectomy with extended lymphadenectomy and omega...

69

2. Neugebauer E, Troidl H, Wood Dauphine S, Bullinger M: **Meran conference on quality-of-life assessment in surgery.** *Theor Surg* 1991, **6**:121–165. 195–220.

3. Rutten LJ, Arora NK, Bakos AD, Aziz N, Rowland J: **Information needs and sources of information among cancer patients: a sytematic review of research.** *Patient Educ Couns* 2005, **57**:250–261.

4. Blazeby JM, Avery K, Sprangers M, Pikhart H, Fayers P, Donovan J: **Health-related quality of life measurement in randomized clinical trials in surgical oncology.** *J Clin Oncol* 2006, **24**:3178–3186.

5. Kaptein AA, Morita S, Sakamoto J: **Quality of life in gastric cancer.** *World J Gastroenterol* 2005, **11**:3189–3196.

6. Sobin LH: In *TNM classification of malignant tumors.* 7th edition. Edited by Gospodarowicz MK, Wittekind Ch. Oxford: Wiley-Blackwell; 2009.

7. Japanese Gastric Cancer Association: **Japanese Classification of Gastric Carcinoma.** *Gastric Cancer* 1998, **1**:10–24. 2nd English Edn.

8. Hoksch B, Ablassmaier B, Zieren J, Mueller J: **Quality of life after gastrectomy: Longmire's reconstruction alone compared with additional pouch reconstruction.** *World J Surg* 2002, **26**:335–341.

9. Therasse P, Arbuck SG, Eisenhauer EA, Wanders J, Kaplan RS, Rubinstein L, Verweij J, van Glabbeke M, van Oosterom AT, Christian MC, Gwyther SG: **New guidelines to evaluate the response to treatment in solid tumors.** *J Nat Cancer Inst* 2000, **92**:205–216.

10. Aaronson NK, Ahmedzai S, Bergman B, Bullinger M, Cull A, Duez NJ, *et al*: **The European Organization for Research and Treatment of Cancer QLQ-C30: A quality-of-life instrument for use in international clinical trials in oncology.** *J Nat Cancer Inst* 1993, **85**:365–376.

11. Aaronson NK, Cull A, Kaasa S, Sprangers MAG: **The EORTC modular approach to quality-of-life assessment in oncology.** *Int J Ment Health* 1994, **23**:75.

12. Fayers P, Aaronson N, Bjordal K, Groenvold M, Aaronson NK: *EORTC QLQ-C30 Scoring Manual.* EORTC Study Group on Quality of Life: Brussels; 1995:31–36.

13. Thybusch-Bernhardt A, Schmidt C, Kuechler T, Schmid A, Henne-Bruns D, Kremer B: **Quality of life following radical surgical treatment of gastric carcinoma.** *World J Surg* 1999, **23**:503–508.

14. de Liaño AD, Martínez FO, Ciga MA, Aizcorbe M, Cobo F, Trujillo R: **Impact of surgical procedure for gastric cancer on quality of life.** *Br J Surg* 2003, **90**:91–94.

15. Langenhoff BS, Krabbe PFM, Wobbes T, Ruers TJM: **Quality of life as an outcome measure in surgical oncology.** *Br J Surg* 2001, **88**:643–652.

16. Rutegard M, Hughes R, Lagergren P, Blazeby JM: **Determinants of global quality of life before and after major cancer surgery: an exploratory study.** *Qual Life Res* 2009, **18**:1131–1136.

17. Matsushita T, Matsushima E, Maruyama M: **Assessment of peri-operative quality of life in patients undergoing surgery for gastrointestinal cancer.** *Support Care Cancer* 2004, **12**:319–325.

18. Huang CC, Lien HH, Wang PC, Yang JC, Cheng CY, Huang CS: **Quality of Life in Disease-Free Gastric Adenocarcinoma Survivors: Impacts of Clinical Stages and Reconstructive Surgical Procedures.** *Dig Surg* 2007, **24**:59–65.

19. Koster R, Gerbbenslerben B, Stutzer H, Salzberger B, Ahrens P, Rohde H: **Quality of life in gastric cancer. Karnofsky's scale and Spitzer's index in comparison at the time of surgery in a cohort of 1081 patients.** *Scand J Gastroenterol* 1987, **22**:102–106.

20. Wu CW, Hsieh MC, Lo SS, Lui WY, P'eng FK: **Quality of life of patients with gastric adenocarcinoma after curative gastrectomy.** *World J Surg* 1997, **21**:777–782.

21. Wu C-W, J-M Chiou JM, Ko FS, Lo SS, Chen JH, Lui WY, Peng JW: **Quality of life after curative gastrectomy for gastric cancer in a randomised controlled trial.** *Br J Cancer* 2008, **98**:54–59.

12

Functional jejunal interposition, a reconstruction procedure, promotes functional outcomes after total gastrectomy

Xuewei Ding[1], Fang Yan[2,3], Han Liang[1], Qiang Xue[1], Kuo Zhang[4], Hui Li[3], Xiubao Ren[3] and Xishan Hao[1*]

Abstract

Background: Functional jejunal interposition (FJI) has been applied as a reconstruction procedure to maintain the jejunal continuity and duodenal food passage after total gastrectomy in patients with gastric cancer. The purpose of this study was to evaluate clinical efficacy of the FJI procedure by comparing the functional outcomes of FJI to Roux-en-Y after total gastrectomy in gastric cancer patients, and investigate physiologic mechanisms by which FJI exerts beneficial outcomes in beagles.

Methods: Patients with stage I-IV gastric cancer without metastasis and recurrence one year after surgery were enrolled in this retrospective study. Seventy one patients received FJI and seventy nine patients received Roux-en-Y after total gastrectomy. We evaluated the nutritional status at three and twelve months and incidence of complications up to twelve months after surgery. Beagles receiving sham operation, FJI, or Roux-en-Y after total gastrectomy were sacrificed forty eight hours postoperatively. Beagles were gavaged with active carbon for evaluating the intestinal transit rate. Intestinal tissues from the duodenojejunal anastomosis were collected for examining interstitial cells of Cajal (ICC), inflammation, and apoptosis.

Results: Compared to the bodyweight before surgery, the bodyweight loss at three and twelve months after surgery in patients receiving FJI was significant less than that in patients with Roux-en-Y. Patients with the FJI procedure showed significant increase of blood hemoglobin and total protein, compared to those at one month after surgery, and the prognostic nutrition index scores at three and twelve months after surgery. The incidence rates of post-operative complications, including reflux esophagitis, dumping syndrome, and Roux-en-Y syndrome were decreased in patients with FJI. Compared to beagles receiving Roux-en-Y, more ICC in the intestinal submuocsa, less intestinal epithelial cell apoptosis, and decreased inflammation in serosal side of the intestine were found in the FJI group. The intestinal transit rate in FJI group was lower than that in Roux-en Y group, indicating that FJI benefits food storage.

Conclusion: The FJI procedure promotes nutritional recovery and decreases post-operative complications in gastric cancer patients after total gastrectomy, which may be through ameliorating intestinal inflammation and damage and reducing ICC loss to preserve food reservoir function and intestinal motility.

Keywords: Gastric cancer, Gastrectomy, Inflammation, Motility, Reconstruction procedure

* Correspondence: haoxishan@tjmuch.com
[1]Department of Gastrointestinal Oncology, National Clinical Research Center for Cancer, Tianjin Cancer Institute and Hospital, Tianjin Medical University, Huanhuxi Road, Ti-Yuan-Bei, Hexi District, Tianjin 300060, P. R. China
Full list of author information is available at the end of the article

Background

Total gastrectomy, a common operation for patients with gastric cancer, is associated with a variety of early and late postoperative complications, leading to malabsorption, reflux oesophagitis, dumping and weight loss. To prevent these post-gastrectomy complications, more than fifty gastric reconstruction procedures have been applied after total gastrectomy in patients with gastric cancer. Currently, the conventional Roux-en-Y procedure is the most widely used procedure [1]. Most of these procedures have the beneficial effects on improving the necessity and efficacy of gastric substitution and duodenal food-passage. However, these reconstruction procedures have limitations for preserving the reservoir function and digestion after total gastrectomy, which result in some common problems such as dietary restriction, early satiety, postprandial fullness, vomiting, heartburn, and diarrhea [2-4]. Studies from randomized control clinical trials have suggested that establishing a jejunal reservoir to create a gastric reservoir function could maintain a low speed of the food passage in the upper intestinal tract and retain the food storage volume, which might improve the post-operation food capacity and nutritional status [5-8]. In our previous clinical practice, we developed a reconstruction procedure, functional jejunal interposition (FJI), which is characterized by maintaining jejunal continuity and duodenal food passage [9]. Our previous clinical studies evaluated effects of six reconstruction procedures on post-operative outcomes and nutritional status after total gastrectomy in patients with gastric cancer, including jejunal continuity (FJI, Braun, modified Braun I and II) and jejunum transection (Roux-en-Y and jejunal interposition) [10]. Among these six procedures, FJI was the only procedure to combine the benefits of jejunal continuity and maintaining the duodenal food passage, which plays a key role in improving nutritional status after total gastrectomy. This clinical observation indicates that FJI may serve as a potential application to improve the quality of patient's life after total gastrectomy.

In this report, we first evaluated the functional outcomes of FJI to the Roux-en-Y procedure with jejunum transection in after total gastrectomy in patients with gastric cancer. Furthermore, we performed a preliminary animal study to investigate the physiologic mechanisms by which FJI exerts beneficial effects after total gastrectomy in beagles. Our results suggest that FJI promotes nutritional recovery and decreases post-operative complications in patients after total gastrectomy. The FJI's beneficial effects are associated with preserving the reservoir function and maintaining intestinal motility. Thus, FJI may serve as a recommended surgical method for total gastrectomy.

Methods

Patients

This clinical research project was approved by the Ethics Committee of Tianjin Cancer Institute and Hospital, Tianjin Medical University, P.R. China, and registered in Tianjin Medical University Cancer Institute and Hospital clinical trial center designated by the Chinese State's Food and Drug Administration. We used AJCC cancer staging manual, sixth edition (2002) to define the cancer stage for patients in this study. Patients with histological diagnosis of gastric adenocarcinoma stage I- IV were enrolled in this retrospective study. These patients did not have metastasis and recurrent tumor after one year of surgery. Patients received total gastrectomy at Tianjin Medical University Cancer Institute and Hospital, Tianjin, China. Patients were randomly selected for FJI or Roux-en-Y after total gastrectomy. Seventy-one patients received FJI and seventy-nine patients received Roux-en-Y in this study. Detailed patient information was shown in Table 1. There is no significant difference about age, sex, and disease stage between FJI and Roux-en-Y groups.

The exclusion criteria for this study were: 1) patients older than 75-year old; 2) patients with liver cirrhosis, cardiovascular diseases, or diabetes; 3) tumors occupied the whole stomach or linitis plastica; 4) advanced cases with obvious invasion to perigastric organ or tissue; 5) cases with positive resected margins confirmed pathologically during operation.

Operation procedures for patients

Specialized gastrointestinal surgeons with more than 10-year experience performed all surgeries in this study. After the standard total gastrectomy and lymph

Table 1 Patient information

	Roux-en-Y	FJI	P value
Male	59	40	p > 0.05
Female	20	31	p > 0.05
Age (mean, years)	58	59	p > 0.05
Stage I-II	14	13	p > 0.05
Stage III-IV	65	58	p > 0.05
Pathology	**Roux-en-Y**	**FJI**	**P value**
Tubular adenocarcinoma	27	7	P < 0.05
Papillary carcinoma	7	5	P > 0.05
Mucinous adenocarcinoma	12	6	P > 0.05
Carcinoma mucocellulare	8	20	P < 0.05
Poorly differentiated adenocarcinoma	22	28	p > 0.05
Diffused carcinoma	3	5	p > 0.05

P values are computed using Wilcoxon rank sum test for continuous data (age) and Fisher's exact test for categorical data (sex, stage, pathology).

node dissection, FJI or Roux-en-Y procedure was performed for patients (Figure 1).

To perform the FJI procedure, an end-to-side esophagojejunostomy was performed at 40 cm anal to Treitz's ligament. Then, an end-to-side duodenojejunostomy was created at the efferent limb at 35 cm distal to the esophagojejunostomy. After these steps, a side-to-side jejunostomy at 5 cm distal to duodenojejunostomy and 20 cm distal to Treitz's ligament was created. Finally, two jejunal ligations were made at 5 cm oral to esophagojejunostomy and 2 cm distal to duodenojejunostomy. The tension applied for ligation was to stop the food transit, but not to induce regional jejunal tissue necrosis.

For the Roux-en-Y procedure, after the standard total gastrectomy, Roux-en-Y procedure was performed by constructing the end-to-side jejunojejunostomy at 40 cm from esophagojejunal anastomosis.

Assessment of post-operative nutritional status and complications

Patients were followed-up every 3 months after surgery and up to 12 months post-operatively. Patients were examined regularly by endoscopy, CT scan and ultrasound. Body weight, blood hemoglobin and total protein levels, and prognostic nutritional index (PNI, the score of PNI = $10 \times$ serum albumin (g/100 ml) + 0.005 × total lymphocytes count/mm^3 in peripheral blood) were used to evaluate postoperative nutritional status. All therapeutic factors other than alimentary reconstruction, such as chemoradiation and other medications, were excluded at the time of investigation.

The incidence of postoperative complications, including reflux esophagitis, dumping syndrome, and Rou-en-Y syndrome, were evaluated. The diagnosis of reflux esophagitis was made by a combination of clinical symptoms, including heartburn, acid dyspepsia, regurgitation, and chest pain, and objective testing with upper endoscopy. Endoscopic examination was assessed using the Los Angeles Classification; one (or more) mucosal break within the tops of two mucosal folds with the size < 5 mm (grade A) and > 5 mm (grade B), and continuous mucosal break

between the tops of two or more mucosal folds which involve < 75% (grade C) and > 75% (grade D) of the circumference. Patients who had the above symptoms and the endoscopic assessment at the level of ≥ grade C were diagnosed as reflux esophagitis.

Dumping syndrome and Roux-en-Y syndrome were evaluated based on patients' medical history using questionnaire and laboratory tests. The questionnaire was asked by an experienced nurse being blinded by the type of the procedure. Dumping syndrome was diagnosed based on symptoms, including abdominal cramps, nausea, diarrhea, tachycardia, sweating, flushing, and dizziness after eating, and oral glucose tolerance test. Roux stasis syndrome was diagnosed based on symptoms, including nausea, vomiting of food but not bile, epigastric fullness, and postprandial pain.

Operation procedures for beagles

All animal experiments were performed according to protocols approved by the Institutional Animal Care and Use Committee at Peking University Health Science Center, Beijing, P. R. China. Beagles (Vital River Laboratories, Beijing, P. R. China) were maintained in a controlled environment at 21° under a 12-h dark/light cycle. All beagles used in this study were at six month old and body weights were between 7 kg and 10 kg.

Beagles were randomly selected for Sham operation (5 beagles), FJI (10 beagles) or Roux-en-Y (7 beagles) after total gastrectomy, performed by the same specialized gastrointestinal surgeon (Figure 1). Beagles were fasting for 12 hours before anesthetized using 2% Pentobarbital Sodium Salt. After the standard total gastrectomy, The Roux-en-Y procedure was performed by constructing the end-to-side jejunojejunostomy at 40 cm from esophagojejunal anastomosis. The ends of the Roux and Y limb were closed (Figure 1). To perform FJI procedure, an end-to-side esophagojejunostomy was performed at 40 cm anal to Treitz's ligament. Then, an end-to-side duodenojejunostomy was created at the efferent limb at 35 cm distal to the esophagojejunostomy, followed by a side-to-side jejunostomy at 5 cm distal

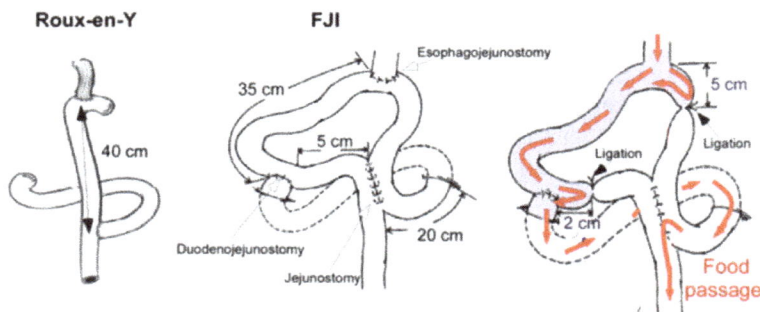

Figure 1 Schematic models of the reconstruction procedures after total gastrectomy performed for patients and for beagles.

to duodenojejunostomy and 20 cm distal to Treitz's ligament. Finally, 2 jejunal proper ligations were made at 5 cm oral to esophagojejunostomy and 2 cm distal to duodenojejunostomy (Figure 1). After surgery, beagles were given 5% glucose and 0.9% saline (1000 ml/day) with restriction of oral food intake.

Measurement of intestinal transit rate

At 47 hours postoperatively, beagles were anesthetized using 2% Pentobarbital Sodium Salt and administered 50 ml of 10% active carbon in water to the esophagojejunal junction through a gavage tube. Beagles were sacrificed 1 hour after gavage and the active carbon migration distance in the small intestine was measured. The intestinal transit rate was calculated as: the active carbon migration distance/the total small intestinal length.

Tissue section preparation

The intestine tissues were collected 48 hours after operation, including 5 cm oral and 5 cm anal to the site of the duodenojejunal anastomosis in beagles receiving FJI, 5 cm oral and 5 cm anal to the site of the jejunojejunostomy in beagles receiving Roux-en-Y, and jejunal tissues from beagles receiving sham operation. Tissue samples were fixed in 10% formalin for preparing and paraffin-embedded intestinal tissue sections.

Analysis of intestinal inflammation

Paraffin-embedded tissue sections were stained with hematoxylin and eosin for light microscopic examination to assess intestinal inflammation. Samples were examined by a pathologist blinded to the treatment condition.

Immunohistochemistry

Antigen retrieval of formalin-fixed sections was performed using the Antigen Unmasking Solution (Vector laboratories, Inc. Burlingame, CA). Sections were blocked using 10% goat serum and stained with anti- c-Kit (for ICC staining, Santa Cruz Biotechnology, Inc., Santa Cruz, CA, USA) antibody at 4°C overnight. Then, FITC-labeled anti-rabbit antibody was incubated with sections at room temperature for 1 hour. For neutrophil and macrophage staining, sections were incubated with FITC-anti-Ly-6C/G (a marker for neutrophil, Invitrogen Corp., Carlsbad, CA) or FITC-anti-F4/80 (a marker for macrophage, Invitrogen) antibody at 4°C overnight, respectively. Sections were mounted using Vectashield™ Mounting Medium containing DAPI (Vector laboratories, Inc. Burlingame, CA) and observed by fluorescence microscopy. FITC and DAPI images were taken from the same field.

The number of ICC per 20X power field and the numbers of neutrophil and macrophage per 10X power field

Table 2 The PNI score in patients after total gastrectomy

	Roux-en-Y	FJI	P value*
3 months	45.85 ± 5.59 (N = 79)	51.74 ± 5.49 (N = 71)	<0.05
12 months	48.14 ± 5.22 (N = 79)	53.70 ± 5.83 (N = 71)	<0.05

*Compared to PNI scores at the same post-operative time.

were determined by counting the number of positive cells in at least 20 fields.

Apoptotic assay

Apoptosis was detected in tissue sections using ApopTag™ *In Situ* Oligo Ligation (ISOL) kit (Intergen Company, Purchase, NY), following manufacturer's guidelines, and observed by differential interference contrast (DIC) microscopy. The number of apoptotic cell per 40X power field was determined by counting the number of positive cells in at least 20 fields.

Statistical analysis

Statistical significance of the difference between FJI and Roux-en-Y groups was determined using *student t test* analysis for nutritional status and x^2 *test* analysis *for* the incidence of postoperative complications. Statistical significance of cell numbers from beagle study was determined by one-way ANOVA followed by Newman-Keuls analysis using Prism 5.0 (GraphPad Software, Inc. San Diego, CA) for multiple comparisons. Data are presented as mean ± S.E.M. A *p* value < 0.05 was defined as statistically significant.

Table 3 The nutritional status of patients after total gastrectomy

Time after surgery	3 months		12 months	
Disease stage	I-II	III-IV	I-II	III-IV
Bodyweight loss (kg)#				
Roux-en-Y	6.03 ± 2.72	6.91 ± 1.84	5.36 ± 2.50	5.87 ± 2.17
FJI	5.36 ± 2.50	5.65 ± 1.72	3.11 ± 2.47	3.52 ± 2.18
P value*	0.01	0.036	0.01	0.041
Hemoglobin increase (g/dL)†				
Roux-en-Y	9.29 ± 5.76	5.92 ± 4.52	9.29 ± 5.76	7.02 ± 4.84
FJI	10.31 ± 5.91	8.97 ± 6.07	10.31 ± 5.91	10.00 ± 6.36
P value*	0.65	0.002	0.65	0.004
Total protein increase (g/dl)†				
Roux-en-Y	4.18 ± 2.59	4.08 ± 2.18	4.96 ± 3.06	5.59 ± 2.79
FJI	5.32 ± 2.75	5.52 ± 2.74	6.67 ± 3.35	7.32 ± 3.29
P value*	0.279	0.002	0.179	0.002

#Shown value = the value at the indicated post-operative time – the value before the surgery# or the value at 1 month after the surgery†.
*Comparison was made between these two groups with the same disease stage and at the same post-operative time.

Table 4 The incidence rates of postoperative complications at 12 months after total gastrectomy

	Roux-en-Y	FJI	X2	P value
Dumping Syndrome	16.5% (13/79)	5.6% (4/71)	6.437	0.040
Reflux Esophagitis	16.55 (13/79)	4.2% (3/71)	7.231	0.027
Roux-en-Y Syndrome	17.7% (14/79)	5.6% (4/71)	6.549	0.038

Results

Beneficial effects of FJI on the functional outcomes in gastric cancer patients after total gastrectomy

We evaluated post-operative nutritional status and complications up to 12 months post-operatively. In this study, all patients in FJI and Roux-en-Y groups survived for 12 months after surgery. First, we evaluated the PNI score, which correlates with the nutritional status in patients after surgery. PNI scores in patients receiving FJI (48.14 ± 5.22 at 3 months and 53.70 ± 5.83 at 12 months after operation) were significant higher than those in patients with Roux-en-Y (45.85 ± 5.59 at 3 months and 51.74 ± 5.49 at 12 months) (Table 2).

Then, we assessed the changes of bodyweight and blood hemoglobin and total protein levels in patients at 3 and 12 months after surgery. Compared to the bodyweight before surgery, the bodyweight loss at three and twelve months after surgery in the FJI groups with stage I-II and II-IV gastric cancer was significant less than that in patients with Roux-en-Y (Table 3). The increases of blood hemoglobin and total protein at three and twelve

months after surgery, as compared to those at 1 month after surgery, were significantly higher in patients with stage III-IV gastric cancer receiving FJI than Roux-en-Y group (Table 3). Although, in patients with stage I-II disease, patients receiving FJI showed higher levels of increases of blood hemoglobin and total protein levels at three and twelve months after operation, as compared those in patients with Roux-en-Y, these changes were not significant (Table 3). These data suggested that retaining duodenal food transit in post-gastrectomy reconstruction supports good nutritional status, which may be more important for patients with late stage gastric cancers.

There are three common postoperative complications of reconstruction after total gastrectomy, reflux esophagitis, dumping syndrome, and Rous-en-Y syndrome. The incidence rates of reflux esophagitis, dumping syndrome, and Roux-en-Y syndrome in patients receiving Roux-en-Y were 16.5%, 16.5%, and 17.7%, respectively, which were significantly decreased to 4.2%, 5.6%, and 5.6% in patients receiving FJI, at 12 months after total gastrectomy (Table 4). Thus, the FJI procedure decreases postoperative complications in gastric cancer patients after total gastrectomy. Our data from patient study showed that FJI promotes nutritional recovery and decreases the risk of subsequent complications after gastrectomy, as compared to Roux-en-Y.

Furthermore, no class II and higher complications defined in Clavien-Dindo classification, such as anastomotic

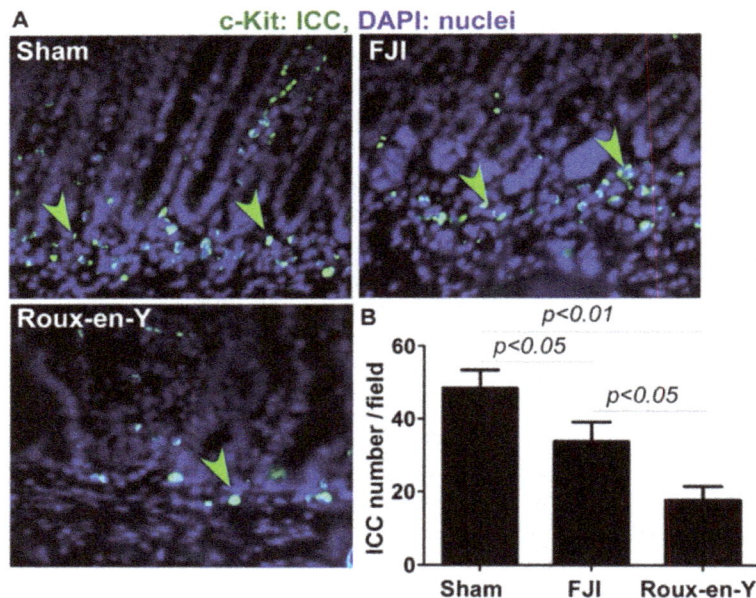

Figure 2 FJI preserves ICC in the small intestine. The intestinal tissues were isolated from beagles at 48 hours postoperatively. Paraffin-embedded tissue sections were stained using an anti-c-Kit (ICC marker) antibody and a FITC-conjugated secondary antibody. Nuclei were stained using DAPI (blue). Fluorescent and DAPI images were taken from the same field **(A)**. Green arrowheads: ICC. The number of ICC per 20X power field is shown **(B)**. Sham = 5 beagles, FJI = 10 beagles, Roux-en-Y = 7 beagles.

leakage, pancreatic fistula and bleeding, were found in patients receiving Roux-en-Y and FJI procedure in this study.

FJI's beneficial effects on ameliorating intestinal inflammation and damage and preserving intestinal motility in beagles

To investigate the physiologic mechanisms underlying FJI benefitting nutritional recovery and decreasing complications, we performed animal studies. We first studied the intestinal transit rate (the active carbon migration distance/the total small intestinal length) in beagles. At 48 hours postoperatively, the intestinal transit rate in sham group was 0.14 ± 0.03. Although the intestinal transit rate in FJI group (0.32 ± 0.11) was significantly higher than that in the sham group ($p < 0.05$), it was significant lower than that in Roux-en-Y group (0.52 ± 0.21,

$p < 0.05$). These data suggested that FJI exerts a reservoir function to benefit food storage.

To study the effects of FJI and Roux-en-Y procedures on preserving intestinal motility, we detected interstitial cells of Cajal (ICC) in the intestine. Immunohistochemistry analysis of ICC showed that there were more ICC in submuocsa of the small intestine in FJI group than those in Roux-en-Y group (Figure 2A and B). Therefore, this result indicates that FJI preserves ICC, which may contribute to maintaining intestinal functional motility.

Inflammation is a major factor to disrupt intestinal motility, including ICC network. Therefore, we evaluated the inflammatory responses after surgery. 60% (6/10) beagles receiving FJI and 100% (7/7) beagles receiving Roux-en-Y showed inflammation in serosal side of the small intestine around anastomosis, including hemorrhage, fibrin

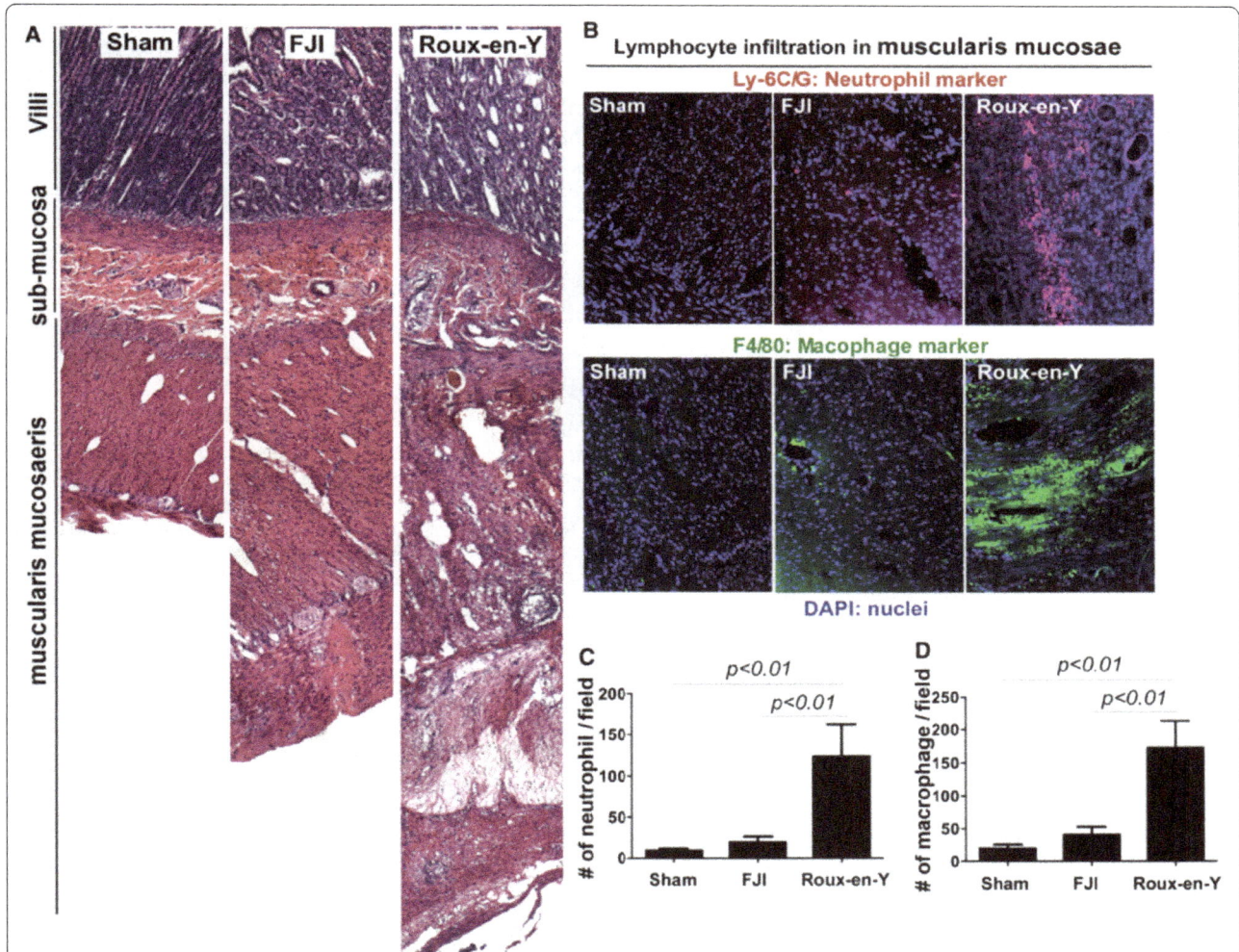

Figure 3 FJI decreases inflammation and neutrophil and macrophage infiltration into the small intestine in beagles. Beagle tissue sections were prepared as described in Figure 2. Tssue sections were stained using hematoxylin and eosin to assess injury and inflammation (**A**). Neutrophil and macrophage were stained using Cy3-conjugated anti-Ly-6C/G (a marker for neutrophil) and FITC-conjugated anti-F4/80 (a marker for macrophage) antibodies, respectively. Nuclei were stained using DAPI (blue) (**B**). The numbers of neutrophil (**C**) and macrophage (**D**) per 10X power field are shown. Sham = 5 beagles, FJI = 10 beagles, Roux-en-Y = 7 beagles.

deposition, and ulceration (Figure 3A). The degree of serosal inflammation was lower in FJI, compared to that in Roux-en-Y group. Inflammatory responses after surgery include significant increase in lymphocyte infiltration and pro-inflammatory cytokine production. We found that the numbers of neutrophil and macrophage infiltration in muscularis mucosae of the small intestine were less in FJI group than that in Roux-en-Y group (Figure 3B-D). We did not find significant inflammation in mucosa of the small intestine in any of these three groups.

Disruption of the integrity of this monolayer is a major defect in intestinal inflammation [11]. Thus, we performed an apoptotic assay to detect apoptosis in the intestine. We found that small intestinal epithelial cell apoptosis was significant reduced in beagles receiving FJI, compared to that in Roux-en-Y group (Figure 4A and B). These data indicate that FJI results in less intestinal tissue injury and inflammation when compared to Roux-en-Y.

Discussion

Gastrointestinal surgery usually results in gastrointestinal tissue injury which leads to inflammatory responses within the tunica muscularis. The present study revealed that FJI benefits food storage and ameliorates intestinal inflammation and damage which may contribute to reducing ICC loss. ICC receives motor neural and mechanical inputs and generate and propagate electrical rhythmicity to control gastrointestinal motility [12-15]. ICC is responsible for generating and propagating electrical slow waves that coordinate the phasic contractions [15,16]. It has been reported that there were loss of acute disruption of ICC networks, slow waves, and phasic contractions five hours after surgery [17]. Thus, we detected ICC in the small intestinal 48 hours after operation. These beneficial effects of FJI may contribute to the improvement of outcomes after total gastrectomy in patients with gastric cancer observed in our clinical studies.

Many techniques for the restoration of intestinal continuity after gastrectomy have been proposed, both to compensate for the lost function of the stomach and in attempts to prevent postgastrectomy syndromes. The continuity of gastrointestinal tract plays a key role in the coordination of intestinal motility. Emerging evidence has shown that surgical manipulation of gastrointestinal

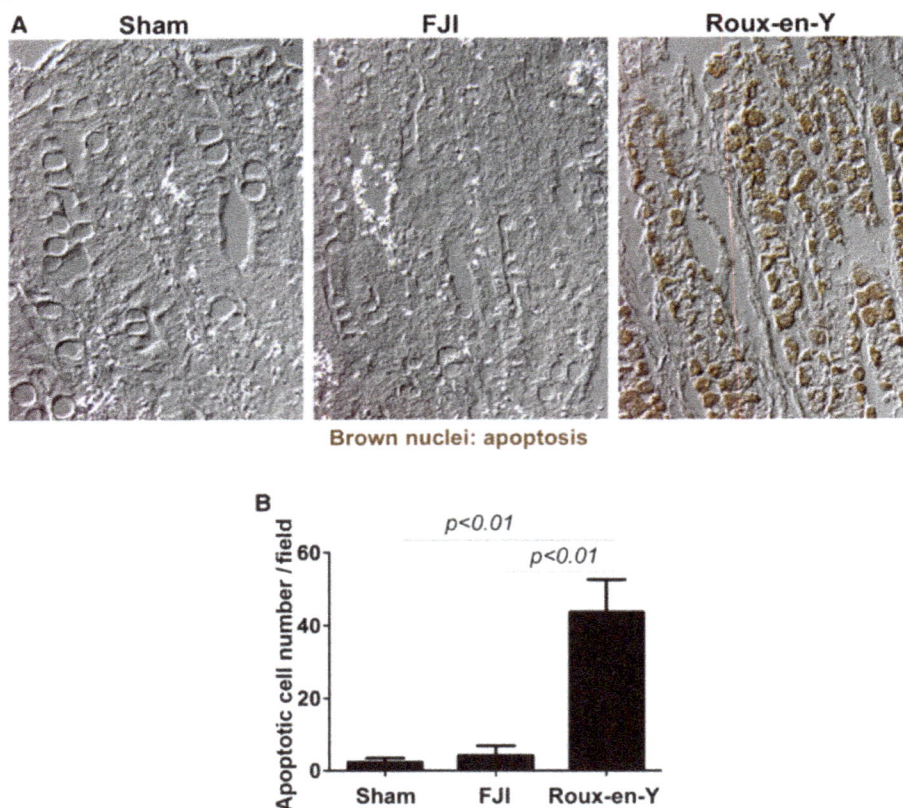

Figure 4 FJI decreases apoptosis in the small intestinal epithelial cells in beagles. Beagle tissue sections were prepared as described in Figure 2. Apoptosis was detected using ISOL kit (brown nuclei) (**A**). The number of apoptotic cells per 40X power field is shown (**B**). Sham = 5 beagles, FJI = 10 beagles, Roux-en-Y = 7 beagles.

tract, such as resection followed by reanastomosis, resulted in disruption of intestinal motility [18]. Roux-en-Y Syndrome represents a syndrome of abdominal pain, nausea, vomiting and fullness [19]. Roux-en-Y Syndrome has been frequently observed in patients who received Roux-en-Y reconstruction after partial gastrectomy with morbidity as higher as 30% [20]. It was suggested that the major cause of Roux-en-Y Syndrome was due to disruption of intestinal integrity and enteric neural continuity, leading to the subsequent disorder of intestinal motility. Furthermore, several studies found that disruption of the motility by gastrointestinal resection was through damage of ICC, the pacemakers for the gastrointestinal tract. Our study showed that FJI preserved ICC compared to Rou-en-Y procedure. Thus, FJI may exert the beneficial effects on reducing Roux-en-Y Syndrome.

The integrity of the intestinal epithelium is critical for maintaining normal intestinal functions while providing a defense against pathogenic microbes and detrimental substances in the intestinal lumen. The degree of inflammation in the muscularis is related to the degree of manipulation of the intestinal tissues. Inflammation may lead to several pathological responses, such as the loss of ICC proximal to intestinal obstructions after gastrointestinal surgery [21]. Therefore, reduced inflammation may mediate preservation of ICC in patients receiving FJI.

Chyme is mixed with bile and pancreatic secretions in duodenum. The passage of food triggers secreting of intestinal hormones such as secretin, cholecystokinin and insulin. Therefore, preserving duodenal food passage should enhance the digestive function. For example, duodenal food passage has been shown to exert beneficial effects on regulating blood sugar level after total gastrectom [3]. It has been reported that the type of reconstruction procedure after total gastrectomy plays a role in regulating postprandial gastrointestinal hormone production [22]. Therefore, facilitating food storage by FJI may contribute to its outcomes to improve nutritional status in patients.

In summary, FJI's clinical beneficial outcomes may be associated with the reservoir function and its effects on preserving intestinal motility. Therefore, FJI has potential clinical application to improve the quality of life for patients after total gastrectomy.

Conclusion

Our clinical studies indicate that the FJI procedure promotes nutritional recovery and decreases post-operative complications in patients with gastric cancer after total gastrectomy. Findings from animal studies further provide insights into understanding the physiologic mechanisms by which FJI exerts beneficial effects on outcomes after total gastrectomy, including preserving reservoir function and maintaining intestinal motility. Based on

the surgical procedure used for FJI, FJI can maintain jejunal continuity and duodenal food passage. Thus, retaining the intestinal integrity by FJI may lead to beneficial clinical outcomes after surgery. However, more clinical studies are needed to further assess FJI to procedures using the conventional jejunal interposition.

Competing interests
The authors declare that they have no competing interests.

Authors' contributions
XD and KZ carried out the experimental studies. HL, QX, HL, XR and XH participated in the design of the study and data analysis, XD and FY drafted the manuscript. All authors read and approved the final manuscript.

Acknowledgements
We thank Dr. Wenfen Cao at Department of Pathology at Tianjin Medical University Cancer Institute and Hospital for her assistance for this study.

Grant support
This work was supported by the grant awarded by the Tianjin Science and Technology Committee (No. 06txtjjc14502), the grant for Key Basic Research Projects awarded by the Ministry of Science and Technology of P. R. China (No.2010CB529301), the grant for Anticancer Major Projects awarded by the Tianjin Municipal Science and Technology Commission (12ZCDZSY16400), and core services performed through Vanderbilt University Medical Center's Digestive Disease Research Center supported by NIH grant P30DK058404.

Author details
[1]Department of Gastrointestinal Oncology, National Clinical Research Center for Cancer, Tianjin Cancer Institute and Hospital, Tianjin Medical University, Huanhuxi Road, Ti-Yuan-Bei, Hexi District, Tianjin 300060, P. R. China. [2]Department of Pediatrics, Division of Gastroenterology, Hepatology and Nutrition, Vanderbilt University Medical Center, Nashville, TN, USA. [3]Department of Immunology, Key Laboratory of Cancer Prevention and Therapy, National Clinical Research Center for Cancer, Tianjin Cancer Institute and Hospital, Tianjin Medical University, Tianjin, P. R. China. [4]Department of Laboratory Animal Science, Peking University Health Science Center, Beijing, P. R. China.

References
1. Lawrence Jr W. Reconstruction after total gastrectomy: what is preferred technique? J Surg Oncol. 1996;63:215–20.
2. Fuchs KH, Thiede A, Engemann R, Deltz E, Stremme O, Hamelmann H. Reconstruction of the food passage after total gastrectomy: randomized trial. World J Surg. 1995;19(698):705–6.
3. Schwarz A, Buchler M, Usinger K, Rieger H, Glasbrenner B, Friess H. Importance of the duodenal passage and pouch volume after total gastrectomy and reconstruction with the Ulm pouch: prospective randomized clinical study. World J Surg. 1996;20:60–6.
4. Svedlund J, Sullivan M, Liedman B, Lundell L. Quality of life after gastrectomy for gastric carcinoma: controlled study of reconstructive procedures. World J Surg. 1997;21:422–33.
5. Kono K, Iizuka H, Sekikawa T, Sugai H, Takahashi A, Fujii H, et al. Improved quality of life with jejunal pouch reconstruction after total gastrectomy. Am J Surg. 2003;185:150–4.
6. Lehnert T, Buhl K. Techniques of reconstruction after total gastrectomy for cancer. Br J Surg. 2004;91:528–39.
7. Liedman B, Bosaeus I, Hugosson I, Lundell L. Long-term beneficial effects of a gastric reservoir on weight control after total gastrectomy: a study of potential mechanisms. Br J Surg. 1998;85:542–7.
8. Svedlund J, Sullivan M, Liedman B, Lundell L. Long term consequences of gastrectomy for patient's quality of life: the impact of reconstructive techniques. Am J Gastroenterol. 1999;94:438–45.
9. Hao XS, Li Q, Yin J. The application of FJI and its comparison with different alimentary reconstructions after total gastrectomy for cancer. Chinese-German J Clin Oncol. 2002;1:79–81.

10. Pan Y, Li Q, Wang DC, Wang JC, Liang H, Liu JZ. Beneficial effects of jejunal continuity and duodenal food passage after total gastrectomy: a retrospective study of 704 patients. Eur J Surg Oncol. 2008;34:17–22.

11. Xavier RJ, Podolsky DK. Unravelling the pathogenesis of inflammatory bowel disease. Nature. 2007;448:427–34.

12. Huizinga JD, Thuneberg L, Kluppel M, Malysz J, Mikkelsen HB, Bernstein A. W/kit gene required for interstitial cells of Cajal and for intestinal pacemaker activity. Nature. 1995;373:347–9.

13. Kobayashi S, Chowdhury JU, Tokuno H, Nahar NS, Iino S. A smooth muscle nodule producing 10–12 cycle/min regular contractions at the mesenteric border of the pacemaker area in the guinea-pig colon. Arch Histol Cytol. 1996;59:159–68.

14. Kobayashi S, Torihashi S, Iino S, Pang YW, Chowdhury JU, Tomita T. The inner sublayer of the circular muscle coat in the canine proximal colon: origins of spontaneous electrical and mechanical activity. Arch Histol Cytol. 1995;58:45–63.

15. Sanders KM, Ordog T, Koh SD, Torihashi S, Ward SM. Development and plasticity of interstitial cells of Cajal. Neurogastroenterol Motil. 1999;11:311–38.

16. Code CF, Marlett JA. The interdigestive myo-electric complex of the stomach and small bowel of dogs. J Physiol. 1975;246(2):289–309.

17. Yanagida H, Yanase H, Sanders KM, Ward SM. Intestinal surgical resection disrupts electrical rhythmicity, neural responses, and interstitial cell networks. Gastroenterology. 2004;127:1748–59.

18. Bassotti G, Chiarinelli ML, Germani U, Chiarioni G, Morelli A. Effect of some abdominal surgical operations on small bowel motility in humans: our experience. J Clin Gastroenterol. 1995;21:211–6.

19. Mathias JR, Fernandez A, Sninsky CA, Clench MH, Davis RH. Nausea, vomiting, and abdominal pain after Roux-en-Y anastomosis: motility of the jejunal limb. Gastroenterology. 1985;88:101–7.

20. van der Mijle HC, Kleibeuker JH, Limburg AJ, Bleichrodt RP, Beekhuis H, van Schilfgaarde R. Manometric and scintigraphic studies of the relation between motility disturbances in the Roux limb and the Roux-en-Y syndrome. Am J Surg. 1993;166:11–7.

21. Won KJ, Suzuki T, Hori M, Ozaki H. Motility disorder in experimentally obstructed intestine: relationship between muscularis inflammation and disruption of the ICC network. Neurogastroenterol Motil. 2006;18:53–61.

22. Kalmar K, Nemeth J, Kelemen D, Agoston E, Horváth OP. Postprandial gastrointestinal hormone production is different, depending on the type of reconstruction following total gastrectomy. Ann Surg. 2006;243:465–71.

13

Overexpression of Cystatin SN positively affects survival of patients with surgically resected esophageal squamous cell carcinoma

You-Fang Chen[1,2], Gang Ma[1,3†], Xun Cao[1,3†], Rong-Zhen Luo[1,4], Li-Ru He[1,5], Jie-Hua He[1,4], Zhi-Liang Huang[1,2], Mu-Sheng Zeng[1] and Zhe-Sheng Wen[1,2*]

Abstract

Background: Cystatin SN is a secreted protein and a cysteine proteinase inhibitor. It has been considered to be a tumor marker for gastrointestinal tract cancer in several functional researches. However, the clinicopathological and prognostic significance of Cystatin SN expression in esophageal squamous cell carcinoma (ESCC) has not been elucidated.

Methods: In our study, the expression of Cystatin SN was detected in 209 surgically resected ESCC tissues and 170 peritumoral normal esophageal mucosae by immunohistochemistry. The prognostic significance of Cystatin SN expression was analysed with Kaplan-Meier plots and the Cox proportional hazards regression models.

Results: The results showed that the immunostaining of Cystatin SN in ESCC tissues was less intense than that in the normal control tissue ($P < 0.001$). Compared with patients with low tumoral Cystatin SN expression, ESCC patients with tumors high-expression Cystatin SN exhibited increased disease-free survival (DFS) and overall survival (OS) ($P < 0.001$ and $P < 0.001$, respectively). Furthermore, the expression level of Cystatin SN could further stratify the ESCC patients by survival (DFS and OS) in the stage II subgroup ($P < 0.001$ and $P < 0.001$, respectively). Multivariate analyses showed that Cystatin SN expression, N status and differentiation were independent and significant predictors of survival.

Conclusions: We concluded that ESCC patients whose tumors express high levels of Cystatin SN have favourable survival compared with those patients with low Cystatin SN expression. Tumoral Cystatin SN expression may be an independent predictor of survival for patients with resectable ESCCs.

Keywords: Esophageal squamous cell carcinoma, Cystatin SN, Immunohistochemistry, Prognosis

Background

Esophageal cancer (EC) is the fourth leading cause of cancer-related death worldwide, and there were approximately 482,300 new esophageal cancer cases and 406,800 EC-related deaths in 2008, with incidence rates varying almost 16-fold throughout the world [1]. China accounts for approximately 53.6% of new cases and 51.7% of EC-related worldwide [2]. In China,

approximately 90% of all esophageal cancers are squamous cell carcinomas [2,3]. The best option for curing esophageal squamous cell carcinoma (ESCC) is surgical resection, but the delayed clinical presentation of symptoms (e.g., dysphagia and odynophagia) may result in the loss of the opportunity to undergo surgery. Even with the development of surgical techniques and better postoperative management, the 5-year survival rate of patients after complete surgical resection only ranges from 10% to 40% [4].

Cysteine proteases are involved in tissue remodeling during development, and they induce the migration of cancer cells [5,6]. The expression, function and location of many proteases are associated with tumor progression

* Correspondence: wenzhsh@sysucc.org.cn
†Equal contributors
[1]State Key Laboratory of Oncology in South China, Cancer Center, Sun Yet-Sen University, No.651, Dongfeng Road East, Guangzhou, China
[2]Department of Thoracic Oncology, Cancer Center, Sun Yet-Sen University, No.651, Dongfeng Road East, Guangzhou, China
Full list of author information is available at the end of the article

[5,7,8]. In the past, researchers have focused their attentions on tumor cells, but efforts have shifted to the role of cathepsins in the progression of tumor cells, with the goal of designing a novel protease-based drug to attenuate the invasive and metastatic capabilities of tumor cells [5]. Simultaneously, recent evidence suggests that lysosomal cysteine proteases play an important role in ESCC growth, invasion and metastasis [7,8].

The *CST1* gene encodes a secretory peptide called Cystatin SN, which is a cysteine proteinase inhibitor [9]. The balance between cathepsins and their cystatins has been reported to influence various pathological processes, including tumor invasion and metastasis [10,11]. Cystatin SN is one of the family 2 cystatins (including cystatins C, D, S, SA, SN, M and F), which are encoded by one subfamily of the *Cystatin* (*CST*) superfamily [12]. There have been reported that most of the family 2 Cystatins (excluding Cystatin SA) are closely associated with tumor metastasis and invasion [6,11,13-21]. In particular, CST1 plays an important role in the regulation of proteolysis and is highly involved in gastric tumorigenesis though TCF-mediated proliferative signalling [6]. At the same time, CST1 was also identified as a tumor marker for colorectal cancer [21] although this finding lacks the support of clinicalpathological data. All previous observations have implied that Cystatin SN may contribute to the process of carcinogenesis and tumor progression. However, the clinicopathological and prognostic significance of Cystatin SN in human ESCC has not yet been elucidated.

Based on these considerations, in our study, we analysed Cystatin SN protein expression in surgically resected ESCCs from a large patient cohort. Furthermore, we have discussed the clinicopathological and prognostic value of Cystatin SN expression in ESCCs.

Methods

Between October 2000 and April 2007, 240 primary ESCC patients underwent complete surgical resection (R0) at the Sun Yat-sen University Cancer Center were eligible for our study. After exclusion of the noninformative samples (e.g., unrepresentative and lost samples), a total of 209 ESCC tissues and 170 peritumoral tissues were included for immunohistochemical analysis. All patients underwent a pretreatment evaluation (e.g., basic personal information, a complete history, a physical examination and a preoperative examination) and provided a complete follow-up data. The data regarding the tumor (e.g., tumor location, differentiation, T stage, N stage, distant metastasis) were collected from the postoperative pathological results and the preoperative examination. The tumor differentiation grades were based on the World Health Organization criteria, and the tumor-node-metastasis classifications

Table 1 Association between Cystatin SN expression and clinicopathological variables in 209 ESCC patients

Variables	Cases	Cystatin SN expression (%)		P value[*]
		Low (−to+) Number. (%)	High (++to+++) Number. (%)	
Age (years)				0.166
Median[†]	57			
Range	32-80			
≤ 57	113	83(73.5)	30(26.5)	
> 57	96	62(64.6)	24(35.4)	
Gender				0.328
Male	150	107(71.3)	43(28.7)	
Female	59	38(64.4)	21(35.6)	
Tumor location				0.699
Upper	15	9(60.0)	6(40.0)	
Middle	96	68(70.8)	28(29.2)	
Lower	98	68(69.4)	30(30.6)	
Differentiation				0.200
G1	56	39(69.6)	17(30.4)	
G2	105	68(64.8)	37(35.2)	
G3	48	38(79.2)	10(20.8)	
pT status				0.133
pT1	4	1(25.0)	3(75.0)	
pT2	62	42(67.7)	20(32.3)	
pT3	143	102(71.3)	41(28.7)	
pN status				0.176
pN0	116	76(65.5)	40(34.5)	
pN1-3	93	69(74.2)	24(25.8)	
pTNM status				0.183
II	133	88(66.2)	45(33.8)	
III	76	57(75.0)	19(25.0)	

[*]Chi-square test; [†]median age was 57 years for 209 enrolled ESCC patients. G grade, *pT* pathologic tumor, *pN* pathologic node, *pTNM* pathologic tumor-node-metastasis.

were defined according to the the American Joint Committee on Cancer (AJCC, 2009). The study was approved by the Medical Ethics Committee of the Cancer Center at Sun Yat-Sen University.

Follow-up data after surgery (e.g., recurrence, metastasis, vital status, death and the causes of death) were obtained from the patients' records. All patients were followed up every 4-6 months during the first 3 years and every year thereafter. All patients' vital statuses were confirmed in January 2012.

Immunohistochemistry (IHC)

A total of 209 ESCC tissues and 170 paired peritumoral normal esophageal tissues were fixed in 10% neutral buffered formalin after complete surgical resection (R0)

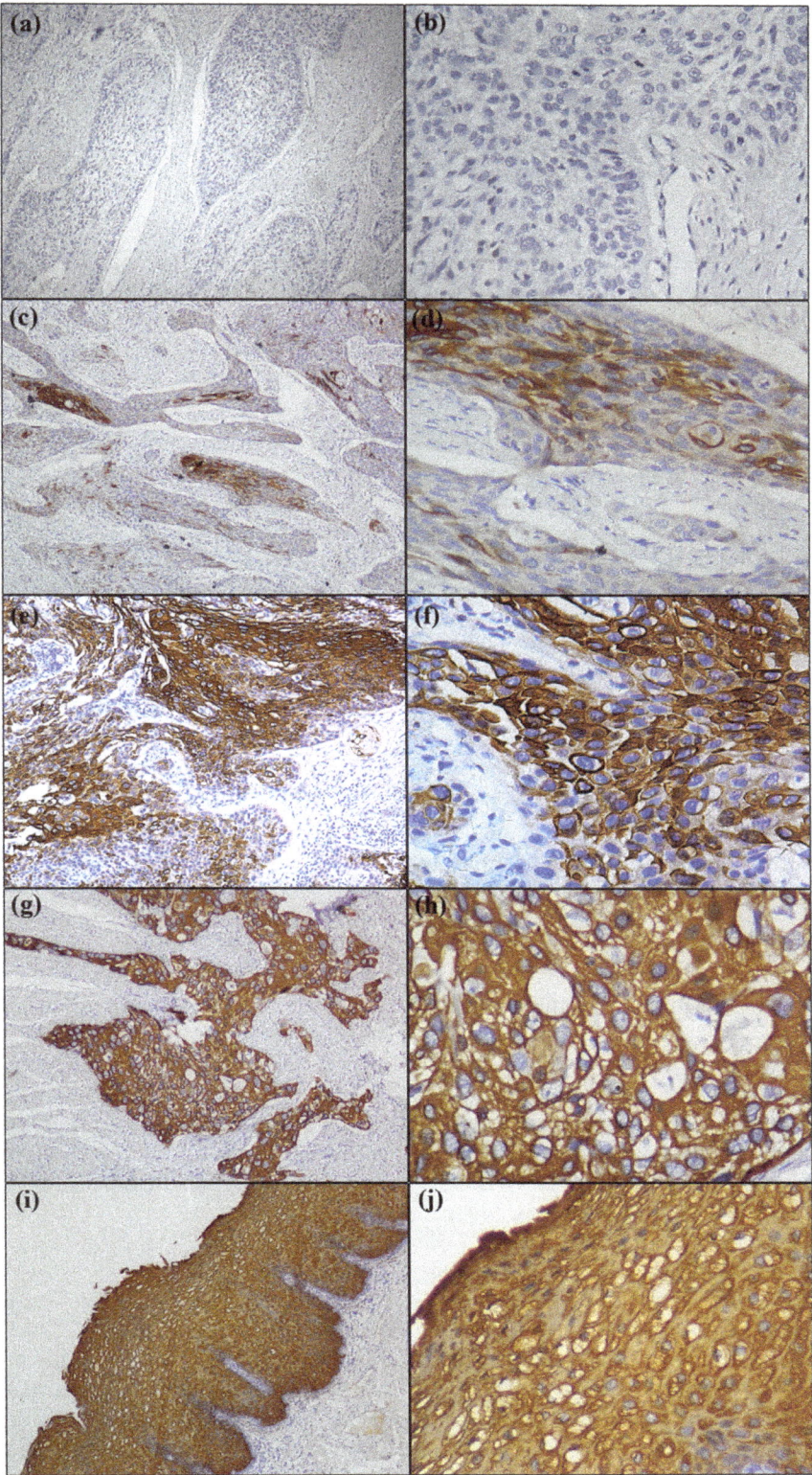

Figure 1 (See legend on next page.)

(See figure on previous page.)

Figure 1 Immunohistochemical staining of esophageal squamous cell carcinoma (ESCC) and peritumoral normal esophageal mucosae with anti-Cystatin SN. Low expression of Cystatin SN were detected in ESCC tissues (**a**, **b** and **c**, **d**), and the IRS grades of (**a**, **b**) and (**c**, **d**) belong to absent(−) and weak(1+), respectively, in which (**a**, **c**) original magnification is × 100, and (**b**, **d**) original magnification is × 400, respectively; High expression of Cystatin SN was detected in ESCC tissues (**e**, **f** and **g**, **h**) and peritumoral normal esophageal mucosae(**i**, **j**), and the IRS grades of (**e**, **f**) and (**g**, **h** and **i**, **j**) belong to moderate (2+) and strong (3+), respectively, in which (**e**, **g**, **i**) original magnification is × 100, and (**f**, **h**, **j**) original magnification is × 400, respectively.

at our cancer centre before being embedded in paraffin and used for pathological evaluation. All paraffin-embedded specimens used in this study were cut into 4 μm sections and baked for 1 h at 65°C. IHC staining was performed using the Dako Envision system (Dako, Carpinteria, CA) following the manufacturer's recommended protocols, which have been described previously [22]. Briefly, all sections were deparaffinised and rehydrated and endogenous peroxidase activity was blocked prior to immunostaining. Then, the slides were processed for antigen retrieval by boiling in 10 mM citrate buffer (pH 6.0) for 5 minutes. After natural cooling, all sections were treated with a rabbit polyclonal cystatin SN antibody (1:800 dilution; NBP1-55,995, Novus, Littleton, USA) overnight at 4°C. Subsequently, the sections were incubated with a biotinylated secondary antibody for 30 min at 37°C. Finally, the sections were incubated with streptavidin-horseradish peroxidase complex and developed with diaminobenzidine (DAB). Mayer's haematoxylin was used as a counterstain. For a negative control, the antibody was replaced with normal rabbit serum.

IHC evaluation

The grading of the cytoplasmic Cystatin SN staining was performed using light microscopy to generate an immunoreactivity score (IRS) [23,24]. The IRS of CST1 was calculated by multiplying the intensity and extent scores. Entire sections were observed to assign the scores. The staining intensity was scored as 0 (no staining), 1 (weak staining, yellow brown), 2 (moderate staining, yellow brown), or 3 (strong staining, brown), and the percentage of positively stained cells was evaluated as 0 (0%), 1 (1% to 10%), 2 (11% to 50%), 3 (51% to 70%), or 4 (71% to 100%). In our study, we used the median of all IRSs

Table 2 Immunohistochemistry results for Cystatin SN in esophageal squamous cell carcinoma (ESCC) compared with peritumoral normal esophageal tissues

Cyatatin SN	ESCC (N = 209)	Peritumoral normal tissues (N = 170)
0	29 (13.9%)	0
1+	116 (55.5%)	0
2+	28 (13.4%)	0
3+	36 (17.2%)	170 (100%)

(4.0) as the cut-off point [25]. The IRS was classified as: − (0 score, absent); 1+ (range from 1 to 4, weak); 2+ (range from 5 to 8 score, moderate); or 3+ (range from 9 to 12, strong). We defined − to 1+ as "Cystatin SN- low expression" and 2+ to 3+ as "Cystatin SN- high expression".

The stained tissue sections were assessed and scored independently by two senior pathologists (Ruo-Zhen Luo and Jie-Hua He), both of whom were blinded to the clinical characteristics of the patients. The final score for Cystatin SN was defined using the average values of the two observers' scores. To ensure the consistency of the scores, discordant cases were reviewed.

Statistical analysis

All statistical analyses were performed using the SPSS 13.0 statistical software package (SPSS, Chicago, IL). The differences in the IRSs between ESCC and peritumoral normal esophageal tissues were calculated using the paired-sample Student test (paired-sample t-test). The Chi-squared test (χ^2 test) was used to analyse the correlations between Cystatin SN expression and the clinico-pathological characteristics of the ESCCs. Survival curves were plotted using Kaplan-Meier plots and Log-rank tests. Multivariate analysis was performed using the Cox proportional hazard method, which was performed for all significant variables using univariate analysis. Overall survival (OS) and disease-free survival (DFS) were calculated from the date of surgery to the date of death or the last follow-up and to the date of recurrence or distant metastasis, respectively. $P < 0.05$ was considered statistically significant.

Results
Patient characteristics

The clinicopathological characteristics of the 209 ESCC patients are summarised in Table 1. Up to the last follow-up visit (January 2012), the 1-, 3-, 5-, and 10-year survival rates for the whole cohort of patients were 83.7%, 56.9%, 50.1% and 0.96%, respectively. None patients received neoadjuvant treatment. Excluding the patients who had KPS < 70 or/and refused chemotherapy, 79 patients have completed systemic adjuvant chemotherapy (cisplatin-based combinations) (OS, 66 months; 5-years survival, 53.8%) after curative-intent surgery.

Cystatin SN expression and its correlations with clinicopathological characteristics

Cystatin SN expression was observed predominantly in the cytoplasm of the tumor cells and normal squamous epithelial cells (Figure 1). Using the criteria described above, strong staining (3+) of Cystatin SN was detected in all of normal squamous epithelial cells, whereas various staining patterns were obtained in the ESCC tissues. There was a statistically significant difference between the Cystatin SN staining of the tumors and the normal tissues ($P < 0.001$, Table 2). However, there was no significant associations between the Cystatin SN expression of the ESCCs and age, gender, tumor location, differentiation, T status, N status, and pathological stage in the Chi-squared test ($P > 0.05$, Table 1).

Correlations between Cystatin SN expression, the patients clinicopathological characteristics and survival

Up to the last follow-up date, 119 cancer-related ESCC deaths were observed. The median observation period was 56 months (range 3 to 134 months). The median DFS and OS were 46 and 63 months, respectively.

In the Kaplan-Meier analysis, the expression of cystatin SN was closely correlated with the DFS and OS of ESCC patients. For the whole cohort, the median DFS and OS were significantly longer for patients with high tumoral expression levels of Cystatin SN than in patients with low tumoural expression levels (both $P < 0.001$, Figure 2, Table 3). Then, we examined the associations between Cystatin SN expression and survival based on the clinicopathological characteristics of the 209 ESCC patients. The results showed that the expression levels of Cystatin SN distinguished the patients with good DFS and OS from patients with poor DFS and OS when the patients were stratified by T status (pT1-2, $P = 0.001$ and $P = 0.001$, respectively; pT3-4, $P = 0.003$ and $P = 0.001$, respectively). This stratification based on the Cystatin SN expression level was also observed for pN0 patients ($P < 0.001$ and $P < 0.001$, respectively), stage II patients ($P < 0.001$ and $P < 0.001$, respectively), tumor grade 1 patients ($P = 0.003$ and $P = 0.001$, respectively) and tumor grade 2 patients ($P = 0.001$ and $P = 0.002$, respectively) (Table 3).

A number of factors, including age, gender, tumor location, surgery, differentiation, T status, N status and cystatin SN expression, were used in the univariate Cox regression analysis to assess their impact on the survival of ESCC patients. The variables that were found to impact survival in the univariate analysis were entered into the multivariate analysis model. In this multivariate analysis model, the results showed that significant and independent predictors of survival were the differentiation, N status and Cystatin SN expression (Table 4).

Discussion

The *CST1* gene, which encodes the S-type Cystatin SN peptide, belongs to the Cystatin (CST) superfamily, the members of which control the proteolytic activities of cysteine proteases [5]. Studies have indicated that proteases are involved in both primary and metastatic tumor growth [26,27]. The *CST1* gene is known to play a crucial role in human gastrointestinal tract cancer, including colon cancer and gastric cancer [6,27]. To the best of our knowledge, our study is the first to systematically evaluate the expression and clinicopathologic significance of Cystatin SN in ESCC. Our findings have

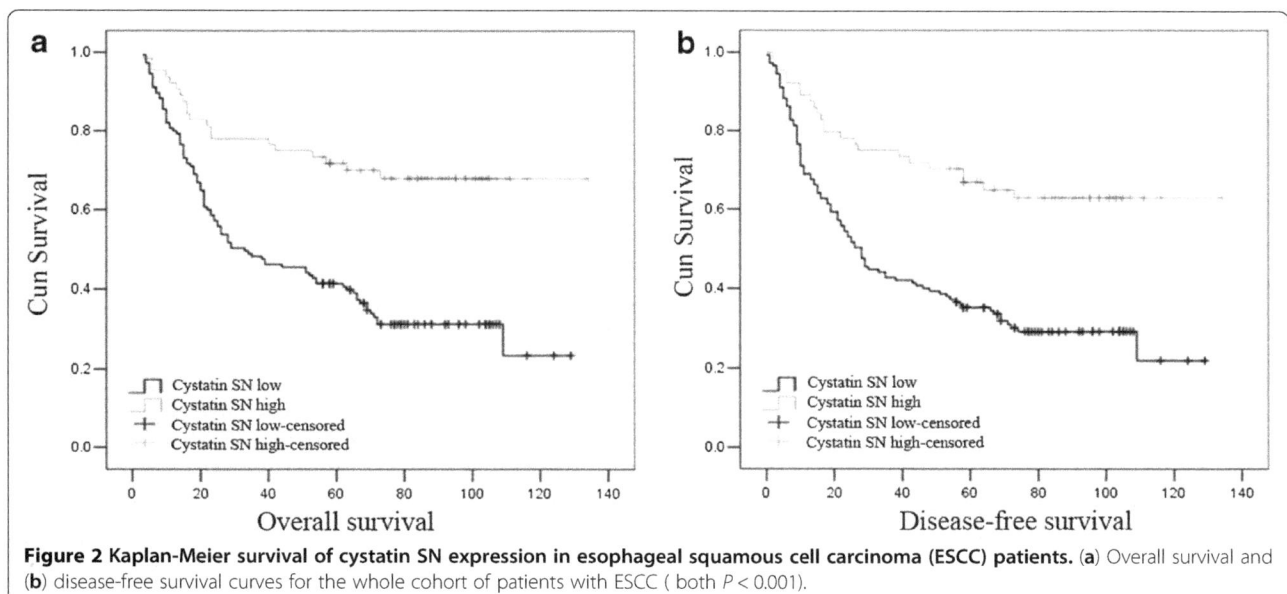

Figure 2 Kaplan-Meier survival of cystatin SN expression in esophageal squamous cell carcinoma (ESCC) patients. (**a**) Overall survival and (**b**) disease-free survival curves for the whole cohort of patients with ESCC (both $P < 0.001$).

Table 3 Prognostic value of Cystatin SN expression in 209 ESCC patients

Cystatin SN expression	Cases	DFS (months)			OS (months)		
		Mean	Median	P-value*	Mean	Median	P-value*
Total	209			< 0.001			< 0.001
Low expression	145	52	28		57	33	
High expression	64	94	NR		100	NR	
pT status				0.001			0.001
pT1-2	66						
Low expression	43	56	29		60	35	
High expression	23	108	NR		110	NR	
pT3-4	143			0.003			0.001
Low expression	102	49	25		54	26	
High expression	41	73	NR		80	NR	
pN status							
pN0	116			< 0.001			< 0.001
Low expression	76	70	67		75	72	
High expression	40	118	NR		118	NR	
PN1-3	93			0.058			0.017
Low expression	69	29	18		34	21	
High expression	24	44	27		53	42	
pTNM							
Stage II	133			< 0.001			< 0.001
Low expression	88	67	56		72	67	
High expression	45	117	NR		117	NR	
Stage III	76			0.336			0.099
Low expression	57	27	11		31	19	
High expression	19	34	26		45	40	
Differentiation							
G1	56			0.003			0.001
Low expression	39	67	66		71	67	
High expression	17	106	NR		110	NR	
G2	105			0.001			0.002
Low expression	68	49	28		54	35	
High expression	37	92	NR		94	NR	
G3	48			0.604			0328
Low expression	38	37	22		43	25	
High expression	10	49	17		60	23	

*Log-rank test.
DFS disease-free survival, *OS* overall survival, *pT* pathologic tumor, *pN* pathologic node, *pTNM* pathologic tumor-node-metastasis, *G* tumor grade, *NR* not reached.

indicated that Cystatin SN serves as an independent prognostic factor in ESCC patients.

In our study, the immunostaining of ESCC samples revealed that Cystatin SN is predominantly located in the cytoplasm. Previous studies showed that Cystatin SN was present primarily in the cytosolic region of gastric cancer cells, [6] but it was detected in the cytomembrane of colorectal cancer cells [21]. Those observations indicate that the expression of Cystatin SN in different cancers may be tissue–specific [9]. However, we failed to show any significant correlations between Cystatin SN expression and patients clinicopathological parameters. In contrast, some studies revealed that overexpression of Cystatin SN correlated with descending pathological TNM stage for gastric and colorectal cancer. We believe that can explained by the following factors. First, the

Table 4 Univariate and multivariate regression analysis for DFS and OS in the whole cohort

Variables	Disease-free survival						Overall survival					
	Univariate analysis			Multivariate analysis			Univariate analysis			Multivariate analysis		
	HR	95% CI	P value[*]	HR	95% CI	P value[*]	HR	95% CI	P value[*]	HR	95% CI	P value[*]
Age[†]	1.258	0.872-1.813	0.219	.....	.....	.....	1.359	0.933-1.981	0.110	.....	.....	.....
Gender[‡]	0.832	0.535-1.295	0.416	.....	.....	.....	0.759	0.478-1.205	0.242	.....	.....	.....
Location[§]	0.763	0.558-1.043	0.090	.....	.....	.....	0.751	0.542-1.040	0.084	.....	.....	.....
Surgery[¶]	1.034	0.851-1.256	0.738	.....	.....	.....	1.052	0.863-1.284	0.615	.....	.....	.....
pT status[ι]	1.133	0.782-1.644	0.509	.....	.....	.....	1.118	0.772-1.618	0.554	.....	.....	.....
Differentiation[£]	1.393	1.065-1.823	0.016	1.411	1.086-1.833	0.010	1.319	1.004-1.734	0.047	1.331	1.020-1.738	0.035
pN status[δ]	3.211	2.198-4.692	< 0.001	3.096	2.131-4.498	< 0.001	3.032	2.056-4.471	< 0.001	2.926	1.998-4.286	< 0.001
Cystatin SN[ζ]	0.431	0.271-0.685	< 0.001	0.426	0.270-0.672	< 0.001	0.377	0.231-0.616	< 0.001	0.378	0.233-0.614	< 0.001

[*]Cox proportional hazards model; [†]Age ≤ 57 vs. Age > 57; [‡]Male vs. Female; [§]Upper thoracic vs. Middle thoracic vs. Lower thoracic; [¶]Left thoracotomy vs. Thoracic-abdominal-cervical incision; [ι]pT1 vs. pT2 vs. pT3 vs. pT4; [£]Tumor grade 1 vs. Tumor grade 2 vs. Tumor grade 3; [δ]pN0 vs. pN1/2/3; [ζ]High expression of Cystatin SN vs. low expression of Cystatin SN. HR hazard ratio, CI confidence interval, pT pathologic tumor, pN pathologic node.

biology character of Cystatin SN may have tissue specificity. Second, the enrolled ESCCs is only II, III stages and belongs to a single institution's database, which may results in a selection bias and low statistical power to detect meaningful relationships. Therefore, this conclud ion merits additional research.

In the studies mentioned above, Cystatin SN, which was proved to contribute to cell proliferation, has been reported as an oncogene in colorectal and gastric caicinoma [6,21]. Howere, in our study, we found that ESCC patients with positive expression of Cystatin SN had significantly longer DFS and OS than those with negative Cystatin SN expression. We believe that can be explained by two particular factors. Firstly, histology differences such as squamous cell carcinoma and adenocarcinoma might explain the observed phenomena. Secondly, the heterogeneity of biomarkers might also result in the discrepancies in the findings between the previous literatures and our study. These results are similar to other members of the CST superfamily in a number of previous reports. Cystatin C is a nonglycosylated 13 kDa basic protein, consisting of 120 amino acids. It belongs to the cystatin superfamily of cysteine proteinase inhibitors. Strojan et al [28] demonstrated significantly longer survival in squamous cell carcinoma of the head and neck patients with high Cystatin C than in those with low Cystatin C. However, in colorectal cance [15], the patients with high levels of Cystatin C exhibited a significantly higher risk of death than those with lower levels. Alterations in secretion may result in higher extracellular and lower intracellular levels of Cystatin C and, therefore, the reverse correlation of Cystatin C with patients' survival is to be expected. On the other hand, one has to be aware that cysteine proteases and consequently their inhibitors are also involved in biological processes other than tissue remodeling during the progression of primary tumors, such as the regulation of

inflammatory and immune responses [29] or apoptosis [30], so that different level of Cystatin C may lead to various clinical outcomes. Moreover, in the subgroup analysis, Cystatin SN expressions distinguish the DFS or OS, especially in the groups of pN0 and stage II patients. Our results suggested that Cystatin SN in ESCC maybe play an significant role in the early stage of carcinogenesis. The underlying mechanism need further study.

The TNM stage is the most powerful and widely accepted predictor of survival for ESCCs [31]. However, many patients with the same stage of disease have different outcomes, indicating the TNM stage may be insufficient to distinguish ESCC patients' survival [32]. An increasing number of studies have focused on the use of biomarkers to predict patients' survival and select patients who will benefit from adjuvant treatments. To date, the metastasis and invasiveness of several tumors have been shown to be associated with members of the CST superfamily, such as Cystatin C (encoded by CST3), CystatinD (encoded by CST5), Cystatin F (encoded by CST7), Cystatin M (encoded by CST6) and Cystatin S (encoded by CST4), which have been described and investigated [11,13-18]. Our study focused on the relationship between one of CST superfamily members and the survival of cancer patients. In our study, Cystatin SN expression, combined with the N status and differentiation, serve as independent and significant predictors in surgically resected ESCCs. Consistent with the findings reported by the previous studies, we also suggested some factors, including age, gender, tumor location, surgery and pT status, were not the independently significant predictive factors for ESCC survival, in spite of some other different points. And some crowd confounding factors may influence the foundings, of course, it needs additional studies. On the other hand, the Cystatin SN expression was shown to distinguish the DFS or OS in a subgroup analysis, especially in the subgroups of pN0 and stage II patients. Therefore, our results indicate that Cystatin SN expression combined with clinicopathological parameters may serve as an extra factor for identifying ESCC patients with a higher risk of tumor recurrence and metastasis.

Unfortunately, one limitation of out study in the lack of confirmation on Cystatin SN expression status by quantitative methods like Reverse Transcription-Polymerase Chain Reaction (RT-PCR), which could, in conjunction with results of IHC, further refine the prognostic value of this biomarker. Also, our study is a retrospective study, relied exclusively on a single-institutional database. Additional mechanistic investigations into this area will be vital to facilitate our understanding of the biological significance of Cystatin SN.

Conclusions

In conclusion, Cystatin SN expressed higher level in peritumoral normal esophageal mucosae than in the ESCC tissues. Compared with the patients with low expressive level of Cystatin SN, high expression patients have more favourable survivals. Our findings have demonstrated that Cystatin SN expression in ESCC tissue may represent as an independent predictor of survival for patients with resectable ESCC.

Competing interests

The authors declare that they have no competing interests.

Authors' contributions

YFC, GM and XC performed the statistical analysis, drafted the manuscript and participated in the sequence alignment. RZL and LRH participated in the design of the study and participated in the sequence alignment. JHH and MSZ participated in the sequence alignment. ZLH carried out data acquisition. ZSW conceived of the study, and participated in its design and coordination and helped to draft the manuscript. All authors read and approved the final manuscript.

Acknowledgements

This study was supported by the Science and Technology Project of Guangdong
Province, China (No. 2010B031600315)

Author details

[1]State Key Laboratory of Oncology in South China, Cancer Center, Sun Yet-Sen University, No.651, Dongfeng Road East, Guangzhou, China. [2]Department of Thoracic Oncology, Cancer Center, Sun Yet-Sen University, No.651, Dongfeng Road East, Guangzhou, China. [3]Department of Critical Care Medicine, Cancer Center, Sun Yet-Sen University, No.651, Dongfeng Road East, Guangzhou, China. [4]Department of Pathology, Cancer Center, Sun Yet-Sen University, No.651, Dongfeng Road East, Guangzhou, China. [5]Department of Radiation Oncology, Cancer Center, Sun Yet-Sen University, No.651, Dongfeng Road East, Guangzhou, China.

References

1. Jemal A, Bray F, Center MM, Ferlay J, Ward E, Forman D: Global cancer statistics. CA Cancer J Clin 2011, 61(2):69–90.
2. Guo P, Li K: Trends in esophageal cancer mortality in China during 1987–2009: age, period and birth cohort analyzes. Cancer Epidemiol 2012, 36(2):99–105.
3. Tran GD, Sun XD, Abnet CC, Fan JH, Dawsey SM, Dong ZW, Mark SD, Qiao YL, Taylor PR: Prospective study of risk factors for esophageal and gastric cancers in the Linxian general population trial cohort in China. Int J Cancer J Int du cancer 2005, 113(3):456–463.
4. Enzinger PC, Mayer RJ: Esophageal cancer. N Engl J Med 2003, 349(23):2241–2252.
5. Koblinski JE, Ahram M, Sloane BF: Unraveling the role of proteases in cancer. Clinica Chimica Acta; Int J Clin Chem 2000, 291(2):113–135.
6. Choi EH, Kim JT, Kim JH, Kim SY, Song EY, Kim JW, Yeom YI, Kim IH, Lee HG: Upregulation of the cysteine protease inhibitor, cystatin SN, contributes to cell proliferation and cathepsin inhibition in gastric cancer. Clinica Chimica Acta; Int J Clin Chem 2009, 406(1–2):45–51.
7. Szumilo J, Burdan F, Zinkiewicz K, Dudka J, Klepacz R, Dabrowski A, Korobowicz E: Expression of syndecan-1 and cathepsins D and K in advanced esophageal squamous cell carcinoma. Folia histochemica et cytobiologica/Polish Academy of Sciences, Polish Histochemical and Cytochemical Society 2009, 47(4):571–578.
8. Andl CD, McCowan KM, Allison GL, Rustgi AK: Cathepsin B is the driving force of esophageal cell invasion in a fibroblast-dependent manner. Neoplasia 2010, 12(6):485–498.
9. Dickinson DP, Thiesse M, Hicks MJ: Expression of type 2 cystatin genes CST1-CST5 in adult human tissues and the developing submandibular gland. DNA Cell Biol 2002, 21(1):47–65.
10. Turk B, Turk D, Turk V: Lysosomal cysteine proteases: more than scavengers. Biochim Biophys Acta 2000, 1477(1–2):98–111.
11. Vigneswaran N, Wu J, Zacharias W: Upregulation of cystatin M during the progression of oropharyngeal squamous cell carcinoma from primary tumor to metastasis. Oral Oncol 2003, 39(6):559–568.
12. Turk B, Turk V, Turk D: Structural and functional aspects of papain-like cysteine proteinases and their protein inhibitors. Biol Chem 1997, 378(3–4):141–150.
13. Coulibaly S, Schwihla H, Abrahamson M, Albini A, Cerni C, Clark JL, Ng KM, Katunuma N, Schlappack O, Glossl J, et al: Modulation of invasive properties of murine squamous carcinoma cells by heterologous expression of cathepsin B and cystatin C. Int J Cancer J Int du Cancer 1999, 83(4):526–531.
14. Cox JL, Sexton PS, Green TJ, Darmani NA: Inhibition of B16 melanoma metastasis by overexpression of the cysteine proteinase inhibitor cystatin C. Melanoma Res 1999, 9(4):369–374.
15. Kos J, Krasovec M, Cimerman N, Nielsen HJ, Christensen IJ, Brunner N: Cysteine proteinase inhibitors stefin A, stefin B, and cystatin C in sera from patients with colorectal cancer: relation to prognosis. Clin Cancer Res: An Official Journal of the American Association for Cancer Research 2000, 6(2):505–511.
16. Morita M, Yoshiuchi N, Arakawa H, Nishimura S: CMAP: a novel cystatin-like gene involved in liver metastasis. Cancer Res 1999, 59(1):151–158.
17. Schagdarsurengin U, Pfeifer GP, Dammann R: Frequent epigenetic inactivation of cystatin M in breast carcinoma. Oncogene 2007, 26(21): 3089–3094.
18. Utsunomiya T, Hara Y, Kataoka A, Morita M, Arakawa H, Mori M, Nishimura S: Cystatin-like metastasis-associated protein mRNA expression in human colorectal cancer is associated with both liver metastasis and patient survival. Clin Cancer Res: An Official J Am Assoc Cancer Res 2002, 8(8):2591–2594.
19. Alvarez-Diaz S, Valle N, Garcia JM, Pena C, Freije JM, Quesada V, Astudillo A, Bonilla F, Lopez-Otin C, Munoz A: Cystatin D is a candidate tumor suppressor gene induced by vitamin D in human colon cancer cells. J Clin Invest 2009, 119(8):2343–2358.
20. Parle-McDermott A, McWilliam P, Tighe O, Dunican D, Croke DT: Serial analysis of gene expression identifies putative metastasis-associated transcripts in colon tumour cell lines. Br J Cancer 2000, 83(6):725–728.
21. Yoneda K, Iida H, Endo H, Hosono K, Akiyama T, Takahashi H, Inamori M, Abe Y, Yoneda M, Fujita K, et al: Identification of Cystatin SN as a novel tumor marker for colorectal cancer. Int J Oncol 2009, 35(1):33–40.
22. Cao X, Li Y, Luo RZ, He LR, Yang J, Zeng MS, Wen ZS: Tyrosine-protein phosphatase nonreceptor type 12 is a novel prognostic biomarker for esophageal squamous cell carcinoma. Ann Thorac Surg 2012, 93(5):1674–1680.
23. Fermento ME, Gandini NA, Lang CA, Perez JE, Maturi HV, Curino AC, Facchinetti MM: Intracellular distribution of p300 and its differential recruitment to aggresomes in breast cancer. Exp Mol Pathol 2010, 88(2):256–264.

24. Jiang S, Li Y, Zhu YH, Wu XQ, Tang J, Li Z, Feng GK, Deng R, Li DD, Luo RZ, *et al*: Intensive expression of UNC-51-like kinase 1 is a novel biomarker of poor prognosis in patients with esophageal squamous cell carcinoma. *Cancer Sci* 2011, **102**(8):1568–1575.

25. Olaussen KA, Dunant A, Fouret P, Brambilla E, Andre F, Haddad V, Taranchon E, Filipits M, Pirker R, Popper HH, *et al*: DNA repair by ERCC1 in non-small-cell lung cancer and cisplatin-based adjuvant chemotherapy. *N Engl J Med* 2006, **355**(10):983–991.

26. Koop S, Khokha R, Schmidt EE, MacDonald IC, Morris VL, Chambers AF, Groom AC: Overexpression of metalloproteinase inhibitor in B16F10 cells does not affect extravasation but reduces tumor growth. *Cancer Res* 1994, **54**(17):4791–4797.

27. Wilson CL, Heppner KJ, Labosky PA, Hogan BL, Matrisian LM: Intestinal tumorigenesis is suppressed in mice lacking the metalloproteinase matrilysin. *Proc Natl Acad Sci USA* 1997, **94**(4):1402–1407.

28. Strojan P, Oblak I, Svetic B, Smid L, Kos J: Cysteine proteinase inhibitor cystatin C in squamous cell carcinoma of the head and neck: relation to prognosis. *Br J Cancer* 2004, **90**(10):1961–1968.

29. Chapman HA, Riese RJ, Shi GP: Emerging roles for cysteine proteases in human biology. *Annu Rev Physiol* 1997, **59**:63–88.

30. Jaattela M: Escaping cell death: survival proteins in cancer. *Exp Cell Res* 1999, **248**(1):30–43.

31. Gaur P, Hofstetter WL, Bekele BN, Correa AM, Mehran RJ, Rice DC, Roth JA, Vaporciyan AA, Rice TW, Swisher SG: Comparison between established and the Worldwide Esophageal Cancer Collaboration staging systems. *Ann Thorac Surg* 2010, **89**(6):1797–1803. 1804 e1791-1793; discussion 1803–1794.

32. Takeno S, Noguchi T, Takahashi Y, Fumoto S, Shibata T, Kawahara K: Assessment of clinical outcome in patients with esophageal squamous cell carcinoma using TNM classification score and molecular biological classification. *Ann Surg Oncol* 2007, **14**(4):1431–1438.

14

Acute mesenteric ischemia and duodenal ulcer perforation: a unique double pathology

Lois Haruna, Ahmed Aber, Farhan Rashid[*] and Marco Barreca

Abstract

Background: Acute mesenteric ischaemia and duodenal perforation are surgical emergencies with serious consequences. Patients presenting with acute mesenteric ischaemia alone face a high mortality rate as high as 60% whereas those presenting with peptic ulcer perforation the mortality rates range from 6-14%. There are very few reported cases of patients presenting with this dual pathology.

Case presentation: We report a unique case of a 53 year old Italian lady who presented with acute mesenteric ischaemia and duodenal perforation. This is the first report of massive bowel ischaemia and duodenal perforation with no apparent underlying common pathophysiology leading to this presentation.

Conclusion: Early management in the intensive care unit and appropriate surgical intervention maximised the patient's chances of survival despite the poor prognosis associated with her dual pathology. The rare pathology of the patient described can be explained by two possible hypotheses: peptic ulcer disease causing duodenal ulceration, which precipitated ischaemic infarction of the small bowel. The second hypothesis is the patient developed a stress related ulcer following ischaemic bowel infarction secondary to arterial thrombosis.

Keywords: Acute mesenteric ischaemia, Duodenal ulcer perforation, Mesenteric venous thrombosis, Ischemic bowel infarction, Bowel necrosis

Background

Acute mesenteric ischemia (AMI) comprises a group of pathophysiologic processes that have a common end point—bowel necrosis. The survival rate has not improved substantially during the past 70 years, and the major reason is the continued difficulty in recognizing the condition before bowel infarction occurs [1,2].

Clinical presentation is nonspecific in most cases and can be characterized by an initial discrepancy between severe abdominal pain and minimal clinical findings. In general, patients with AMI have an acute onset of symptoms and a rapid deterioration in their clinical condition. Complications such as ileus, peritonitis, pancreatitis, and gastrointestinal bleeding may also mask the initial signs and symptoms of AMI [2].

Acute mesenteric ischemia can be categorized into 4 specific types based on its cause. The most frequent cause is arterial emboli. They are responsible for approximately 40% to 50% of cases [1,3]. Most mesenteric emboli originate from a cardiac source. The second most common cause is acute mesenteric thrombosis accounts for 25% to 30% of all ischemic events [4,5]. Most of the reported cases of mesenteric ischemia due to arterial thrombosis occur with a background of severe atherosclerotic disease, the most common site near the origin of the Superior Mesenteric Artery [6]. Commonly, patients with this condition can tolerate major visceral artery obstruction because the slow progressive nature of atherosclerosis allows the development of important collaterals. The third major cause is non-occlusive mesenteric ischemia. The pathogenesis of is poorly understood but often involves a low cardiac output state associated with diffuse mesenteric vasoconstriction. Splanchnic vasoconstriction in response to hypovolemia, decreased cardiac output, hypotension, or vasopressors best explain the difference between this entity and other forms of AMI [7,8]. Mesenteric venous thrombosis is the least common cause of mesenteric ischemia, representing up to 10% of all patients with mesenteric ischemia and 18% of those with AMI. Most cases are thought to be secondary to other intra-abdominal pathologic

* Correspondence: farhan_rashid@hotmail.com
Department of General Surgery, Luton and Dunstable Hospital, Lewsey Road, Luton, Bedfordshire LU4 ODZ, UK

conditions (such as malignancy, intra-abdominal sepsis, or pancreatitis) or were classified as idiopathic [9].

Mesenteric venous thrombosis is usually segmental, with oedema and hemorrhage of the bowel wall and focal sloughing of the mucosa. Thrombi usually originate in the venous arcades and propagate to involve the arcuate channels. Hemorrhagic infarctions occur when the intramural vessels are occluded [2]. Involvement of the inferior mesenteric vein and large bowel is uncommon. The transition from normal to ischemic intestine is more gradual with venous embolism than with arterial embolism or thrombosis.

Case presentation

A 53-year-old lady presented following a collapse at home. In the ambulance she became unresponsive with a temperature 33.4oC, heart rate of 95 beats per minute and un-recordable blood pressure. On arrival active resuscitation commenced and a brief history of three days of severe, intermittent abdominal pain, absolute constipation, and reduced urine output was noted. Prior to this recent deterioration the patient had been well, with no weight loss or change in appetite. She had a past medical history of hypertension, osteoporosis, a previous appendicectomy; and a 20-pack year smoking history. She denied any dyspeptic symptoms prior to her admission, and had never taken any antacids. Her medications on admission were regular beta blocker, regular long term bisphosphonates and paracetamol on as required basis. On inspection the patient appeared of a normal body habitus, with a BMI of 22 and examination revealed a peritonitic abdomen.

Blood tests from admission revealed grossly elevated inflammatory markers (CRP>500mg/L), neutrophilia and acute kidney failure. Her blood gas showed metabolic acidosis with a high lactate (12.7mmol/L), and low base excess (−21.8 mmol/L) and bicarbonate (6.9mmol/L).

Due to her severe acute renal impairment no contrast was initially used for imaging. CT scan of her abdomen performed on admission revealed extensive free peritoneal fluid and also fluid adjacent to the right kidney in the retro peritoneum (Figure 1). There was no evidence of any free air, obstruction, perforation or abdominal aortic aneurysm, with no evidence for small bowel ischaemia. Furthermore an ascitic tap was performed which revealed a clear straw coloured fluid with a very high lactate dehydrogenase, and normal protein. It did not yield growth of any organisms.

Despite optimal management in the intensive care unit the patient's inflammatory markers, creatinine and alanine aminotranserase all continued to rise, and urine output remained minimal. In light of her clinical deterioration, 12 hours after admission the patient underwent an urgent diagnostic laparoscopy.

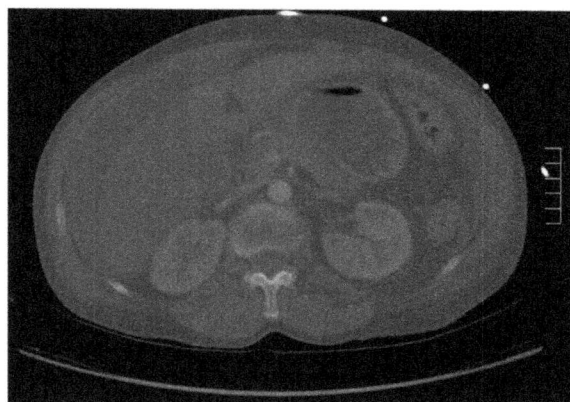

Figure 1 CT scan of the abdomen showing free peritoneal fluid.

Intraoperatively approximately 3 litres of free intraperitoneal purulent bile stained fluid filled the abdomen, and multiple fibrinous exudates surrounded the entire small bowel. A 162 cm section of distal small bowel appeared ischemic, and an anterior duodenal (D1) perforation was identified. The procedure was converted to a laparotomy in view of the findings. The D1 perforation was repaired using an omental patch, and the ischemic bowel wrapped in warm saline-soaked packs, with minimal benefit. The distal 162cm of dead small bowel was resected, and because of her critical condition the neodistal small bowel had a few viable slightly dusky patches left behind for a relook the following day. A washout was performed and a laparostomy using a saline bag was applied.

One day post-operatively the patient was dialysed and kept intubated due to unresolving metabolic acidosis. During the second laparotomy another 50cm of small bowel appeared ischaemia and was resected. 2 meters of healthy small bowel was left in situ. An ileocaecal anastomosis was made, a washout performed, and the abdominal wound closed.

Two weeks after her initial laparotomy the patient had an endoscopy for a nasojejunal tube insertion. The omental patch repair was performed during laparotomy for duodenal perforated ulcer. However, once endoscopy was performed few days after the first laparotomy for naso-jejunal feeding tube insertion, a small hole was identified near the D1 repair site and was clipped (Figure 2). A repeat endoscopy a week later showed closure of the duodenal defect and a 1cm healing ulcer. The patient made a slowly recovery and she was discharged few weeks later.

Histology showed haemorrhagic infarction in sections of small bowel with ischaemic changes throughout the submucosa and muscle coat, with normal appearing Mesenteric vessels.

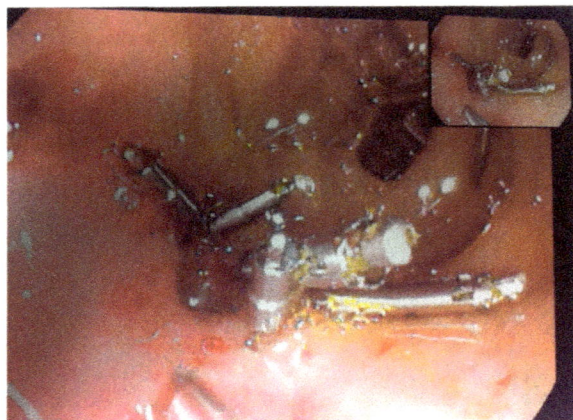

Figure 2 Endoscopic clipping of anterior duodenal perforation.

Discussion and conclusion

The unusual presentation of this patient raised an important question regarding her dual pathology: which occurred first? Did she have a perforated duodenal ulcer, causing sepsis and hypotension leading to small bowel ischemia, or did she suffer from ischaemic bowel, and subsequently developed a stress-related perforated ulcer?

After performing a through literature search, we did identify a single case report that described a patient presenting with acute abdomen and the subsequent intervention revealed exactly the same double pathology of Small bowel ischaemia and duodenal ulcer. However the histopathology of the bowel in that particular case did show evidence of polyarteritis nodosa explaining the cause of the acute bowel ischaemia [10].

In order to explain this double pathology it is vital to note that in peptic ulcer disease the two major precipitating factors are Helicobacter pylori infection and non-steroidal anti-inflammatory drugs (NSAIDs). Ulcer incidence increases with age and therapy with drugs such as corticosteroids, anticoagulants and bisphoshonates. Complications (bleeding, perforation, obstruction) can occur in patients with peptic ulcers of any aetiology. Perforation occurs in about 5% to 10% of patients with active ulcer disease [11].

With this background we are proposing two explanations for this pathology. The first is that the patient had been on long term bisphosphonates and this increased her risk for peptic ulcer disease. If we assume that the perforation of the duodenal ulcer occurred first, it was likely that it led to mesenteric venous thrombosis causing ischaemic infarction of the small bowel. The histology results favour this theory as the patient had segmental involvement of the small bowel with the sparing of the large bowel and this commonly present in acute ischaemia of the bowel that is associated with mesenteric venous thrombosis.

The second hypothesis is that the patient developed a stress related duodenal ulcer post ischaemic bowel infarction and eventually this ulcer perforated. The cause of the ischaemia is likely due to arterial thrombosis with a background of severe atherosclerotic disease caused by the patient's long history of hypertension and smoking. Patients with this type of bowel ischaemia present later as they can tolerate major visceral artery obstruction because the slow progressive nature of atherosclerosis allows the development of important collaterals. The patient had 3 days history of feeling unwell and constipation with minimal urine output before she collapsed.

Abbreviations
AMI: Acute mesenteric ischaemia; NSAIDS: Non-steroidal anti-inflammatory drugs.

Competing interests
The authors declare that they have no competing interests. No financial support has been received.

Authors' contribution
LH drafted the manuscript, and conducted a literature search. AA, FR and MB conducted a literature search and contributed to drafting the manuscript. FR monitored the drafting and assisted with the research. MB performed the operation and reviewed the manuscript and gave final approval for publication. All authors read and approved the final manuscript.

References
1. Lock G: **Acute intestinal ischaemia.** *Best Pract Res Clin Gastroenterol* 2001, 15:83–98.
2. Oldenburg WA, Lau LL, Rodenburg TJ, Edmonds HJ, Burger CD: **Acute mesenteric ischaemia: a Clinical Review.** *Arch Intern Med* 2004, 164:1054–1062.
3. Bradbury AW, Brittenden J, McBride K, Ruckley CV: **Mesenteric ischaemia: a multidisciplinary approach.** *Br J Surg* 1995, 82:1446–1459.
4. Sitges-Serra A, Mas X, Roqueta F, Figueras J, Sanz F: **Mesenteric infarction: an analysis of 83 patients with prognostic studies in 44 cases undergoing a massive small-bowel resection.** *Br J Surg* 1988, 75:544–548.
5. Mansour MA: **Management of acute mesenteric ischemia.** *Arch Surg* 1999, 134:328–330.
6. Kaleya RN, Boley SJ: **Acute mesenteric ischemia: an aggressive diagnostic and therapeutic approach: 1991 Roussel Lecture.** *Can J Surg* 1992, 35:613–623.
7. Wilcox MG, Howard TJ, Plaskon LA, Unthank JL, Madura JA: **Current theories of pathogenesis and treatment of nonocclusive mesenteric ischemia.** *Dig Dis Sci* 1995, 40:709–716.
8. Howard TJ, Plaskon LA, Wiebke EA, Wilcox MG, Madura JA: **Nonocclusive mesenteric ischemia remains a diagnostic dilemma.** *Am J Surg* 1996, 171:405–408.
9. Abdu RA, Zakhour BJ, Dallis DJ: **Mesenteric venous thrombosis: 1911 to 1984.** *Surgery* 1987, 101:383–388.
10. Tun M, Malik AK: **Massive small bowel infarction and duodenal perforation due to abdominal polyarteritis nodosa: a case report.** *Malays J Path* 1994, 16(1):75–78.
11. Gunshefski L, Flancbaum L, Brolin RE, Frankel A: **Changing patterns in perforated peptic ulcer disease.** *Am Surg* 1990, 56:270.

15

Feasibility of enhanced recovery after surgery in gastric surgery: a retrospective study

Takanobu Yamada[1,2]*, Tsutomu Hayashi[1,2], Toru Aoyama[1,2], Junya Shirai[1,2], Hirohito Fujikawa[1,2], Haruhiko Cho[1], Takaki Yoshikawa[1], Yasushi Rino[2], Munetaka Masuda[2], Hideki Taniguchi[3], Ryoji Fukushima[4] and Akira Tsuburaya[1]

Abstract

Background: Enhanced recovery after surgery (ERAS) programs have been reported to be feasible and useful for maintaining physiological function and facilitating recovery after colorectal surgery. The feasibility of such programs in gastric surgery remains unclear. This study assessed whether an ERAS program is feasible in patients who undergo gastric surgery.

Methods: The subjects were patients who underwent gastric surgery between June 2009 and February 2011 at the Department of Gastrointestinal Surgery, Kanagawa Cancer Center. They received perioperative care according to an ERAS program. All data were retrieved retrospectively. The primary end point was the incidence of postoperative complications. The secondary end point was postoperative outcomes.

Results: A total of 203 patients were studied. According to the Clavien-Dindo classification, the incidence of ≥ grade 2 postoperative complications was 10.8% and that of ≥ grade 3 complications was 3.9%. Nearly all patients did not require delay of meal step-up (95.1%). Only 6 patients (3.0%) underwent reoperation. The median postoperative hospital stay was 9 days. Only 4 patients (2.0%) required readmission. There was no mortality.

Conclusions: Our results suggest that our ERAS program is feasible in patients who undergo gastric surgery.

Keywords: Enhanced recovery after surgery, Gastric cancer, Gastrectomy, Feasibility, Postoperative complications

Background

Gastric cancer is the second leading cause of cancer-related death worldwide [1]. Complete surgical resection plays the most important role in the cure of gastric cancer; however, surgery for gastric cancer remains a high-risk procedure with clinically significant postoperative stress, complications, and sequelae. Morbidity and mortality from radical gastrectomy range from 9.1-46.0% and 0-13%, respectively [2-7].

Enhanced recovery after surgery (ERAS) programs have been proposed to maintain physiological function and facilitate postoperative recovery [8]. In the following studies, ERAS was considered to reduce rates of morbidity, shorten length of hospital stay [9-11]. ERAS programs have many elements, including preoperative education, preoperative carbohydrate loading, omission of bowel preparation, epidural analgesia without opioids, early postoperative enteral feeding, early mobilization of patients, and thrombotic prophylaxis. In colorectal surgery, several studies have reported that ERAS programs are feasible and useful [9-11].

We previously demonstrated that an ERAS protocol is useful in patients who undergo elective radical gastrectomy [12]. Other studies have reported that ERAS programs or fast-track surgery in gastric surgery can accelerate postoperative rehabilitation [13-18]. However, the number of patients assessed in these studies was small. In addition, some studies found that the incidence of some postoperative complications, especially nausea, vomiting, and postoperative ileus, tended to be higher in the ERAS group than in the conventional group, suggesting that ERAS programs might increase the risk of some complications after gastric surgery. Because of these controversial results, it is necessary to confirm the feasibility of ERAS programs in gastric surgery.

The present study evaluated whether an ERAS program was feasible in more than 200 patients who underwent

* Correspondence: takay0218@yahoo.co.jp
[1]Department of Gastrointestinal Surgery, Kanagawa Cancer Center, 1-1-2 Nakao, Asahi, 241-0815 Yokohama, Kanagawa, Japan
[2]Department of Surgery, Yokohama City University, Yokohama, Japan
Full list of author information is available at the end of the article

gastric surgery. Emphasis was placed on postoperative gastrointestinal complications.

Methods
Patients
Between June 2009 and February 2011, a total of 256 patients with gastric cancer underwent surgery at the Department of Gastrointestinal Surgery, Kanagawa Cancer Center. The inclusion criteria for this study were (1) a histologically confirmed diagnosis of adenocarcinoma of stomach and (2) the receipt of elective distal gastrectomy or total gastrectomy with lymphadenectomy. We excluded patients who preoperatively received any chemotherapy or radiotherapy. We also excluded patients who underwent proximal gastrectomy or laparoscopy-assisted total gastrectomy because these procedures are not standard in Japan and are mainly used in patients enrolled in clinical trials. These surgeries themselves have not been confirmed safe and feasible yet.

All patients received perioperative care according to our ERAS program. Operations were performed by the same team of surgeons (three specialists and four trainees). In principle, patients with a preoperative diagnosis of stage I disease received laparoscopic surgery with D1+ dissection, and the others received open surgery with D2 dissection [19].

ERAS program
In their Cochrane review, Spanjersberg *et al.* regard ERAS protocols as programs that include 7 or more of 17 ERAS items [10]. Our ERAS program included 13 items.

Preoperative
Preoperative counseling was held in the outpatient clinic before hospitalization and in the ward after admission. Patients could eat a normal diet until dinner of the day before surgery. Magnesium oxide and a New Lecicarbon* suppository (Zeria Pharmaceutical Co., Ltd., Tokyo, Japan) were administered on the day before surgery (Table 1).

Perioperative
Patients, excluding those who had gastric obstruction with decreased output, could drink two 500-ml plastic bottles of OS-1* (2.5% carbohydrate, Otsuka Pharmaceutical, Tokushima, Japan) 3 h before surgery. Premedication was not administered. Anesthesia consisted of a combination of epidural analgesia (Th 7-11) and general anesthesia. In principle, no drain was used in distal gastrectomy, and one or two drains were used in total gastrectomy. The nasogastric tube was removed immediately after surgery (Table 1).

Postoperative
Day of surgery: A continuous thoracic epidural infusion of analgesics was given for 2 days after surgery. To prevent postoperative pain, a nonsteroidal anti-inflammatory drug (50 mg flurbiprofen axetil) was administered intravenously twice daily after surgery until the resumption of oral intake. Postoperative day (POD) 1: Patients were encouraged to sit out of bed for more than 6 h. POD 2: Oral intake was started with water and a can of oral nutrition supplement (250 ml Ensure Liquid *, Abbott Japan Co., Ltd., Tokyo, Japan). After the resumption of oral intake, 300 mg of acetaminophen was administered orally three times daily. The patients were encouraged to walk the length of the ward. An antithrombotic agent (enoxaparin sodium 2 000 IU twice daily or fondaparinux 2.5 mg daily) was injected for 2 days 6 h after removal of the epidural catheter. POD 3: The patients started to eat soft food and were stepped up to regular food every 2 days (3 steps). The criteria for discharge were as follows: adequate pain relief, soft diet intake, return to preoperative mobility level, and normal laboratory data on POD 7 (Table 1).

The ERAS program evaluated in the present study was developed by a team of surgeons and anesthesiologists working in close cooperation with a data safety monitoring committee (DSMC). The feasibility and safety audit was completed by the DSMC in September 2009, when 50 patients had been treated according to the ERAS program. Our ERAS program in practice was approved both by the institutional clinical pathway committee and the DSMC. This study, a retrospective analysis, have been performed upon the approval of the institutional review board of Kanagawa Cancer Center. Informed consent for the ERAS program and using the clinical date without identifying personal information were taken before surgery.

Data collection (end points)
All data were retrieved retrospectively from the patients' database and clinical records. The primary end point was the incidence of postoperative complications. Complications were defined as ≥ grade 2 complications according to Clavien-Dindo classification within 30 days after surgery [20]. Secondary end points were postoperative outcomes such as onset of walking, onset of oral intake, onset of flatus, onset of defecation, delay of meal step-up, reoperation, postoperative hospital stay, readmission, and mortality. We delayed meal step-up if the patient ate 40 percent or less of meals for 2 days.

Pathological findings were categorized according to the 7th edition of UICC-TNM [21]. Continuous data are expressed as medians (range).

Results
A total of 203 patients were studied.

Table 1 Time table of the modified ERAS program

Operative day	-1	0	+1	+2	+3 +4 +5 +6 +7
Preoperative counseling	Preoperative counseling was held in the outpatient clinic before hospitalization and in the ward after admission.				
Pre-medication	Patients do not receive any sedation.				
Oral intake	Normal diet until midnight	Oral hydration solution (OS-1®) 3 h before surgery		Drink a water and oral nutrition supplement (Endure Liquid®)	Liquid diet (3 steps up to a soft diet every 2 days)
Bowel preparation	1 g magnesium oxide and a New Lecicarbon® suppository				
Anesthesia and Analgesics		Combination of epidural analgesia (TH7-11) and general anesthesia during surgery			
		Continuous thoracic epidural infusion of analgesics after surgery	→	Removing epidural catheter	
		Nonsteroidal anti-inflammatory drug intravenously after surgery twice daily	→	Acetoaminophen three times a daily orally	→ → →
Drain and NGT		No drain in distal gastrectomy, one or two drains in total gastrectomy		Removing drain(s)	
		NGT was removed immediately after surgery			
Urinary catheter				Removing	
ADL			Encourage to sit out of bed for more than 6 h	Encourage to walk the length of the ward	→ → → → →
Antithromboprophylaxis			None	Subcutaneous injection of antithrombotic agent (enoxaparin sodium or fondaparinux)	→ → None → →
X-ray and blood exam.	○		○		○ (Check discharge creiteria)

NGT: Nasogastric tube, ADL: Activity of daily life.

Patients' characteristics

There were 133 men and 70 women. Ten patients diagnosed non-adenocarcinoma or having other cancer simultaneously, sixteen patients received preoperative chemotherapy, Twenty two patients undergoing laparoscopy-assisted total gastrectomy, four patients undergoing remnant total gastrectomy, and one patient undergoing proximal gastrectomy were excluded. The median age was 67 (32-84) years. Performance status was good in most patients. Mean body mass index (BMI) was 22.2 (16.2-31.4) (Table 2).

Surgical procedures

Laparoscopic surgery was performed in 76 patients (37.4%), and total gastrectomy in 60 patients (29.6%). 83 patients (40.9%) underwent D2 lymph node dissection. Combined organ resection was performed in 34 patients, among whom 29 (85.3%) additionally underwent splenectomy (including pancreatico-splenectomy in 1 patient). Billroth I reconstruction was performed in 116 (57.1%) patients, and Roux-en-Y reconstruction was done in 83 (40.9%). The median operation time was 179 (80-577) minutes. The estimated median blood loss was 110 (0-1620) ml (Table 2).

Pathological characteristics

Early gastric cancer (T1) was confirmed in 121 patients (59.6%). 131 patients (64.5%) had no evidence of lymph node metastasis. Final disease stage was stage I in 128 patients (63.1%), stage II in 35 (17.2%), stage III in 31 (15.3%), and stage IV in 9 (4.4%) (Table 2).

Complications and postoperative course

Grade 2 or higher complications developed in 23 (11.3%) patients, and grade 3 or higher complications developed

Table 2 Clinicopathological features

		Patients (N = 203)	
Age (years old)*		67(32-84)	
Gender	Male	133	(65.5%)
	Female	70	(34.5%)
BMI (kg/m2)*		22.2(16.2-31.4)	
ECOG-PS	0	177	(87.2%)
	1	26	(12.8%)
	2	0	(0.0%)
ASA-PS	I	99	(48.8%)
	II	103	(50.7%)
	III	1	(0.5%)
Procedure	Open distal gastrectomy	67	(33.0%)
	Laparoscopy-assisted distal gastrectomy	76	(37.4%)
	Open total gastrectomy	60	(29.6%)
Lymph node dissection	D1,D1+	120	(59.1%)
	D2	83	(40.9%)
Reconstruction	Billroth I	116	(57.1%)
	Billroth II	4	(2.0%)
	Roux-en Y	83	(40.9%)
Combined organ resection	yes	34	(16.7%)
	no	169	(83.3%)
Operation time (min.)*		179(80-577)	
Bleeding (ml)*		110(0-1620)	
T categories	T1	121	(59.6%)
	T2	27	(13.3%)
	T3	19	(9.4%)
	T4	36	(17.7%)
N categories	N0	131	(64.5%)
	N1	22	(10.8%)
	N2	19	(9.4%)
	N3	31	(15.3%)
Stage (UICC TNM 7th)	I	128	(63.1%)
	II	35	(17.2%)
	III	31	(15.3%)
	IV	9	(4.4%)

BMI; Body mass index, ECOG-PS; Eastern cooperative oncology group performance status, ASA-PS; American society of anesthesiologists physical status, *median (range).

in 8 (3.9%). Anastomotic leakage occurred in 3 patients (1.5%), ileus in 2 patients (1.0%), and anastomotic stenosis in 2 patients (1.0%). The incidence of ≥ grade 2 complications in patients who underwent open distal gastrectmy, laparoscopy-assisted distal gastrectomy, or open total gastrectomy were 1.9%, 3.4%, or 5.4% respectively (p = 0.069). The incidence of ≥ grade 2 complications in patients who

Table 3 Complications

	Clavien-Dindo classification	
	≥grade 2 n (%)	≥grade 3 n (%)
Pancreas fistula	7(3.4%)	2(1.0%)
Anastomotic leakage	3(1.5%)	3(1.5%)
Ileus	2(1.0%)	0(0%)
Anastomotic stenosis	2(1.0%)	1(0.5%)
Surgical site infection	2(1.0%)	0(0%)
Obstruction	1(0.5%)	1(0.5%)
Pyothorax	1(0.5%)	1(0.5%)
Bleeding	1(0.5%)	0(0%)
Pleural effusion	1(0.5%)	0(0%)
Cholangitis	1(0.5%)	0(0%)
Ascites	1(0.5%)	0(0%)
Toxicoderma	1(0.5%)	0(0%)
Total	23(11.3%)	8(3.9%)

underwent D1 or D1+ dissection was 5.8%, as compared with 18.1% in patients who underwent D2 dissection (p = 0.010). The median onsets of oral intake, flatus, and defecation were POD 2 (1-5), 2 (0-5), and 4 (2-9), respectively. The step-up schedule for meals was delayed in 10 (4.9%) patients. Five of these patients (2.4%) had inadequate oral caloric or fluid intake because of nausea or vomiting. Reoperation was performed in 6 (3.0%) patients. The reasons for reoperation were leakage of the duodenal stump in 2 patients, leakage of the gastroduodenal anastomosis in 1, bowel obstruction in 1, anastomotic stenosis in 1, and pyothorax in 1. The median postoperative hospital stay was 9 (7-53) days. 4 (2.0%) patients were readmitted within 30 days after surgery. The reasons for readmission were ascites, fever, poor oral intake, and surgical site infection in 1 patient each. There was no mortality. No patient had postoperative pneumonia or required replacement of a nasogastric tube, with exception of 3 patients who had postoperative ileus (Tables 3 and 4).

Table 4 Postoperative outcomes

Onset of walk (POD*)	2(1-4)
Onset of oral intake (POD*)	2(1-5)
Onset of flatus (POD*)	2(0-5)
Onset of defecation (POD*)	4(2-9)
Delay of meal step up (n(%))	10(4.9%)
Complication CD ≥ grade2 (n(%))	23(11.3%)
Reoperation (n(%))	6(3.0%)
Postoperative hospital stay(days)*	9(7-53)
Readmission (n(%))	4(2.0%)
Mortality (n(%))	0(0%)

POD; Post operative day, CD; Clavien-Dindo classification, *median (range).

Discussion

This is the first large study to evaluate the feasibility of a comprehensive ERAS program in gastric surgery. In our study, the overall incidence of morbidity (i.e., ≥grade 2 complications) was 10.8%, and the incidence of clinically significant events (≥grade 3 complications) was only 3.9%. These results obtained with our ERAS program are good as compared with complication rates of conventional perioperative care group in our previous report (12.0%) as well as other reported complication rates without ERAS program (10.5-46.0%) [2-7,12]. Although T1 tumors and D1 dissection were dominant in our study, the morbidity rate in the D2 group (18.1%) was comparable to that in a large randomized controlled trial performed in Japan (JOCG9501 study, 20.9%) [5].

Among the many elements of ERAS programs, one of the utmost concerns for surgeons is that early postoperative feeding can induce postoperative ileus or anastomosis leakage. Because of these concerns, oral intake of food was previously not allowed for several days after gastrectomy in Japan [22]. In some European countries, food is also withheld for several postoperative days [23], but this practice is not supported by adequate evidence. In fact, in our study the incidences of postoperative ileus and anastomotic leakage were very low (1.0% and 1.5%, respectively), as compared with previous studies (0-12.5% and 0-4.2%, respectively) [2-7]. The incidences of those in conventional prieoperative care of our hospital (0% and 2%, respectively) were similar with these results [12]. Furthermore, meal step-up did not have to be delayed in nearly all patients (95.1%), and this is also similar with previous reported our internal control (96.0%) [12]. Several studies have also demonstrated that early oral feeding is feasible and beneficial in gastric surgery [13-18,24,25], but this point remains controversial. Heslin et al. reported that early enteral feeding was not beneficial after surgery for upper gastrointestinal malignancies [26]. On the other hand, Lewis et al. found in their meta-analysis that keeping patients 'nil by mouth' is without benefit; in contrast, early enteral feeding was suggested to reduce mortality [27]. There were six complications that need reoperation in current study. Among those, possibility of relation between the leakage of the gastroduodenal anastomosis and ERAS program could not be denied. But others seem to be unlikely. Our results and the findings of previous studies suggest that early oral or enteral feeding is at least feasible and does not increase the risk of postoperative ileus or anastomotic leakage.

Our study had several limitations. 1) It was conducted retrospectively in a single hospital, and the analyses and endpoints were not preplanned. 2) Most patients had good performance status. Patients with poor performance status (e.g. Eastern cooperative oncology group performance status ≥3, severe dementia, and swallowing difficulty) could not be treated in our hospital, because we specialize in cancer treatment. These could be selection bias. 3) More than half of the patients had T1 disease and underwent limited lymph node dissection (D1+), whichmight account for the good results of our study. In particular, D2 or more radical lymph node dissection has been repeatedly reported to increase the risk of surgery-related complications [2-5]. Consistent with the previous findings, the incidence of complications was higher after D2 dissection than after D1 dissection in our study. Finally, 4) our ERAS program did not include fluid management, which is one of the key elements of ERAS programs. There was not robust evidence of perioperative fluid management in gastric surgery at the time we introduced ERAS.

Conclusions

In conclusion, our results suggest that our ERAS program is feasible in at least early-staged and relatively young patients undergoing elective gastric surgery. Further studies, for which population ERAS program can be applied and whether ERAS programs have potential benefits, are necessary.

Abbreviations
ERAS: Enhanced recovery after surgery; POD: Postoperative day; DSMC: Data safety monitoring committee; BMI: Body mass index.

Competing interests
The authors declare that they have no competing interests.

Authors' contributions
TY, TH, TA, JS, HF, HC, TY, HT, RF, and AT conceived and coordinated the study, collected patients' data and participated in the statistical analysis. RY, MM, and AT participated in preparing and drafting the manuscript. All authors read and approved the final manuscript.

Acknowledgement
This study was supported in part by a Grant-in-Aid from the Kanagawa Health Fundation.

Author details
[1]Department of Gastrointestinal Surgery, Kanagawa Cancer Center, 1-1-2 Nakao, Asahi, 241-0815 Yokohama, Kanagawa, Japan. [2]Department of Surgery, Yokohama City University, Yokohama, Japan. [3]Department of Anesthesiology, Kanagawa Cancer Center, 1-1-2 Nakao, Asahi, 241-0815 Yokohama, Kanagawa, Japan. [4]Department of Surgery, Teikyo University School of Medicine, 2-11-1 Kaga, 173-8605 Itabashi, Tokyo, Japan.

References
1. Parkin DM, Bray F, Ferlay J, Pisani P: Global cancer statistics, 2002. *CA Cancer J Clin* 2005, 55:74–108.
2. Bonenkamp JJ, Songun I, Hermans J, Sasako M, Welvaart K, Plukker JT, van Elk P, Obertop H, Gouma DJ, Taat CW, Lanschot J, Meyer S, Graaf PW, Meyenfeldt MF, Tilanus H: Randomised comparison of morbidity after D1 and D2 dissection for gastric cancer in 996 Dutch patients. *Lancet* 1995, 345:745–748.
3. Cuschieri A, Fayers P, Fielding J, Craven J, Bancewicz J, Joypaul V, Cook P: Postoperative morbidity and mortality after D1 and D2 resections for gastric cancer: preliminary results of the MRC randomised controlled surgical trial. The Surgical Cooperative Group. *Lancet* 1996, 347:995–999.

4. Degiuli M, Sasako M, Calgaro M, Garino M, Rebecchi F, Mineccia M, Scaglione D, Andreone D, Ponti A, Calvo F: Morbidity and mortality after D1 and D2 gastrectomy for cancer: interim analysis of the Italian Gastric Cancer Study Group (IGCSG) randomised surgical trial. Eur J Surg Oncol 2004, 30:303–308.

5. Sano T, Sasako M, Yamamoto S, Nashimoto A, Kurita A, Hiratsuka M, Tsujinaka T, Kinoshita T, Arai K, Yamamura Y, Okajima K: Gastric cancer surgery: morbidity and mortality results from a prospective randomized controlled trial comparing D2 and extended para-aortic lymphadenectomy-Japan Clinical Oncology Group study 9501. J Clin Oncol 2004, 22:2767–2773.

6. Kim HH, Hyung WJ, Cho GS, Kim MC, Han SU, Kim W, Ryu SW, Lee HJ, Song KY: Morbidity and mortality of laparoscopic gastrectomy versus open gastrectomy for gastric cancer: an interim report–a phase III multicenter, prospective, randomized trial (KLASS Trial). Ann Surg 2010, 251:417–420.

7. Katai H, Sasako M, Fukuda H, Nakamura K, Hiki N, Saka M, Yamaue H, Yoshikawa T, Kojima K: Safety and feasibility of laparoscopy-assisted distal gastrectomy with suprapancreatic nodal dissection for clinical stage I gastric cancer: a multicenter phase II trial (JCOG 0703). Gastric Cancer 2010, 13:238–244.

8. Lassen K, Soop M, Nygren J, Cox PB, Hendry PO, Spies C, von Meyenfeldt MF, Fearon KC, Revhaug A, Norderval S, Ljungqvist O, Lobo DN, Dejong CH, Enhanced Recovery After Surgery (ERAS) Group: Consensus review of optimal perioperative care in colorectal surgery: Enhanced Recovery After Surgery (ERAS) Group recommendations. Arch Surg 2009, 144:961–969.

9. Varadhan KK, Neal KR, Dejong CH, Fearon KC, Ljungqvist O, Lobo DN: The enhanced recovery after surgery (ERAS) pathway for patients undergoing major elective open colorectal surgery: a meta-analysis of randomized controlled trials. Clin Nutr 2010, 29:434–440.

10. Spanjersberg WR, Reurings J, Keus F, van Laarhoven CJ: Fast track surgery versus conventional recovery strategies for colorectal surgery. Cochrane Database Syst Rev 2011, 2:CD007635.

11. Gustafsson UO, Scott MJ, Schwenk W, Demartines N, Roulin D, Francis N, McNaught CE, MacFie J, Liberman AS, Soop M, Hill A, Kennedy RH, Lobo DN, Fearon K, Ljungqvist O, Enhanced Recovery After Surgery Society: Guidelines for perioperative care in elective colonic surgery: Enhanced Recovery After Surgery (ERAS®) Society recommendations. Clin Nutr 2012, 31:783–800.

12. Yamada T, Hayashi T, Cho H, Yoshikawa T, Taniguchi H, Fukushima R, Tsuburaya A: Usefulness of enhanced recovery after surgery protocol as compared with conventional perioperative care in gastric surgery. Gastric Cancer 2012, 15:34–41.

13. Wang D, Kong Y, Zhong B, Zhou X, Zhou Y: Fast-track surgery improves postoperative recovery in patients with gastric cancer: a randomized comparison with conventional postoperative care. J Gastrointest Surg 2010, 14:620–627.

14. Chen Hu J, Xin Jiang L, Cai L, Tao Zheng H, Yuan Hu S, Bing Chen H, Chang Wu G, Fei Zhang Y, Chuan LZ: Preliminary experience of fast-track surgery combined with laparoscopy-assisted radical distal gastrectomy for gastric cancer. J Gastrointest Surg 2012, 16:1830–1839.

15. Liu XX, Jiang ZW, Wang ZM, Li JS: Multimodal optimization of surgical care shows beneficial outcome in gastrectomy surgery. J Parenter Enteral Nutr 2010, 34:313–321.

16. Grantcharov TP, Kehlet H: Laparoscopic gastric surgery in an enhanced recovery programme. Br J Surg 2010, 97:1547–1551.

17. Dorcaratto D, Grande L, Pera M: Enhanced Recovery in Gastrointestinal Surgery: Upper Gastrointestinal Surgery. Dig Surg 2013, 30:70–78.

18. Sakakshev BE: Enhanced Recovery after Surgery for Gastric Cancer. J Gastrointest Dig Syst 2013, S12:003. doi: 10.4172/2161-069X.S12-003.

19. Japanese Gastric Cancer Association: Japanese gastric cancer treatment guidelines 2010 (ver. 3). Gastric Cancer 2011, 14:113–123.

20. Dindo D, Demartines N, Clavien PA: Classification of surgical complications: a new proposal with evaluation in a cohort of 6336 patients and results of a survey. Ann Surg 2004, 240:205–213.

21. JSobin LH, Gospodarowicz MK, Witterkind CH: International Union Against Cancer (UICC) TNM Classification of Malignant Tumors. 7th edition. Oxford, UK: Wiley-Black-well; 2009.

22. Hirao M, Tsujinaka T, Takeno A, Fujitani K, Kurata M: Patient-controlled dietary schedule improves clinical outcome after gastrectomy for gastric cancer. World J Surg 2005, 29:853–857.

23. Lassen K, Dejong CH, Ljungqvist O, Fearon K, Andersen J, Hannemann P, von Meyenfeldt MF, Hausel J, Nygren J, Revhaug A: Nutritional support

and oral intake after gastric resection in five northern European countries. Dig Surg 2005, 22:346–352.

24. Suehiro T, Matsumata T, Shikada Y, Sugimachi K: Accelerated rehabilitation with early postoperative oral feeding following gastrectomy. Hepatogastroenterology 2004, 51:1852–1855.

25. Jo DH, Jeong O, Sun JW, Jeong MR, Ryu SY, Park YK: Feasibility study of early oral intake after gastrectomy for gastric carcinoma. J Gastric Cancer 2011, 11:101–108.

26. Heslin MJ, Latkany L, Leung D, Brooks AD, Hochwald SN, Pisters PW, Shike M, Brennan MF: A prospective, randomized trial of early enteral feeding after resection of upper gastrointestinal malignancy. Ann Surg 1997, 226:567–577.

27. Lewis SJ, Andersen HK, Thomas S: Early enteral nutrition within 24 h of intestinal surgery versus later commencement of feeding: a systematic review and meta-analysis. J Gastrointest Surg 2009, 13:569–575.

16

Sutureless jejuno-jejunal anastomosis in gastric cancer patients: a comparison with handsewn procedure in a single institute

Luigi Marano[*], Bartolomeo Braccio, Michele Schettino, Giuseppe Izzo, Angelo Cosenza, Michele Grassia, Raffaele Porfidia, Gianmarco Reda, Marianna Petrillo, Giuseppe Esposito, Natale Di Martino

Abstract

Background: The biofragmentable anastomotic ring has been used to this day for various types of anastomosis in the gastrointestinal tract, but it has not yet achieved widespread acceptance among surgeons. The purpose of this retrospective study is to compare surgical outcomes of sutureless with suture method of Roux-and-Y jejunojejunostomy in patients with gastric cancer.

Methods: Two groups of patients were obtained based on anastomosis technique (sutureless group versus hand sewn group): perioperative outcomes were recorded for every patient.

Results: The mean time spent to complete a sutureless anastomosis was 11±4 min, whereas the time spent to perform hand sewn anastomosis was 23±7 min. Estimated intraoperative blood loss was 178±32ml in the sutureless group and 182±23ml in the suture-method group with no significant differences. No complications were registered related to enteroanastomosis. Intraoperative mortality was none for both groups.

Conclusions: The Biofragmentable Anastomotic Ring offers a safe and time-saving method for the jejuno-jejunal anastomosis in gastric cancer surgery, and for this purpose the ring has been approved as a standard method in our clinic. Nevertheless currently there are few studies on upper gastrointestinal sutureless anastomoses and this could be the reason for the low uptake of this device.

Background

The concept of compression anastomosis was introduced for the first time in February 1826 at the meeting of the Societe Royale de Medicine de Marseilles by Felix-Nicholas Denans who performed an end-to-end anastomosis using a metallic (silver or zinc) ring in a canine model [1]. At that time, this technique was still evolving, and in 1892 Murphy developed a new device of compression anastomosis in humans [2-6], which has been called "Murphy's button", that was extensively used. However, its clinical success was limited for relatively common anastomotic stenosis [7]. Approximately one century after Murphy, in 1985, Hardy et al [8] described the biofragmentable anastomotic ring (BAR). This device has been used so far for various types of anastomosis in the upper and lower gastrointestinal tract [6-14], for elective and emergency surgery [8,10-18], but it has not yet achieved widespread acceptance among surgeons [19]. The purpose of this retrospective study is to compare surgical outcomes of BAR with suture method of Roux-and-Y jejunojejunostomy in patients with gastric cancer who have undergone to total or partial gastrectomy.

Material and methods

From April 2002 to June 2010, 131 patients with a mean age of 64 years (range 37-89), 87 males and 44 females with a diagnosis of gastric cancer referred to the 8th

* Correspondence: marano.luigi@email.it
Institution: VIII General and Gastrointestinal Surgery (Chief Prof. N. Di Martino) - School of Medicine - Second University of Naples - Piazza Miraglia 2, 80138 Naples, Italy

General and Gastrointestinal Surgery of the Second University of Naples. Six of these 131 patients (3 males and 3 females) were not resectable in the course of surgery due to local extent of the tumor; one patient was not operable due to the presence of restrictive lung disease and aortic aneurysm, and one refused the operation. The patients who underwent gastric surgery were 123 (82 males and 41 females). 112 patients had a diagnosis of gastric adenocarcinoma, 10 non-Hodgkin lymphoma and 1 gastric carcinoid. Two groups of patients were obtained based on anastomosis technique: in the first group of 64 patients (43 males and 21 females, mean age 64.9) an end-to-side Roux-and-Y jejunojejunostomy was performed using a BAR after 57 total gastrectomy and 7 gastric resections. In the second group of 59 patients (37 males and 22 females, mean age 63.95) an end-to-side Roux-and-Y jejunojejunostomy suture method anastomosis was performed after 57 total gastrectomy and 2 gastric resections. BAR is made of 2 identical rings, each composed of 87.5% absorbable polyglycolic acid and 12.5% barium sulfate acting as a "radiopaque dye" to enhance x-ray imaging (abdominal X-ray examination showed BAR fragmentation approximately between 2 and 3 weeks after surgery [20]) . The rings have an internal lumen that varies from 11 to 20 mm in diameter, depending on the size and are placed into the cut bowel ends. When the device is closed a 1.5- to 2.5-mm gap remains between the 2 rings to prevent extensive tissue ischemia. The appropriate size of BAR device is crucial for a successful anastomosis; the ring must be compatible with the diameter of the bowel and the thickness of the bowel wall [17-19]. If the gap between the 2 rings is too large, a proper seroserosal approximation of the bowel ends will not be achieved, whereas if the compression zone is too narrow, the closing dynamics of the BAR can be altered and the tissue grasped in the gap can be subjected to extensive ischemic necrosis, leading to early detachment of the BAR [21]. An external diameter of 28 mm was preferred in all our patients for enteric anastomosis, whereas that of 31 mm or more was used in colonic or rectal anastomosis [19]. During the procedure, excessive snap pressure should be avoided since the BAR material is relatively friable [18]. The BAR anastomosis was performed by using a standard technique: after a total gastrectomy with an end-to-side esophagojejunostomy or a partial gastrectomy with side-to-end gastrojejunostomy, monofilament not- absorbable pursestring suture is placed, before bowel resection, at the jejunal wall along the pursestring clamp applied tangentially to antimesenterical fold, approximately 60 cm down from esophagojejunostomy or gastrojejunostomy. After bowel resection, a BAR of 28 mm is introduced into the proximal jejunum first by means of the inserter and then the pursestring suture is tied (Figure 1). After removal of the inserter, the other side of the BAR is inserted into the end jejunal wall and

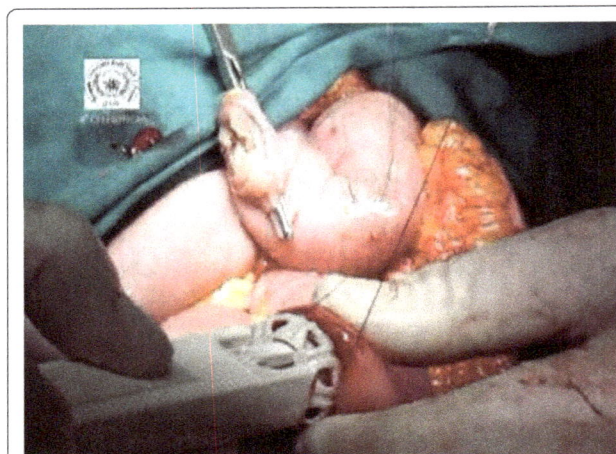

Figure 1 Introduction of 28mm BAR into the proximal jejunum.

the second pursestring is tied (Figures 2 and 3). The BAR is snapped shut by index finger and thumb pressure of two hands, forming a serosa-to-serosa inverted sutureless anastomosis (Figure 4). Before closing the ring the possible rotational error at the anastomosis is corrected. The manually sutured jejunojejunal anastomosis, following the same procedures as described for sutureless anastomosis, is achieved by continuous 3-0 polyglycolic acid multifilament in two layers with inversion technique. Patient demographics, operative procedure, type and location of the anastomosis, overall operating time, intraoperative blood loss, postoperative course and complications, if observed, were recorded for every patient. Postoperative completeness of the BAR anastomosis and fragmentation of the BAR ring were confirmed by abdominal x-ray at 7th and 30th day after surgery. The study was approved by the ethics committee of Second University of Naples and

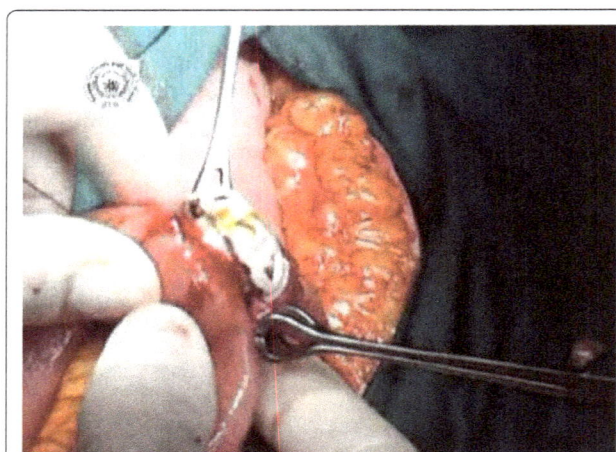

Figure 2 The other side of the BAR is inserted into the end jejunal wall.

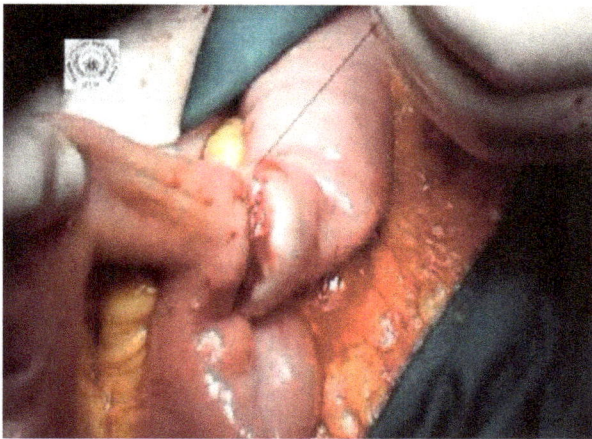

Figure 3 The second purse-string is tied.

conducted according to the ethical standards of the Helsinki declaration. Each patient gave informed written consent.

Results

64 end-to-side Roux-and-Y jejunojejunostomy were performed using a BAR after 57 total gastrectomy and 7 gastric resections. 59 end-to-side Roux-and-Y jejunojejunostomy suture method anastomosis were performed after 57 total gastrectomy and 2 gastric resections for gastric cancer. The mean time spent to complete a BAR anastomosis was 11±4 min, being the time spent to perform hand sewn anastomosis 23±7 min (p=0.030). In the BAR group the estimated operative blood loss was lower compared to the suture-method group (178±32ml and 182±23ml respectively), however the difference didn't reach a statistical significance (p=0.065). The postoperative course was uneventful in 75% (n=44)

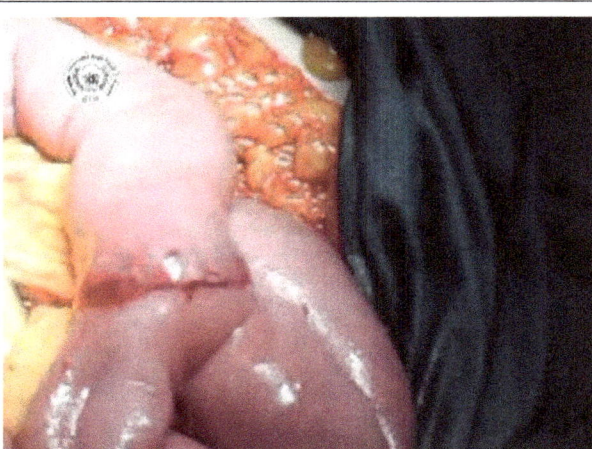

Figure 4 The BAR is snapped forming a serosa-to-serosa inverted sutureless anastomosis.

patients in the suture group and in 95.1% (n=61) the patients in the BAR group. No intraoperative mortality for both groups was found. The assessment of surgical morbidity revealed a complication rate of about 7.8% for the compression anastomosis group (2 intestinal obstructions treated with surgery; 1 duodenal fistula treated with medical therapy; 2 wall infections treated with medical therapy) compared to 8.5% for the sutured anastomosis group (1 duodenal fistula treated with medical therapy; 1 pancreatic fistula treated with medical therapy; 1 intestinal obstruction treated with surgery; 2 esophago-jejunal anastomotic leakages, respectively, treated with medical and surgical therapy) even if the complications are independents of the enteroanastomosis. The non-surgical morbidity was 16.8% for the BAR group and about 14.1% for the hand sewn group (p=0.183). No significant differences were noted between the groups in the starting time to oral feeding and intestinal canalization (Table 1). The duration of the postoperative hospital stay was also similar in both groups (10±2days in the BAR group; 10±3 in the suture group; p=0.137).

Discussions

The usefulness of BAR is well established in colonic anastomoses, but the effectiveness of a compression ring in small bowel anastomoses after gastric cancer surgery has not yet been well proven. Encouraged by little but favorable experiences with the device in colonic surgery we decided to analyze the outcomes of jejuno-jejunal BAR anastomosis compared with jejuno-jejunal hand sewn anastomosis. Our results demonstrate that patients with a jejuno-jejunal BAR anastomosis recover from upper gastrointestinal resections with no delay when compared to those with a manually sutured, conventional anastomosis. The most significant complication associated with anastomosis is anastomotic leakage [19]: although the occurrence of severe complications was lightly more frequent in the suture group (8.5%) when compared with sutureless group (7.8%), they were independent of the enteroanastomosis. In particular, the none overall jejuno-jejunal leak rate in the present study, as exhibited also by other Authors (2-4.2%) [10-14,17,18,22,23], probably indicate that the compression anastomosis is effective and a safe surgical procedure. Furthermore the surgical technique of BAR anastomosis represents a standardized approach with a very low period of the learning curve. Selection of the appropriate size of the ring and gap width is thought to be one of the critical determinants for a successful BAR anastomosis [19]. In the present study, for ease of use, we preferred to use the ring with external diameter of 28 mm. without any resistance at introduction into bowel lumen for all patients. Another advantage of BAR anastomosis is that it is a faster procedure than hand sewn method, because the mean time of

Table 1 Perioperative outcomes of 64 compression end-to-side Roux-and-Y jejunojejunostomy and 59 handsewn end-to-side Roux-and-Y jejunojejunostomy

	Compression anastomosis (n=64)	Handsewn anastomosis (n=59)	p
Estimated intraoperative blood loss	178±32 ml	182±23 ml	.065
Mean jejunojejunostomy time	11±4 min	23±7 min	<0.05
Intraoperative mortality	0%	0%	N.E.
Surgical morbidity	7.8%	8.5%	N.E.
Intestinal obstruction	2 (n)	1 (n)	N.E.
Duodenal fistula	1 (n)	1 (n)	N.E.
Pancreatic fistula	/	1 (n)	N.E.
Esophago-jejunal leakage	/	1 (n)	N.E.
Wall infections	2 (n)	/	N.E.
Non-surgical morbidity	16.8%	14.1%	.183
Starting time to oral feeding	7th day	7th day	/
Intestinal canalization	2.1±0.6 min	2.3±0.5 min	.321
Mean hospital stay	10±2 days	10±3 days	.137

N.E. Not evaluated

compression procedure is approximately 50% less than the suture procedure, as resulting from our data (11±4 min of BAR anastomoses versus 23±7 min of suture anastomoses (p<0.05)). Therefore it can be applied more preferably to patients with comorbidities where both rapidity and security of the anastomosis is required [14,16,17,22,23].

Conclusions

In our opinion the Biofragmentable Anastomotic Ring offers a safe and time-saving method for the jejuno-jejunal anastomosis in gastric cancer surgery, and for this purpose the ring has been approved as a standard method in our clinic. Nevertheless, currently there are few studies on upper gastrointestinal BAR anastomoses and this could be the reason for the low uptake of this device.

List of abbreviations used
BAR: Biofragmentable Anastomotic Ring.

Acknowledgements
The authors thank Dr Francesco Torelli for participating at some surgical intervention as surgeon's assistant.
This article has been published as part of *BMC Surgery* Volume 12 Supplement 1, 2012: Selected articles from the XXV National Congress of the Italian Society of Geriatric Surgery. The full contents of the supplement are available online at http://www.biomedcentral.com/bmcsurg/supplements/12/S1.

Authors' contributions
All authors approved the final manuscript. *Study concept and design*: NDM and LM; *Acquisition of data*: BB, MS, RP; *Analysis and interpretation of data*: AC, LM, GI, GR, MP; *Drafting of the manuscript*: LM, BB; *Critical revision of the manuscript for important intellectual content*: NDM, LM, GI; *Statistical analysis*: MG, GE, AC; *Study supervision*: NDM, LM.

Competing interests
Authors have no conflicts of interest or financial ties to disclose.

References

1. Kaidar-Person O, Rosenthal RJ, Wexner SD, Szomstein S, Person B: Compression anastomoses: history and clinical considerations. *Am J Surg* 2008, 195:818-26.
2. Booth CC: What has technology done to gastroenterology? *Gut* 1985, 26:1088-94.
3. Amat C: Appareils a sutures: Les viroles de denans; les points de Bonnier: Les boutons de Murphy. *Arch Med Pharmacie Militaires Paris* 1895, 25:273-85.
4. Murphy JB: Cholecysto-intestinal, gastro-intestinal, entero-intestinal anastomosis, and approximation without sutures. *Med Rec N Y* 1892, 42:665-76.
5. Gordon RC, John B: Murphy: unique among American surgeons. *J Invest Surg* 2006, 19:279-81.
6. McCue JL, Phillips RK: Sutureless intestinal anastomoses. *Br J Surg* 1991, 78:1291-6, Sutureless intestinal anastomoses.
7. Senn N: Enterorrhaphy: its history, technique and present status. *JAMA* 1893, 21:215-35.
8. Hardy TG Jr, Pace WG, Maney JW, Katz AR, Kaganov AL: A biofragmentable ring for sutureless bowel anastomosis. An experimental study. *Dis Colon Rectum* 1985, 28:484-90.
9. Kanshin NN, Lytkin MI, Knysh VI, Klur VIu, Khamidov AL: First experience with application of compression anastomoses with the apparatus AKA-2 in operations on the large intestine. *Vestn Khir Im I I Grek* 1984, 132:52-7.
10. Bubrick MP, Corman ML, Cahill CJ, Hardy TG Jr, Nance FC, Shatney CH: Prospective, randomized trial of the biofragmentable anastomotic ring. The BAR InvestigationalGroup. *Am J Surg* 1991, 161:136-42.
11. Cahill CJ, Betzler M, Gruwez JA, Jeekel J, Patel JC, Zederfeldt B: Sutureless large bowel anastomosis: European experience with the biofragmentable anastomosis ring. *Br J Surg* 1989, 76:344-7.
12. Corman ML, Prager ED, Hardy TG Jr, Bubrick MP: Comparison of the Valtrac biofragmentable anastomosis ring with conventional suture and stapled anastomosis in colon surgery. Results of a prospective randomized clinical trial. *Dis Colon Rectum* 1989, 32:183-7.
13. Gullichsen R, Ovaska J, Rantala A, Havia T: Small bowel anastomosis with the biofragmentable anastomosis ring and manual suture: a prospective, randomized study. *World J Surg* 1992, 16:1006-9.
14. Pahlman L, Ejerblad S, Graf W, Kader F, Kressner U, Lindmark G, et al: Randomized trial of a biofragmentable bowel anastomosis ring in high-risk colonic resection. *Br J Surg* 1997, 84:1291-4.
15. Seow-Choen F, Eu KW: Circular staplers versus the biofragmentable ring for colorectal anastomosis: a prospective randomized study. *Br J Surg* 1994, 81:1790-1.

Sutureless jejuno-jejunal anastomosis in gastric cancer patients: a comparison...

101

16. Fansler RF, Mero K, Steinberg SM, McSwain NE, Flint LM, Ferrara JJ: **Utility of the biofragmentable anastomotic ring in traumatic small bowel injury.** *Am Surg* 1994, **60**:379-83.

17. Thiede A, Geiger D, Dietz UA, Debus ES, Engemann R, Lexer GC, *et al*: **Overview on compression anastomoses: biofragmentable anastomosis ring multicenter prospective trial of 1666 anastomoses.** *World J Surg* 1998, **22**:78-86.

18. Choi HJ, Kim HH, Jung GJ, Kim SS: **Intestinal anastomosis by use of the biofragmentable anastomotic ring: is it safe and efficacious in emergency operations as well?** *Dis Colon Rectum* 1998, **41**:1281-6.

19. Kim SH, Choi HJ, Park KJ, Kim JM, Kim KH, Kim MC, *et al*: **Sutureless intestinal anastomosis with the biofragmentable anastomosis ring: experience of 632 anastomoses in a single institute.** *Dis Colon Rectum* 2005, **48**(11):2127-32.

20. Aggarwal R, Darzi A: **Compression anastomoses revisited.** *J Am Coll Surg* 2005, **201**:965-71.

21. Galizia G, Lieto E, Castellano P, Pelosio L, Imperatore V, Canfora F, *et al*: **Comparison between the biofragmentable anastomosis ring and stapled anastomoses in the extraperitoneal rectum: a prospective, randomized study.** *Int J Colorectal Dis* 1999, **14**:286-90.

22. Di Castro A, Biancari F, Brocato R, Adami EA, Truosolo B, Massi G: **Intestinal anastomosis with the biofragmentable anastomosis ring.** *Am J Surg* 1998, **176**:472-4.

23. Ghitulescu GA, Morin N, Jetty P, Belliveau P: **Revisiting the biofragmentable anastomotic ring: is it safe in colonic surgery?** *Can J Surg* 2003, **46**:92-8.

17

Laparoscopic versus open wedge resection for gastrointestinal stromal tumors of the stomach: a single-center 8-year retrospective cohort study of 156 patients with long-term follow-up

Jia-Qin Cai[†], Ke Chen[†], Yi-Ping Mou[*], Yu Pan, Xiao-Wu Xu, Yu-Cheng Zhou and Chao-Jie Huang

Abstract

Background: The aim of this study was to compared laparoscopic (LWR) and open wedge resection (OWR) for the treatment of gastric gastrointestinal stromal tumors (GISTs).

Methods: The data of 156 consecutive GISTs patients underwent LWR or OWR between January 2006 and December 2013 were collected retrospectively. The surgical outcomes and the long-term survival rates were compared. Besides, a rapid systematic review and meta-analysis were conducted.

Results: Clinicopathological characteristics of the patients were similar between the two groups. The LWR group was associated with less intraoperative blood loss (67.3 vs. 142.7 ml, $P < 0.001$), earlier postoperative flatus (2.3 vs. 3.2 days, $P < 0.001$), earlier oral intake (3.2 vs. 4.1 days, $P < 0.001$) and shorter postoperative hospital stay (6.0 vs. 8.0 days, $P = 0.001$). The incidence of postoperative complications was lower in LWR group but did not reach statistical significance (4/90, 4.4% vs. 8/66, 12.1%, $P = 0.12$). No significant difference was observed in 3-year relapse-free survival rate between the two groups (98.6% vs. 96.4%, $P > 0.05$). The meta-analysis revealed similar results except less overall complications in the LWR group (RR = 0.49, 95% CI, 0.25 to 0.95, $P = 0.04$). And the recurrence risk was similar in two group (RR = 0.80, 95% CI, 0.28 to 2.27, $P > 0.05$).

Conclusions: LWR is a technically and oncologically safe and feasible approach for gastric GISTs compared with OWR. Moreover, LWR appears to be a preferable choice with mini-invasive benefits.

Keywords: Gastrointestinal stromal tumor, Laparoscopy, Meta-analysis, Survival

Background

Gastrointestinal stromal tumors (GISTs), the most common mesenchymal tumor of the gut, are often characterized by high expression of KIT [1,2]. The most common sites for GIST include the stomach (60%) and jejunum or ileum (30%) followed by duodenum (5%), colon and rectum (less than 5%), esophagus (less than 1%), and appendix (less than 1%) [2]. GISTs have malignant potential, and it is reported that recurrence of GISTs often occured at the peritoneal surface or liver [3]. Surgical resection is the mainstay management for primary localized GISTs. As submucosal and lymphatic spread are rare, the surgical principles are composed of an R0 resection with a normal mucosa margin, no systemic lymph node dissection, and avoidance of perforation, which results in peritoneal seeding even in cases with otherwise low risk profiles [2-4].

Since the development of minimally invasive surgical approaches, laparoscopic surgery for gastrointestinal tumors has evolved rapidly over the past decade. Various types of laparoscopic approaches for GISTs have been described, including wedge resection of the stomach, intragastric tumor resection, and combined endoscopic-laparoscopic resection [5-8]. For gastric GISTs, lymph node metastases are rare and localised resection with a

---

* Correspondence: mouyiping2002@163.com
[†]Equal contributors
Department of General Surgery, Sir Run Run Shaw Hospital, School of Medicine, Zhejiang University, 3 East Qingchun Road, Hangzhou 310016, Zhejiang Province, China

clear margin of 1 to 2 cm appears to be an adequate treatment [9,10]. Besides, recent evidence has shown that survival depends on the tumor size and histological features rather than the extent of resection [3]. Therefore, gastric GISTs can be treated without major anatomical resections [11] and are suitable for laparoscopic wedge resection (LWR). Several case series have proved the safety and feasibility of LWR for gastric GISTs, however, the oncologic benefits of LWR have not been widely reported and the sample size of those researches were relatively small. In the current study, we retrospectively reviewed data for GIST patients who underwent LWR and traditional open wedge resection (OWR) at our hospital between 2006 and 2013. The clinical data, benefits of operation, perioperative outcomes, and oncologic outcomes were reviewed. Besides, a rapid systematic review with a meta-analysis was conducted to further assess accurately the current status of LWR for gastric GIST.

Methods

Patients

Between January 2006 and December 2013, 177 consecutive patients with suspected gastric GIST underwent laparoscopic or open wedge resection in the Department of General Surgery at the Sir Run Run Shaw Hospital, China. The exclusion criteria included: (1) patients concomitant with tumors outside stomach; (2) patients with metastatic disease at the time of operation; (3) patients diagnosed as other types of submucosal tumor after immunohistochemical examination. Blood tests, chest X-rays, enhanced computed tomography scans of the abdomen and pelvis, and endoscopic ultrasonography were performed before operation. This study protocol was prospectively approved by ethics committee of Sir Run Run Shaw Hospital, School of Medicine, Zhejiang University and conducted in accordance with the ethical guidelines of the Declaration of Helsinki. Informed consent was signed prior to surgery by each case.

Surgical procedure

The patient is placed in the supine position under general anesthesia. The surgeon stood on the right side of the patient. One assistant stood on the right side of the patient and held the laparoscope, and another stood on the left side of the patient. Carbon dioxide pneumoperitoneum was established through the Veress needle and set at 15 mmHg. One initial 10-mm trocar was inserted for laparoscopy below the umbilicus and another four trocars (one of 12 mm, three of 5 mm) were inserted into the left upper flank, left flank, right upper flank, and right flank quadrants; a total of five trocars were inserted, and arranged in a V-shape.

Mobilizing the tumor before excised were usually as fellows: Tumor in anterior wall of the gastric body and pylorus was excised directly. If tumor was in anterior wall near lesser curvature, the hepatogastric ligament was dissected firstly to free it. If it was in anterior wall near great curvature, parts of gastrocolic ligament and gastrosplenic ligament were dissected firstly. For tumor located in posterior wall, the gastrocolic and gastrosplenic ligament were dissected, then lifted up the stomach to expose the tumor. Those in fundus, the gastrocolic and gastrosplenic ligament was also dissected as well as left gastroepiploic vessels and short gastric vessels, so the fundus can be mobilized and the tumor can be expose. Gastroscopy was used intraoperatively to evaluate tumor localization if necessary. Tumor was excised using ultrasonic scalpel or endoscopic linear stapler with at least 1-2 cm surgical margin. The defect left by excision using ultrasonic scalpel in the gastric wall was reinforced using laparoscopic hand-suturing technique. If the tumors were near the cardia or pylorus, excision using ultrasonic scalpel was preferred, as it can reduce the risk of cardiac or pyloric stricture. While the tumors were in the gastric fundus, excision using endoscopic linear stapler was preferred, for tumor had a good mobility to perform this procedure easily. For tumors located near the esophagogastric junction, especially those with intraluminal growth, we used laparoscopic transgastric wedge resection to avoid deformity or stenosis in the gastric inlet. A summary of the detailed transgastric resection were described in our published article [6].

Data collection and follow-up evaluation

The patients' demographic data, surgical outcomes, and complications were reviewed, and the survival rate was analyzed. The prognostic indicators of GISTs were based on tumor size and mitotic index, according to the risk assessment classification proposed by Fletcher et al. [12] Gastric GISTs were categorized for malignant potential as very low risk (<2 cm and <5 mitoses/50 high-power fields, HPFs), low risk (2–5 cm and <5 mitoses/50 HPFs), intermediate risk (<5 cm and 6–10 mitoses/50 HPFs or 5–10 cm and <5 mitoses/50 HPFs), and high risk (>5 cm and >5 mitoses/50 HPFs, >10 cm and any mitotic rate, any size, or >10 mitoses/50 HPFs). The immunohistochemical analysis included detection of CD117, CD34, smooth muscle actin protein (SMA), S-100, and desmin expression. Follow-up results were obtained from patients' medical records and telephone calls, and recurrence was determined by endoscopy, computed tomography, positron emission tomography, etc, and the last follow-up day was January 30, 2014.

A rapid systematic review and meta-analysis

We searched PubMed, Cochrane Library, Web of Science and BIOSIS Previews for literature comparing LWR and OWR published between January 1995 and April 2014.

The following keywords were used: "gastrointestinal stromal tumor", "GIST", "laparoscopy", "laparoscopic", "minimally invasive surgery", "gastric resection", "gastric surgery", and "comparative study". The language of the publications was confined to English. The papers containing any of the following were excluded: (1) concomitant with tumors outside stomach; (2) not wedge resection; (3) if there was overlap between authors or centers, the higher quality or more recent literature were selected. Two investigators reviewed the titles and abstracts, and assessed the full text to establish eligibility. The Newcastle-Ottawa Quality Assessment Scale (NOS) was used for quality assessment of observational studies. A threshold of six stars or above has been considered indicative of high quality.

Statistical analysis

Quantitative data are given as the means ± standard deviations (SDs). The differences in the measurement data were compared using the Student's t test, and comparisons between groups were tested using the χ^2 test or the Fisher exact probability test. Relapse-free survival (RFS) rates were calculated by the Kaplan-Meier method using SPSS software, version 18.0 (SPSS Inc, Chicago, United States). Relapse-free survival was calculated from the day of surgery to the day of recurrence. $P < 0.05$ was considered statistically significant.

The meta-analysis was performed in line with recommendations from the Cochrane Collaboration and the Quality of Reporting of Meta-Analyses guidelines [13,14]. Continuous variables were assessed using the weighted mean difference (WMD), and dichotomous variables were analyzed using the risk ratio (RR). If the study provided medians and ranges instead of means and standard deviations (SDs), we estimated the means and SDs as described by Hozo et al. [15]. To account for clinical heterogeneity, which refers to diversity in a sense that is relevant for clinical situations, we used the random effects model based on DerSimonian and Laird's method. Potential publication bias was determined by conducting informal visual inspection of funnel plots based on the complications. Data analyses were performed using Review Manage version 5.1 (RevMan 5.1) software downloaded from the Cochrane Library. $P < 0.05$ was considered statistically significant.

Results

Demographic and clinicopathologic characteristics

Among the 177 patients, 21 were excluded. Five patients with coexistence of any other malignancies were excluded. Fourteen patients were excluded because diagnosed as other types of submucosal tumor instead of GIST. Two patients with metastatic disease were also excluded. Finally, 156 patients were enrolled into this study. Among them, 90 patients underwent laparoscopic wedge resection (LWR group) for gastric GISTs, while 66 patients received open wedge resection (OWR group).

The LWR group included 31 males (34.4%), and the mean age was 58.6 ± 10.7 years. The OWR group included 29 males (43.9%), and the mean age was 56.8 ± 11.9 years. Mean body mass index (BMI) for the LWR was 22.8 ± 3.1 kg/m2 compared with 23.3 ± 3.7 kg/m2 among the OWR. The ASA score for each patient was: ASA I [LWR, 44 (48.9%); OWR, 33 (50.0%)], ASA II [LWR, 41 (45.6%); OWR, 30 (45.5%)], and ASA III [LWR, 5 (5.6%); OWR, 3 (4.5%)]. No statistical differences were observed between the group's demographic characteristics, ASA scores, comorbidities, and BMI (Table 1). The mean preoperative hemoglobin and albumin levels were 12.8 ± 1.9 g/dL and 42.2 ± 4.2 g/L in LWR group, and 12.7 ± 2.4 g/dL and 42.9 ± 4.5 g/L in OWR group.

The pathological variables of the patients are summarized in Table 2. The mean tumor size in the LWR group was 3.5 cm and in the OWR group it was 4.3 cm. The mean tumor size in the LWR group was smaller than OWR group (P = 0.02). However, for properties, there was no statistically significant difference between the two groups according to Fletcher's criteria ($P > 0.05$). In all GIST patients, 84.6% had a mitotic rate of fewer than 5 mitoses per 50 high-power field (HPF), 9.6% had a mitotic rate between 5 and 10 mitoses per 50 HPF, and 5.8% had more than 10 mitoses per 50 HPF. The two groups were comparable with respect to tumor location, with the majority of patients having tumors located in the gastric body or fundus (77.7% in the LWR and 63.6% in the OWR group).

Operative outcomes and postoperative recovery

The outcomes associated with surgery and postoperative recovery are shown in Table 3. In the OWR group, the mean amount of estimated intraoperative bleeding was more than in the LWR (67.3 ± 80.5 ml vs. 142.7 ± 102.0;

Table 1 Clinical characteristics of patients

Variable(%)	LWR(n = 90)	OWR(n = 66)	P value
Gender (male/female)	31/59	29/37	0.79
Age (years)	58.6 ± 10.7	56.8 ± 11.9	0.33
BMI (kg/m2)	22.8 ± 3.1	23.3 ± 3.7	0.29
ASA classification (I/II/III)	44/41/5	33/30/3	1.00
Comorbidities (yes)	35(38.9)	26(39.4)	0.77
Hypertension	29(32.2)	17(25.8)	
Diabetes mellitus	9(10)	7(10.6)	
Cardiovascular	5(5.6)	4(6.1)	
Pulmonary	2(2.2)	1(1.5)	
Previous abdominal surgery	22(24.4)	20(30.3)	0.42
Preoperative hemoglobin	12.8 ± 1.9	12.7 ± 2.4	0.91
Preoperative albumin	42.2 ± 4.2	42.9 ± 4.5	0.31

Table 2 Pathologic features of patients

Variable(%)	LWR(n = 90)	OWR(n = 66)	P value
Tumor size (cm)	3.5 ± 1.9	4.3 ± 2.4	0.02
Tumor location			0.08
Cardia	14(15.6)	10(15.2)	
Fundus	29(32.2)	16(24.2)	
Body near lesser curvature	11(12.2)	4(6.1)	
Body near greater curvature	30(33.3)	22(33.3)	
Antrum	6(6.7)	14(21.2)	
Mitotic rate (per 50 HPF)			0.20
<5	80(88.9)	52(78.8)	
5 ~ 10	7(7.8)	8(12.1)	
>10	3(3.3)	6(9.1)	
Immunohistochemistry			
CD117(+)	86(95.6)	66(100)	0.11
CD34(+)	87(96.7)	63(95.5)	0.20
DOG-1(+)	72(80.0)	58(87.9)	0.19
SMA	30(33.3)	17(25.8)	0.31
S-100	16(17.8)	14(21.2)	0.59
Desmin	9(10)	6(9.1)	0.95
Fletcher classification			0.51
Very low risk	20(22.2)	13(19.7)	
Low risk	46(51.1)	28(42.4)	
Intermediate risk	16(17.8)	16(24.2)	
High risk	8(8.9)	9(13.6)	

$P < 0.01$). Mean operative time was similar between groups (106.6 ± 40.1 min vs. 119.9 ± 59.9; $P > 0.05$). There were 21 cases in the LWR group used intraoperative endoscopy to locate the tumors.

Mean times to postoperative flatus and oral intake were significantly shorter in the LWR group than in the

Table 3 Operative findings and postoperative clinical courses

Variable	LWR(n = 90)	OWR(n = 66)	P value
Operation time (min)	106.6 ± 40.1	119.9 ± 59.9	0.12
Blood loss (ml)	67.3 ± 80.5	142.7 ± 102.0	0.000
Intraoperative endoscopy	21(23.3)	0(0.0)	
Time to first flatus (days)	2.3 ± 0.9	3.2 ± 0.8	0.000
Time to oral intake (days)	3.2 ± 1.0	4.1 ± 0.9	0.000
Postoperative hospital stay (days)	6.0 ± 2.1	8.0 ± 5.1	0.001
Postoperative complications	4(4.4)	8(12.1)	0.08
Anastomotic hemorrhage	0	2	
Abdominal abscess	0	1	
Delayed gastric emptying	3	3	
Wound infection	0	2	
Pulmonary infection	1	0	

OWR group (2.3 days vs. 3.2 days, $P < 0.01$, and 3.2 days versus 4.1 days, $P < 0.01$). The mean duration of postoperative hospital stay was two days longer in the OWR group (6.0 days vs. 8.0 days, $P < 0.01$).

The incidence of postoperative complications was higher for the OWR group than the LWR group. But the difference did not reach statistical significance (4.4% vs. 12.1%, $P = 0.08$). Incidences of morbidity in LWR group included three cases of delayed gastric emptying and one case of pulmonary infection. Complications in OWR group included two cases of anastomotic hemorrhage, one case of abdominal abscess, three cases of delayed gastric emptying and two cases of wound infection. All these complications were controlled with conservative treatment.

Follow-up results

Of the 156 identified patients, 149 (95.5%) were followed up and 7 were lost to follow-up. Follow-up data were available for 87 (96.6%) and 62 (93.9%) of patients treated with LWR and OWR, respectively. The median follow-up was 21.0 months (range, 1-90 months) in the LWR group and 44.5 months (range, 1-96 months) in the OWR group.

One patient in the LWR group diagnosed with low risk of disease recurrence developed metachronous liver metastasis 9 months after operation. Two patients in the OWR group developed liver metastasis 11 months and 24 months after operation, respectively. They were both diagnosed with high risk of recurrence and were still alive at the end of last follow-up. One patient of low risk of recurrence in the LWR group dead of breast cancer 42 months after gastric surgery. However, there was no evidence of GIST recurrence before her death. The 3-year RFS rates was 98.6% in LWR group and 96.4% in OWR group. There were no significant differences between the two groups ($P > 0.05$) (Figure 1).

A rapid systematic review and meta-analysis

The initial search strategy retrieved 972 publications in English. After the titles and abstracts were reviewed, papers without comparison of LWR and OWR were excluded, which left 20 comparative studies, fourteen [9,16-28] of which did not meet the inclusion criteria and were excluded. This left a total of six comparative observational studies [29-34]. A flow chart of the search strategies is illustrated in Figure 2. Including the present data, a total of 525 patients were included in the analysis with 264 undergoing LWR (50.3%) and 261 undergoing OWR (49.7%). According to the NOS, one out of the six observational studies got 7 stars, two articles got 8 stars, and the remaining three got 9 stars. The characteristics and methodological quality assessment scores of the included studies are shown in Table 4.

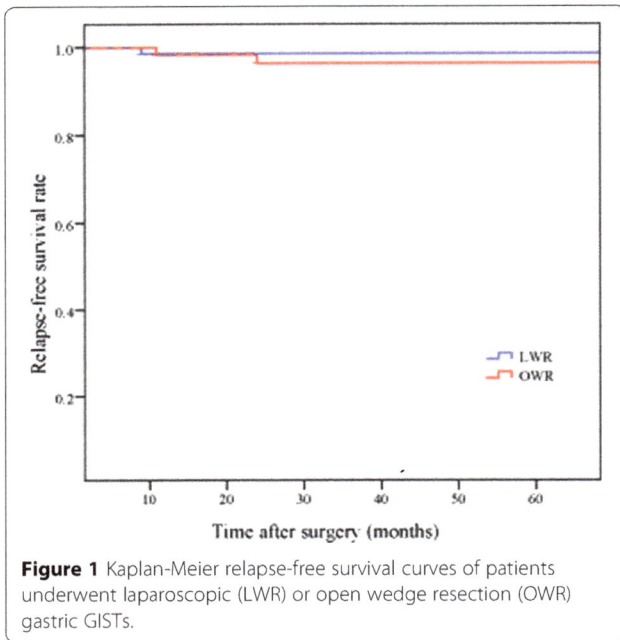

Figure 1 Kaplan-Meier relapse-free survival curves of patients underwent laparoscopic (LWR) or open wedge resection (OWR) gastric GISTs.

All studies reported operative time [29-34]. The present analysis showed no statistically significant difference in the operative time of the two groups (WMD = 4.08 min; 95% CI, -20.23 to 28.39; $P = 0.74$) (Figure 3A). Two studies reported blood loss [30,34]. Intraoperative blood loss was significantly lower in the LWR compared with the OWR group (WMD = -60.02 ml; 95% CI, -76.90 to -43.14 ml; $P < 0.01$) (Figure 3B). All studies reported overall complications [29-34]. There were significantly fewer overall complications in the LWR than the OWR group (RR = 0.49, 95% CI, 0.25 to 0.95, $P = 0.04$) (Figure 3C). Visual inspection of the funnel plot revealed symmetry, indicating no serious publication bias (Figure 4). Morbidity was specified in two studies [31,34]. One study reported a wound infection in OWR group [31]. Another reported one wound infection and one anastomosis site bleeding in LWR group and one

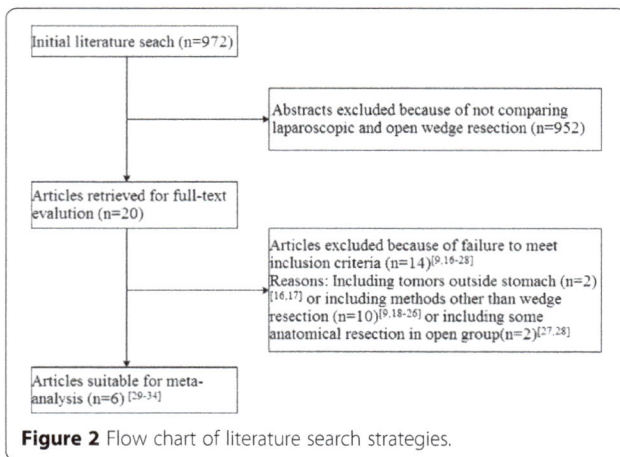

Figure 2 Flow chart of literature search strategies.

wound infection, one wound dehiscence and four pyrexia in OWR group [34].

All studies reported duration of hospital stay [29-34]. Patients in the LWR group had a shorter postoperative hospital stay (WMD = -2.21 days; 95% CI, -3.09 to -1.34, $P < 0.01$) (Figure 3D). Four studies reported time to first flatus [29,30,32,33] and five studies reported time to oral intake [29,30,32-34]. Patients in the LWR group were able to pass flatus (WMD = -1.28 days; 95% CI, -1.61 to -0.96, $P < 0.01$) (Figure 3E) and resume oral intake earlier (WMD = -1.51 days; 95% CI, -2.07 to -0.95, $P < 0.01$) (Figure 3F).

During the follow-up period, recurrence was observed in four studies [29,31,32,34]. Including our study, the recurrence risk in LWR was 2.3% (6/264) and 3.1% (8/261) in OWR, but the difference between LWR and OWR was not significant (RR = 0.80, 95% CI, 0.28 to 2.27, $P = 0.67$) (Figure 3G). Wan et al. [34] have reported that there was no significant difference in the 5-year RFS between LWR and OWR (93.7% in LWR, 95.5% in OWR). Goh et al. [32] also have reported that there was no significant differences in RFS between groups.

Discussion

Adenocarcinomas are the most common tumors of the stomach, whereas submucosal tumors of the stomach such as GISTs are rare. Unlike adenocarcinomas of gastrointestinal tract, GISTs showed that negative macroscopic margins only may portends a survival benefit [3]. Lymphatic spread is quite uncommon, and as such, systemic lymphadenectomy has been deemed unnecessary [2,3]. These characteristics, along with GISTs' tendency to grow in an exophytic manner, led many surgeons prefer wedge resection rather than formal gastrectomy for gastric GISTs whenever feasible. Though laparoscopic wedge resection is expected to be a preferable choice for GISTs compared with traditional open wedge resection as previously reported [27,29-33,35,36], more convincing evidence is still needed to prove its safety and feasibility. This manuscript summarizes the outcomes of LWR of gastric GISTs in the relatively larger series of patients to date. Our data demonstrate that the patients who underwent LWR for gastric GISTs results in effective control of the disease with minimal perioperative morbidity and no mortality. Besides, a rapid systematic review with a meta-analysis was conducted to summarize all the published information. We believe this could help surgeons to share the optimal individualized decision for patients.

Our series of patients who underwent LWR had less intraoperative blooding than that in the OWR group. The reduced length of incision wound, accurate operation and the application of energy-dividing devices, contributed to the reduction of blood loss. Pain after surgery was milder in LWR than in OWR, reflecting as

Table 4 Summary of studies included in the meta-analysis

Author	Nation	Study type	Publication year	Study period	Sample size		Follow-up (months)		Quality scores
					LWR	OWR	LWR	OWR	
Ishikawa [29]	Japan	Retro	2006	1993-2004	14	7	60(5–119)	61(3–130)	8
Mochizuki [30]	Japan	Retro	2006	2000-2004	12	10	26 (6–53)	NR	8
Catena [31]	Italy	Pros	2008	1995-2006	21	25	35(5–58)	91(80–136)	9
Goh [32]	Singapore	Retro	2010	2001-2009	14	39	8(3–60)	21(2–72)	7
Lee [33]	Korea	Retro	2011	2001-2008	50	50	21(0–64)	22(0–93)	9
Wan [34]	China	Retro	2012	2004-2011	63	64	NR	NR	9

Retro: retrospective observational study; Pros: prospective observational study; NR: not reported.

the shorter duration or the lower dosage of analgesic application [29,32]. The time to first flatus was also earlier in LWR than in OWR, which indicated more rapid recovery of gastrointestinal function after LWR. Reduced use of analgesic drugs, shortened time of abdominal cavity exposure, alleviated inflammatory reactions, and earlier postoperative activities are considered to be the main reasons for earlier gastrointestinal recovery from LWR; all of which may also contribute to shortening the duration of postoperative hospital stay. The meta-analysis also revealed these mini-invasive advantages of the LWR. Interestingly, the operative time in the LWR group did not longer than OWR which is different from many other type of laparoscopic surgery [37-42]. This is because the time-consuming laparoscopic lymphadenectomy is unnecessary for GISTs resection due to the fact that the lymphatic metastasis of GISTs is quite rare. As time spending on the establishment of pneumoperitoneum and the closure of the trocar incision and minilaparotomy is likely to shorter than the open and closure of laparotomy, it is possible that the operative time for the LWR will be shorter than OWR with the development of the surgical techniques and laparoscopic instruments.

Regarding the postoperative complication, the incidence was higher in the OWR group than the LWR group, but the difference did not reach statistical significance in our study. However, the meta-analysis indicated a significant reduction in the LWR group ($P = 0.04$). In our study, there was a high incidence of wound problem in the OWR group. This is also true in included trials which specified the morbidity [31,34]. It was conceivable that complications other than wound problem were similar between groups because LWR results in the same organ and tissue resection as OWR.

LWR for gastric GISTs seems to have become a popular technique, the indications for this procedure in relation to tumor size are still controversial. Large lesions increase the difficulty to resect using endoscopic linear staplers and the risk of tumor spillage when removal. It was previously suggested by the NCCN Guidelines updated in 2007 for Optimal Management of Patients with GIST that laparoscopic techniques could be approached

for tumors less than 5 cm [2]. However, many investigators have reported successful and safe removal of larger GISTs [26,43-45]. In our series, 12 cases with tumor size larger than 5 cm underwent LWR successfully with no conversion, demonstrating its feasibility, though the mean tumor size of OWR group was slightly larger than LWR group (4.3 versus 3.5 cm). This observation was mainly biased by the inherent selection process for patients to undergo a laparoscopic approach. patients with smaller tumors may be more amenable to laparoscopy versus larger tumors, which may tend to treat with laparoscopy or laparotomy. There were 20 cases in our series with tumor located near the esophagogastric junction or the pylorus who were considered inappropriate to undergo LWR. Performing this procedure has a high possibility of stenosis or deformity in the gastric inlet or outlet because it is associated with excessive resection of the healthy tissue of the gastric wall by laparoscopic stapling [46]. If the tumor was extraluminal growth, we resected the tumor using ultrasonic scalpel, then used laparoscopic intracorporeal handsewn method to close the incision. With those intraluminal growth, the laparoscopic transgastric wedge resection, which provided direct vision of the lesion and inner stomach, and allows better control of the surgical margin, was introduced. Whereas, if the tumor was large, laparoscopic distal or total gastrectomy was performed instead of LWR which is impossible in such situation. After tumors removal, all these cases were confirmed by intraoperative gastroscope examination to avoid gastric inlet or outlet narrowing. Currently, there are still no clear consensus guidelines for gastric GISTs laparoscopic approach based on tumor size and location. We advocate that tumor size and location should not be an absolute contraindication to laparoscopic techniques. However, one thing should be in mind that regardless laparoscopy or open surgery, it must be avoid direct tumor manipulation in an effort to eliminate the incidence of tumor rupture since tumor spillage can results in shortened disease-free survival [47].

With recent trials confirming the short-term surgical safety and long-term survival efficacy of laparoscopic techniques in other gastrointestinal malignancy [48-53],

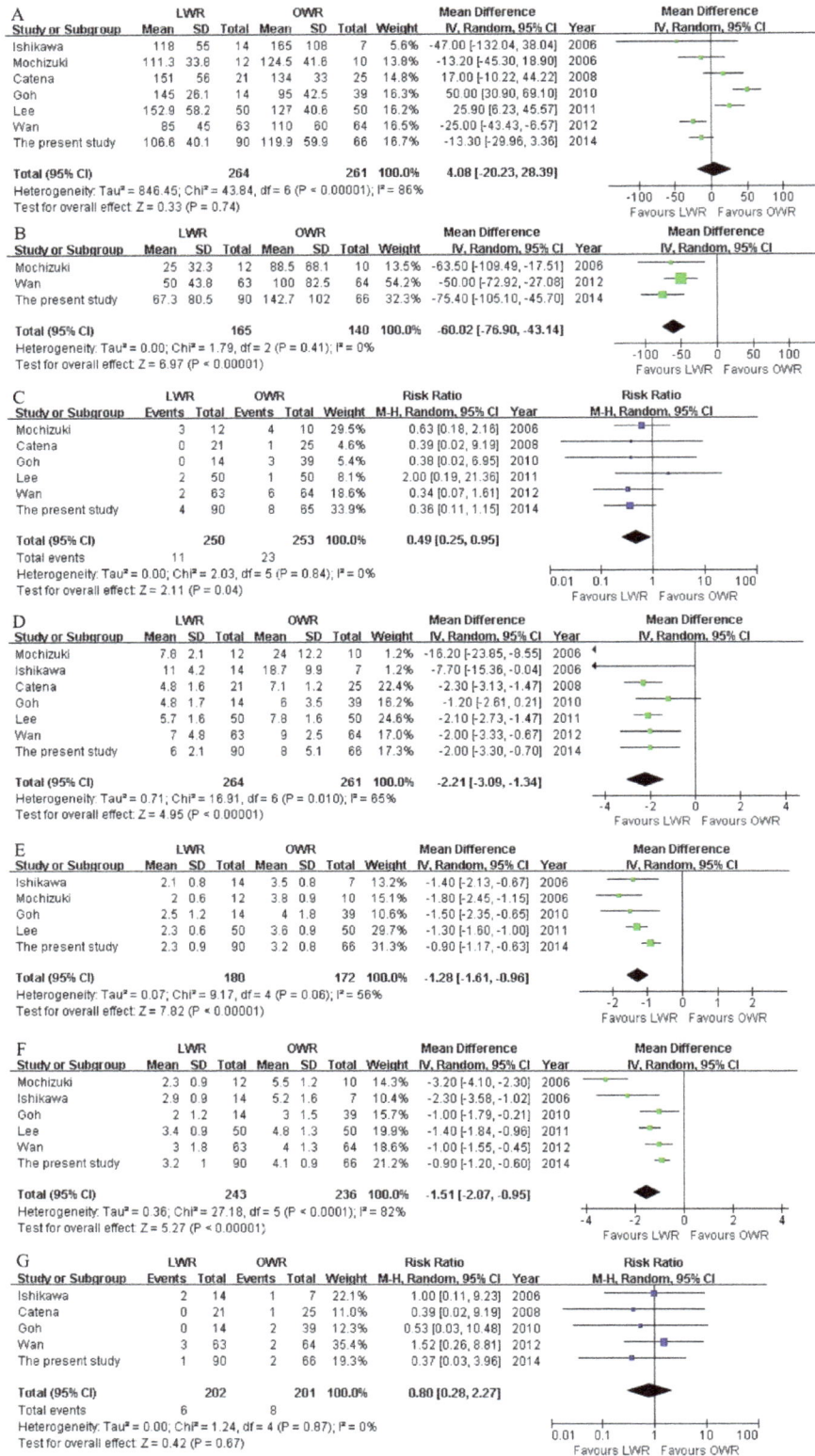

Figure 3 Meta-analysis of the pooled data. **(A)** Operative time. **(B)** Intraoperative blood loss. **(C)** Overall complications. **(D)** Postoperative hospital stay. **(E)** First flatus. **(F)** Oral intake. **(G)** recurrences.

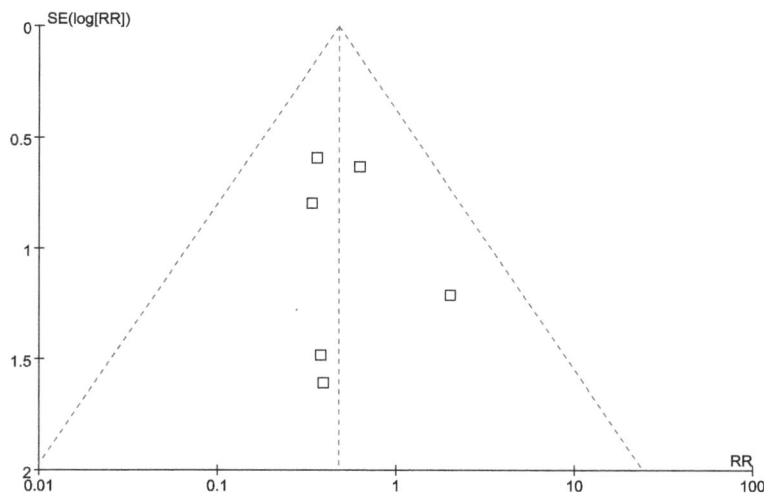

Figure 4 Funnel plot of the overall postoperative complications.

the role of laparoscopic surgery in resection of GISTs of the stomach should be clarified. Long-term survival remain critical for all patients with GISTs regardless of a benign or malignant designation since these tumors have an uncertain biologic behavior. It is widely accepted that the tumor size and mitotic index are two key factors on GISTs long-term outcomes. Several recent reports have also detailed recurrence rates of patients with gastric GISTs after laparoscopic surgery ranging from 4.8 to 18% [11,26,29,54,55]. In our study, LWR group had a lower recurrence rate (1.1%) compared to previous reports. This result was mainly due to most of patients in LWR group with tumors at very low, or low malignant risk (73.1%), whose recurrence may be delayed for as long as 10 years [56]. Moreover, in our center patients with tumors at moderate, or high malignant risk are routinely recommended to continue treatment with imatinib after surgery, which can effectively improved recurrence-free survival and overall survival of GIST patients with a high risk of GIST recurrence [57,58]. Despite the fact that tumor size of OWR group was larger than LWR group, two groups were comparable with no significant difference according to Fletcher's criteria. Our series demonstrates the oncologic safety of the laparoscopic approach, with efficacy and recurrence rates similar to open surgical controls. All the tumor-recurrent cases in our study developed recurrence in 2 years after surgery, once more proving that most of the GISTs recurrence occurs within the first 2 years after surgery [3,11,59].

As nonadenocarcinomas in the stomach are uncommon, the sample of 156 patients is considered large. But it is still small for definitive conclusions on the safety and effectiveness of LWR. Thus, our rapid systematic review and meta-analysis synthesized the existing observational studies with strictly limiting inclusion and exclusion criteria. The included studies were primarily derived from the countries with the most widespread use of laparoscopic gastrectomy (two from Japan, one from Korea, one from China, one from Singapore, and one from Italy), and the total number of cases incorporated in the study was 525. The larger the number of patients in a meta-analysis, the greater its power to detect a possible treatment effect. Therefore, our comprehensive meta-analysis will contribute to a more systematic and objective evaluation for the safety and effectiveness of LWR.

There are some limitations to our study. The major bias was derived from retrospective nature and lack of prospectively defined inclusion criteria for those undergoing LWR. Also, the majority of cases in our study are in the past 3 years, which is short for the low risk GISTs to develop recurrence, and the follow up will continue. Although the meta-analysis confirmed the mini-invasive benefits of LWR and the similar postoperative and oncological outcomes between LWR and OWR, the simple size of some articles included was quite small and there was no prospective or randomized study that can markedly undermine the strength of the analysis. Our results should be confirmed by further randomized controlled trials that compare the open versus laparoscopic approach for the treatment GISTs.

Conclusions
This study demonstrates laparoscopic wedge resection is a technically and oncologically safe and feasible approach for GISTs compared with open wedge resection. Moreover, laparoscopic wedge resection appears to be a preferable choice with mini-invasive benefits based on our data and a rapid systematic review with a meta-analysis.

Abbreviations

LWR: Laparoscopic wedge resection; OWR: Open wedge resection; GISTs: Gastrointestinal stromal tumors; RR: Risk ratio; WMD: Weighted mean differences; CI: Confidence intervals; NOS: Newcastle-Ottawa Quality Assessment Scale; SD: Standard deviation; RFS: Relapse-free survival; HPFs: High-power fields; SMA: Smooth muscle actin; BMI: Body mass index.

Competing interests

The authors declare that they have no competing interests.

Authors' contributions

CJQ designed the study; CK, XXW and MYP performed the operation; ZYC, CJQ and HCJ collected literatures and conducted the analysis of pooled data; CJQ, CK and PY wrote the manuscript; MYP proofread and revised the manuscript; all authors have approved the version to be published.

Acknowledgements

This study was supported by Zhejiang Key Subject of Medical Science Foundation (grant No.11-CX-21).

References

1. Miettinen M, Majidi M, Lasota J. Pathology and diagnostic criteria of gastrointestinal stromal tumors (GISTs): a review. Eur J Cancer. 2002;38 Suppl 5:S39–51.
2. Demetri GD, von Mehren M, Antonescu CR, DeMatteo RP, Ganjoo KN, Maki RG, et al. NCCN Task Force report: update on the management of patients with gastrointestinal stromal tumors. J Natl Compr Canc Netw. 2010;8 Suppl 2:S1–41.
3. DeMatteo RP, Lewis JJ, Leung D, Mudan SS, Woodruff JM, Brennan MF. Two hundred gastrointestinal stromal tumors: recurrence patterns and prognostic factors for survival. Ann Surg. 2000;231:51–8.
4. Rutkowski P, Wozniak A, Dębiec-Rychter M, Kąkol M, Dziewirski W, Zdzienicki M, et al. Clinical utility of the new American Joint Committee on Cancer staging system for gastrointestinal stromal tumors: current overall survival after primary tumor resection. Cancer. 2011;117:4916–24.
5. Lee CH, Hyun MH, Kwon YJ, Cho SI, Park SS. Deciding laparoscopic approaches for wedge resection in gastric submucosal tumors: a suggestive flow chart using three major determinants. J Am Coll Surg. 2012;215:831–40.
6. Xu X, Chen K, Zhou W, Zhang R, Wang J, Wu D, et al. Laparoscopic transgastric resection of gastric submucosal tumors located near the esophagogastric junction. J Gastrointest Surg. 2013;17:1570–5.
7. Kang WM, Yu JC, Ma ZQ, Zhao ZR, Meng QB, Ye X. Laparoscopic-endoscopic cooperative surgery for gastric submucosal tumors. World J Gastroenterol. 2013;19:5720–6.
8. Valle M, Federici O, Carboni F, Carpano S, Benedetti M, Garofalo A. Gastrointestinal stromal tumors of the stomach: the role of laparoscopic resection: single-centre experience of 38 cases. Surg Endosc. 2014;28:1040–7.
9. Matthews BD, Walsh RM, Kercher KW, Sing RF, Pratt BL, Answini GA, et al. Laparoscopic vs open resection of gastric stromal tumors. Surg Endosc. 2002;16:803–7.
10. Cuschieri A. Laparoscopic gastric resection. Surg Clin North Am. 2000;80:1269–84.
11. Novitsky YW, Kercher KW, Sing RF, Heniford BT. Long-term outcomes of laparoscopic resection of gastric gastrointestinal stromal tumors. Ann Surg. 2006;243:738–47.
12. Fletcher CD, Berman JJ, Corless C, Gorstein F, Lasota J, Longley BJ, et al. Diagnosis of gastrointestinal stromal tumors: a consensus approach. Int J Surg Pathol. 2002;10:81–9.
13. Stroup DF, Berlin JA, Morton SC, Olkin I, Williamson GD, Rennie D, et al. Meta-analysis of observational studies in epidemiology: a proposal for reporting. JAMA. 2000;283:2008–12.
14. Clarke M, Horton R. Bringing it all together: Lancet-Cochrane collaborate on systematic reviews. Lancet. 2001;357:1728.
15. Hozo SP, Djulbegovic B, Hozo I. Estimating the mean and variance from the median, range, and the size of a sample. BMC Med Res Methodol. 2005;5:13.
16. Basu S, Balaji S, Bennett DH, Davies N. Gastrointestinal stromal tumors (GIST) and laparoscopic resection. Surg Endosc. 2007;21:1685–9.

17. Chen YH, Liu KH, Yeh CN, Hsu JT, Liu YY, Tsai CY, et al. Laparoscopic resection of gastrointestinal stromal tumors: safe, efficient, and comparable oncologic outcomes. J Laparoendosc Adv Surg Tech A. 2012;22:758–63.
18. Nishimura J, Nakajima K, Omori T, Takahashi T, Nishitani A, Ito T, et al. Surgical strategy for gastric gastrointestinal stromal tumors: laparoscopic vs. open resection. Surg Endosc. 2007;21:875–8.
19. Pitsinis V, Khan AZ, Cranshaw I, Allum WH. Single center experience of laparoscopic vs. open resection for gastrointestinal stromal tumors of the stomach. Hepatogastroenterol. 2007;54:606–8.
20. Silberhumer GR, Hufschmid M, Wrba F, Gyoeri G, Schoppmann S, Tribl B, et al. Surgery for gastrointestinal stromal tumors of the stomach. J Gastrointest Surg. 2009;13:1213–9.
21. Wu JM, Yang CY, Wang MY, Wu MH, Lin MT. Gasless laparoscopy-assisted versus open resection for gastrointestinal stromal tumors of the upper stomach: preliminary results. J Laparoendosc Adv Surg Tech A. 2010;20:725–9.
22. De Vogelaere K, Hoorens A, Haentjens P, Delvaux G. Laparoscopic versus open resection of gastrointestinal stromal tumors of the stomach. Surg Endosc. 2013;27:1546–54.
23. Pucci MJ, Berger AC, Lim PW, Chojnacki KA, Rosato EL, Palazzo F. Laparoscopic approaches to gastric gastrointestinal stromal tumors: an institutional review of 57 cases. Surg Endosc. 2012;26:3509–14.
24. Lee PC, Lai PS, Yang CY, Chen CN, Lai IR, Lin MT. A gasless laparoscopic technique of wide excision for gastric gastrointestinal stromal tumor versus open method. World J Surg Oncol. 2013;11:44.
25. Shu ZB, Sun LB, Li JP, Li YC, Ding DY. Laparoscopic versus open resection of gastric gastrointestinal stromal tumors. Chin J Cancer Res. 2013;25:175–82.
26. Kim KH, Kim MC, Jung GJ, Kim SJ, Jang JS, Kwon HC. Long term survival results for gastric GIST: is laparoscopic surgery for large gastric GIST feasible? World J Surg Oncol. 2012;10:230.
27. Karakousis GC, Singer S, Zheng J, Gonen M, Coit D, DeMatteo RP, et al. Laparoscopic versus open gastric resections for primary gastrointestinal stromal tumors (GISTs): a size-matched comparison. Ann Surg Oncol. 2011;18:1599–605.
28. Melstrom LG, Phillips JD, Bentrem DJ, Wayne JD. Laparoscopic versus open resection of gastric gastrointestinal stromal tumors. Am J Clin Oncol. 2012;35:451–4.
29. Ishikawa K, Inomata M, Etoh T, Shiromizu A, Shiraishi N, Arita T, et al. Long-term outcome of laparoscopic wedge resection for gastric submucosal tumor compared with open wedge resection. Surg Laparosc Endosc Percutan Tech. 2006;16:82–5.
30. Mochizuki Y, Kodera Y, Fujiwara M, Ito S, Yamamura Y, Sawaki A, et al. Laparoscopic wedge resection for gastrointestinal stromal tumors of the stomach: initial experience. Surg Today. 2006;36:341–7.
31. Catena F, Di Battista M, Fusaroli P, Ansaloni L, Di Scioscio V, Santini D, et al. Laparoscopic treatment of gastric GIST: report of 21 cases and literature's review. J Gastrointest Surg. 2008;12:561–8.
32. Goh BK, Chow PK, Chok AY, Chan WH, Chung YF, Ong HS, et al. Impact of the introduction of laparoscopic wedge resection as a surgical option for suspected small/medium-sized gastrointestinal stromal tumors of the stomach on perioperative and oncologic outcomes. World J Surg. 2010;34:1847–52.
33. Lee HH, Hur H, Jung H, Park CH, Jeon HM, Song KY. Laparoscopic wedge resection for gastric submucosal tumors: a size-location matched case-control study. J Am Coll Surg. 2011;212:195–9.
34. Wan P, Yan C, Li C, Yan M, Zhu ZG. Choices of surgical approaches for gastrointestinal stromal tumors of the stomach: laparoscopic versus open resection. Dig Surg. 2012;29:243–50.
35. Bédard EL, Mamazza J, Schlachta CM, Poulin EC. Laparoscopic resection of gastrointestinal stromal tumors: not all tumors are created equal. Surg Endosc. 2006;20:500–3.
36. Sexton JA, Pierce RA, Halpin VJ, Eagon JC, Hawkins WG, Linehan DC, et al. Laparoscopic gastric resection for gastrointestinal stromal tumors. Surg Endosc. 2008;22:2583–7.
37. Chen K, Xu XW, Zhang RC, Pan Y, Wu D, Mou YP. Systematic review and meta-analysis of laparoscopy-assisted and open total gastrectomy for gastric cancer. World J Gastroenterol. 2013;19:5365–76.
38. Law WL, Lee YM, Choi HK, Seto CL, Ho JW. Impact of laparoscopic resection for colorectal cancer on operative outcomes and survival. Ann Surg. 2007;245:1–7.
39. Ito K, Ito H, Are C, Allen PJ, Fong Y, DeMatteo RP, et al. Laparoscopic versus open liver resection: a matched-pair case control study. J Gastrointest Surg. 2009;13:2276–83.

40. Teh SH, Tseng D, Sheppard BC. Laparoscopic and open distal pancreatic resection for benign pancreatic disease. J Gastrointest Surg. 2007;11:1120–5.

41. Xie K, Zhu YP, Xu XW, Chen K, Yan JF, Mou YP. Laparoscopic distal pancreatectomy is as safe and feasible as open procedure: a meta-analysis. World J Gastroenterol. 2012;18:1959–67.

42. Kercher KW, Heniford BT, Matthews BD, Smith TI, Lincourt AE, Hayes DH, et al. Laparoscopic versus open nephrectomy in 210 consecutive patients: outcomes, cost, and changes in practice patterns. Surg Endosc. 2003;17:1889–95.

43. Lee JS, Kim JJ, Park SM. Totally laparoscopic resection for a large gastrointestinal stromal tumor of stomach. J Gastric Cancer. 2011;11:239–42.

44. Jeong IH, Kim JH, Lee SR, Kim JH, Hwang JC, Shin SJ, et al. Minimally invasive treatment of gastric gastrointestinal stromal tumors: laparoscopic and endoscopic approach. Surg Laparosc Endosc Percutan Tech. 2012;22:244–50.

45. De Vogelaere K, Van Loo I, Peters O, Hoorens A, Haentjens P, Delvaux G. Laparoscopic resection of gastric gastrointestinal stromal tumors (GIST) is safe and effective, irrespective of tumor size. Surg Endosc. 2012;26:2339–45.

46. Tagaya N, Mikami H, Kubota K. Laparoscopic resection of gastrointestinal mesenchymal tumors located in the upper stomach. Surg Endosc. 2004;18:1469–74.

47. Ng EH, Pollock RE, Munsell MF, Atkinson EN, Romsdahl MM. Prognostic factors influencing survival in gastrointestinal leiomyosarcomas: implications for surgical management and staging. Ann Surg. 1992;215:68–77.

48. Clinical Outcomes of Surgical Therapy Study Group. A comparison of laparoscopically assisted and open colectomy for colon cancer. N Engl J Med. 2004;350:2050–9.

49. Kitano S, Shiraishi N, Uyama I, Sugihara K, Tanigawa N, Japanese Laparoscopic Surgery Study Group. A multicenter study on oncologic outcome of laparoscopic gastrectomy for early cancer in Japan. Ann Surg. 2007;245:68–72.

50. Pak KH, Hyung WJ, Son T, Obama K, Woo Y, Kim HI, et al. Long-term oncologic outcomes of 714 consecutive laparoscopic gastrectomies for gastric cancer: results from the 7-year experience of a single institute. Surg Endosc. 2012;26:130–6.

51. Chen K, Xu XW, Mou YP, Pan Y, Zhou YC, Zhang RC, et al. Systematic review and meta-analysis of laparoscopic and open gastrectomy for advanced gastric cancer. World J Surg Oncol. 2013;11:182.

52. Wang W, Chen K, Xu XW, Pan Y, Mou YP. Case-matched comparison of laparoscopy-assisted and open distal gastrectomy for gastric cancer. World J Gastroenterol. 2013;19:3672–7.

53. Singh RK, Pham TH, Diggs BS, Perkins S, Hunter JG. Minimally invasive esophagectomy provides equivalent oncologic outcomes to open esophagectomy for locally advanced (stage II or III) esophageal carcinoma. Arch Surg. 2011;146:711–4.

54. Amin AT, Kono Y, Shiraishi N, Yasuda K, Inomata M, Kitano S. Long-term outcomes of laparoscopic wedge resection for gastrointestinal stromal tumors of the stomach of less than 5 cm in diameter. Surg Laparosc Endosc Percutan Tech. 2011;21:260–3.

55. Matsuhashi N, Osada S, Yamaguchi K, Okumura N, Tanaka Y, Imai H, et al. Long-term outcomes of treatment of gastric gastrointestinal stromal tumor by laparoscopic surgery. Hepatogastroenterol. 2013;60:2011–5.

56. Pidhorecky I, Cheney RT, Kraybill WG, Gibbs JF. Gastrointestinal stromal tumors: current diagnosis, biologic behavior, and management. Ann Surg Oncol. 2000;7:705–12.

57. Joensuu H, Eriksson M, Sundby Hall K, Hartmann JT, Pink D, Schütte J, et al. One vs three years of adjuvant imatinib for operable gastrointestinal stromal tumor: a randomized trial. JAMA. 2012;307:1265–72.

58. Dematteo RP, Ballman KV, Antonescu CR, Maki RG, Pisters PW, Demetri GD, et al. Adjuvant imatinib mesylate after resection of localised, primary gastrointestinal stromal tumour: a randomised, double-blind, placebo-controlled trial. Lancet. 2009;373:1097–104.

59. Nowain A, Bhakta H, Pais S, Kanel G, Verma S. Gastrointestinal stromal tumors: clinical profile, pathogenesis, treatment strategies and prognosis. J Gastroenterol Hepatol. 2005;20:818–24.

18

Risk factors for lymph node metastasis in early gastric cancer patients: Report from Eastern Europe country– Lithuania

Rimantas Bausys[1,2], Augustinas Bausys[1,2*], Indre Vysniauskaite[3], Kazimieras Maneikis[2], Dalius Klimas[2], Martynas Luksta[4], Kestutis Strupas[2,4] and Eugenijus Stratilatovas[1,2]

Abstract

Background: Current risk factors for lymph node metastasis in early gastric cancer have been primarily determined in Asian countries; however their applicability to Western nations is under discussion. The aim of our study was to identify risk factors associated with lymph node metastasis in Western cohort patients from the Eastern European country - Lithuania.

Methods: A total of 218 patients who underwent open gastrectomy for early gastric cancer were included in this retrospective study. After histolopathological examination, risk factors for lymph node metastasis were evaluated. Overall survival was evaluated and factors associated with long-term outcomes were analyzed.

Results: Lymph node metastases were present in 19.7% of early gastric cancer cases. The rates were 5/99 (4.95%) for pT1a tumors and 38/119 (31.9%) for pT1b tumors. Submucosal tumor invasion, lymphovascular invasion, and high grade tumor differentiation were identified as independent risk factors for lymph node metastasis. Submucosal tumor invasion and lymphovascular invasion were also associated with worse 5-year survival results.

Conclusion: Our study established submucosal tumor invasion, lymphovascular invasion, and high grade tumor differentiation as risk factors for lymph node metastasis.

Keywords: Early gastric cancer, Lymph node metastasis, Risk factors, Mucosal tumor, T1a

Background

Gastric cancer is one of the leading causes of cancer death worldwide. It is believed that early detection and appropriate treatment can reduce mortality caused by gastric cancer. After the detection of cancer, preoperative disease staging must be performed to plan an ideal treatment for each individual patient. Next, the absence or presence of lymph node metastasis (LNM) must be confirmed to apply the treatment strategy. Lymph node status has great significance to the path of care chosen in early gastric cancer (EGC). It is not only important for proper treatment, but also for the prognosis of survival [1, 2]. Additionally, confirmation of LNM is crucial

when an endoscopic approach is considered, because such a procedure does not cure the disease in lymph nodes. One obstacle in determining lymph node status has been the uncertainty of radiological tests. Staging of gastric cancer typically utilizes a variety of imaging modalities, such as computed tomography (CT), magnetic resonance imaging (MRI), endoscopic ultrasounds and combined positron tomography, as well as, laparoscopic staging and cytogenetic analysis of peritoneal fluid in appropriate patients [3, 4]. The evaluation of metastatic infiltration of lymph nodes is mostly based on CT and MRI imaging. However, neither have the correct high sensitivity and specificity for the detection of LNM in gastric cancer [5, 6]. The lack of accurate radiological imaging calls for research of risk factors for LNM in EGC, which are used when endoscopic treatments of EGC are considered. According to the European Society for Medical Oncology (ESMO) guidelines, gastric

* Correspondence: abpelikanas@gmail.com
[1]Department of Abdominal Surgery and Oncology, National Cancer Institute, Santariskiu str. 1, Vilnius 08660, Lithuania
[2]Faculty of Medicine, Vilnius University, Ciurlionio str. 21, Vilnius 03101, Lithuania
Full list of author information is available at the end of the article

adenocarcinomas staged as T1a, well-differentiated, less than 2 cm diameter and not ulcerated have very low or no risks for LNM. Those that fall under such standard criteria are eligible for endoscopic mucosal resection (EMR)/ endoscopic submucosal dissection (ESD) [7–10]. These guidelines are based on known risk factors for LNM, which have been determined in Asia. However, recently published data has revealed race as an independent risk factor for LNM, raising concern whether such risk factors can be considered in Western countries [11, 12].

The aim of our study was to integrate our experience of treating early gastric cancer with open gastrectomy to identify risk factors for LNM in EGC in Western populations.

Methods

This retrospective study included 218 patients who underwent surgical treatment for EGC in the Department of General and Abdominal Surgery and Oncology, National Cancer Institute, Vilnius, Lithuania between January 2005 and December 2015. In total, 1654 patients with gastric adenocarcinoma were operated on at the institution during the study period. 1436 (86,8%) patients underwent surgery for advanced gastric cancer and 218 (13,2%) for EGC.EGC was defined as a cancer that does not invade past the submucosa, irrespective of regional lymph node metastasis (T1 any N). None of the patients received neoadjuvant chemotherapy or radiotherapy prior to surgery. All patients had morphological gastric cancer verification before surgery, except in a few cases when it was not possible due to technical feasibility. Depending on cancer localization in the stomach and histological characteristics of the tumor, the type of surgery - total or subtotal gastrectomy- was determined before the operation. Reconstruction after a total gastrectomy was performed with esophagojejunostomy using a jejunal loop and Braun's side-to-side enteroanastomosis (m.Omega). Reconstruction after subtotal gastrectomy consisted of an antecolic end-to-side gastrojejunostomy with Braun's jejunojejunostomy (m.Balfur).The standard lymphanodectomy in our institution was a D2 lymph node dissection and was performed in accordance with the guidelines of the Japanese Research Society for Gastric Cancer. D1 lymphanodectomy was an alternative option based on the surgeon's individual decision. R0 resection was defined as no tumor remaining macroscopically and microscopically, and was achieved in all cases. Specimens' histological examination was performed in the National Center of Pathology, Vilnius, Lithuania. Standard histological examination protocol included entire lesion examination with 5 mm wide slices. All of the dissected lymph nodes were analyzed, each lymph node was

embedded in paraffin, and at least two sections were prepared and visualized. Immunohistochemistry was performed using an anti-podoplanin antibody (D2–40) and CD34 antibody to identify and distinguish the lymphatic endothelium. The rate of LNM was calculated after histological evaluation. Various clinicopathological parameters such as gender, age, primary tumor invasion, tumor differentiation grade, lymphatic and vascular invasion, tumor type according to Lauren classification, ulceration, tumor size and localization were evaluated as possible risk factors for LNM. Analysis of postoperative morbidity and intra-hospital 30- and 90-day mortality rates were performed. Surgical complications were classified by Clavien-Dindo classification.

Outcomes of interest included the overall survival (OS) rates. OS was defined as the duration from the date of surgery to the date of death. Data on survival and death were obtained from Lithuania's Cancer register and Lithuania's death register. The date of the last follow up was 31 December 2016. 6 (2.7%) patients were lost during the follow-up period. Mean and median follow-up periods were 68 and 63 months (range from 0 to 142) respectively.

Statistical analysis

All statistical analyses were conducted using the statistical program SPSS 16.0 (SPSS, Chicago, IL, USA). Clinicopathological characteristics were analyzed by a 2-tailed t test, one-way ANOVA test, Chi-square test, or Fisher exact test. The risk factors found to be significant in univariate analysis were included in subsequent multivariate logistic regression analyses to identify the independent variables associated with lymph node metastasis in patients with gastric cancer. Overall survival was analyzed by the Kaplan–Meier method, and the curves drawn were compared by the log-rank test. Multivariate survival analysis was performed using the Cox proportional-hazards model (hazard ratio and 95% confidence intervals). In all statistical analyses, a p value of <0.05 was considered to be significant.

Results

From January 2005 to December 2015, 218 patients undergoing total or subtotal gastrectomy for EGC were included in this study. All of the patients were of Caucasoid race. Baseline characteristics of all patients are shown in Table 1.

There were 117 (53.7%) men and 101 (46.3%) women, with a mean age of 65.58 ± 12.33 years. Total gastrectomy was performed in 38 cases and subtotal gastrectomy in 180 cases. Forty-five of 220 patients had postoperative complications, with four of them lethal. Postoperative mortality and morbidity rates were 1.8 and

Table 1 Baseline characteristics of all patients

Variable		
Age (mean ± SD, range) (min.-max. Years)		65.58 ± 12.33 (27–88)
BMI (mean ± SD, range) (kg/m²)		26.31 ± 5.41
Count of retrieved lymph nodes (mean ± SD, range) (min.-max.)		19.89 ± 9.69 (3–70)
Gender	Male	117 (53.7%)
	Female	101 (46.3%)
ASA score	I	23 (10.6%)
	II	105 (48.2%)
	III	87 (39.9%)
	IV	3 (1.4%)
Tumor localization	Lower third	79 (36.2%)
	Middle third	125 (57.3%)
	Upper third	14 (6.4%)
Tumor invasion	Mucosal	99 (45.4%)
	Sub-mucosal	119 (54.6%)
Lymph node status	Positive	43 (19.7%)
	Negative	175 (80.3%)
Tumor differentiation grade	G1	44 (20.2%)
	G2	70 (32.1%)
	G3	104 (47.7%)
Type of surgery	Total gastrectomy	38 (17.4%)
	Subtotal gastrectomy	180 (82.6%)
Type of lymphanodectomy	D1	23 (10.6%)
	D2	195 (89.4%)

20.6% respectively. The vast majority of complications (29 of 45, 64.4%) were not life threatening and did not require any surgical, endoscopic, or radiological interventions. According to Clavien-Dindo classification they were either grade I or II complications. Grade III complications occurred in 8 cases (3.6%), and reoperation was indicated for 5 (2.3%) patients. Complications requiring intensive care unit management (grade IV) were rare – 4 cases (1.8%). Four patients (1.8%) died during the intra-hospital period after postoperative complications had occurred. Causes of death for these patients were as follows. One patient had anastomotic leakage and peritonitis, while three patients died from nonsurgical complications: pulmonary embolism – 1 case, pneumonia and sepsis - 1 case and acute cardiovascular insufficiency – 1 case. Mean hospitalization time was 17.34 ± 5.90 days and mean postoperative period was 13.00 ± 5.39 days. 30 day mortality rates were higher when compared to intra-hospital mortality rates and involved 6 (2,8%) cases. Three additional deaths were registered between the 31st and 90th postoperative day. 90 day postoperative mortality rates reached 4.1%.

Higher 90 days mortality rates were associated with elderly age (≥75 years; 12.5% vs 1.2%, $p = 0.010$). Other factors such as gender, smoking status, obesity (BMI > 30), ASA score, extent of lymphanodectomy, type of surgery, and tumor localization did not impact mortality rate, $p > 0.05$.

Majority of the patients underwent a D2 lymphadenectomy – 195 (89.4%). The average number of removed lymph nodes was 19.89 ± 9.69. After performing histological examination of operative material, LNM were revealed in 43 (19.7%) cases. Factors associated with LNM were evaluated by univariate analysis. There was a significantly higher risk for LNM in tumors with submucosal layer infiltration (compared to mucosal infiltration, $p = 0.001$), lymphovascular invasion (LV+ vs LV-, $p = 0.001$), high grade differentiation (G3 vs G1&G2, $p = 0.047$), diffuse or mix type according to Lauren classification (compared to intestinal type, $p = 0.012$), and diameter exceeding 2 cm (compared to tumors ≤ 2 cm, $p = 0.026$). Age, gender, tumor localization, ulceration, and signet ring cell carcinoma had no significance in the presence of LNM (Table 2).

The multivariate analysis showed that submucosal tumor invasion, lymphovascular invasion, and high tumor differentiation grade were independent risk factors for lymph node metastasis (Table 3).

Survival analysis

5-year overall survival was 83.3% in patients without LNM and 54.2% in patients with LNM, $p = 0.001$ (Fig. 1). In the univariate analysis, LNM (p = 0.001), higher ASA classification (ASA III/IV p = 0.001), D1 lymphanodectomy ($p = 0.049$), and lymphovascular invasion (p = 0.001) had a negative effect on 5-year survival (Fig. 2). In multivariate analysis, lymphovascular invasion ($p = 0.028$; HR 2.19; 95% CI 1.08–4.42) and age ($p = 0.020$; HR 1.04; 95% CI 1.01–1.08) were discovered as independent factors with negative influences on the postoperative overall survival rate.

Discussion

The definition of EGC was established by the Japanese Gastroenterological Endoscopic Society in 1962, originally characterizing EGC as gastric cancer that invades no deeper than the submucosa regardless of lymph node metastasis. EGC is more commonly diagnosed in Asia compared with Western countries. In Japan, EGC comprises approximately 60% of all diagnosed gastric cancers, whereas in Western countries the incidence of EGC varies from 10% to 20%. Such differences could be explained by the presence of more screening programs in Asian countries and also by different interpretations of histological changes. Western pathologists consider

Table 2 Clinicopathological data of patients with EGC and univariate analysis of risk factors for lymph node metastasis

		LNM-	LNM+	p	Odds ratio (95% CI)
Gender	Male	99 (84.6%)	18 (15.4%)	p = 0.090	1.80 (0.92–3.55)
	Female	76 (75.2%)	25 (24.8%)		
Age		65.26 ± 12.17	66.91 ± 13.03	p = 0.433	–
Tumor localization	Lower 1/3	62 (78.5%)	17 (21.5%)	p = 0.457	–
	Middle1/3	100 (80.0%)	25 (20.0%)		
	Upper 1/3	13 (92.9%)	1 (7.1%)		
Tumor invasion	T1a	94 (94.9%)	5 (5.1%)	p = 0.001	8.82 (3.31–23.46)
	T1b	81 (68.1%)	38 (31.9%)		
Tumor differentiation	G1 & G2	100 (87.7%)	14 (12.3%)	p = 0.006	2.76 (1.36–8.57)
	G3	75 (72.1%)	29 (22.4%)		
Lymphovascular invasion	LV+	12 (40%)	18 (60%)	p = 0.001	9.78 (4.20–22.72)
	LV-	163 (86.7%)	25 (13.3%)		
Lauren classification	Diffuse & mix	59 (71.1%)	24 (28.9%)	p = 0.012	2.09 (1.20–3.64)
	Intestinal	106 (86.2%)	17 (13.8%)		
Tumor size	≤2 cm	91 (86.7%)	14 (13.3%)	p = 0.026	2.27 (1.12–4.59)
	>2 cm	83 (74.1%)	29 (25.9%)		
Ulceration	Ulcerated	58 (74.4%)	20 (25.6%)	p = 0.114	1.73 (0.88–3.42)
	Non-ulcerated	116 (83.5%	23 (16.5%)		
Signet ring cell	Yes	11 (73.3%)	4 (26.7%)	p = 0.513	1.46 (0.44–4.86)
	No	149 (80.1%)	37 (19.9%)		

invasion into the lamina propria of the mucosa mandatory characteristics for the diagnosis of carcinoma, whereas nuclear and structural features are more important in Japan. Therefore, EGC lesions diagnosed in Japan are potentially diagnosed as high grade dysplasia in Western countries. This distinction could partly explain the higher incidence of EGC in the Asian population and be responsible for better patient prognoses when compared to Western counterparts [11]. Several studies in Asian countries have declared excellent 5-year survival rates for EGC patients with overall survival exceeding 90%. Comparatively, our study presents worse results with the 5-year overall survival rate reaching only 77,6%. Since there is a disparity in histological

Table 3 Multivariate analysis of risk factors for lymph node metastasis

Factor	p value	Odds Ratio (95% CI)
Submucosal tumor invasion (T1b)	p = 0.001	6.55 (2.28–18.81)
Tumor differentiation grade G3	p = 0.045	2.01 (1.03–14.66)
Lymphovascular invasion	p = 0.001	6.06 (2.28–16.07)
Tumor size >2 cm	p = 0.155	1.82 (0.79–4.19)
Diffuse type according to Lauren classification	p = 0.693	1.29 (0.35–4.69)

interpretations and a difference in average life expectancy amongst distinct regions, it is difficult to compare data of several studies using the same statistical indicators [2, 13]. Disagreement between Asian and Western interpretations of pre-cancerous lesions and EGC could also influence results of studies analyzing risk factors and rate of LNM in EGC patients. During the last 5 years, 17 studies investigating factors associated with LNM in EGC were published. Eleven studies came from Asian countries and six from Western countries (Table 4).

Rates of LNM reported in various Asian and Western countries were varying. In Asia LNM rates ranged from 2.8% to 15.5% for patients with tumors invading only the mucosal layer [14, 15] and from 18.3% to 56.2% for patients with tumors invading the submucosal layer [16, 17]. Respectively, in Western countries, rates of LNM varied from 1.9% to 16.7% when the tumor was localized to the mucosa and from 18.2% to 42.9% when the tumor invaded the submucosal layer [17, 18]. Our study results were similar; rates of LNM for patients with T1a and T1b cancer were 5.1 and 22.4%, respectively. Risk factors for LNM determined in various studies were also differing. In Asian studies, the most frequently mentioned factors were depth of invasion (9 of 11 studies), tumor size (7 of 11 studies), and lymphatic or lymphovascular invasion (7 of 11 studies). In Western studies, lymphovascular invasion has been of recent focus in five of six studies with our

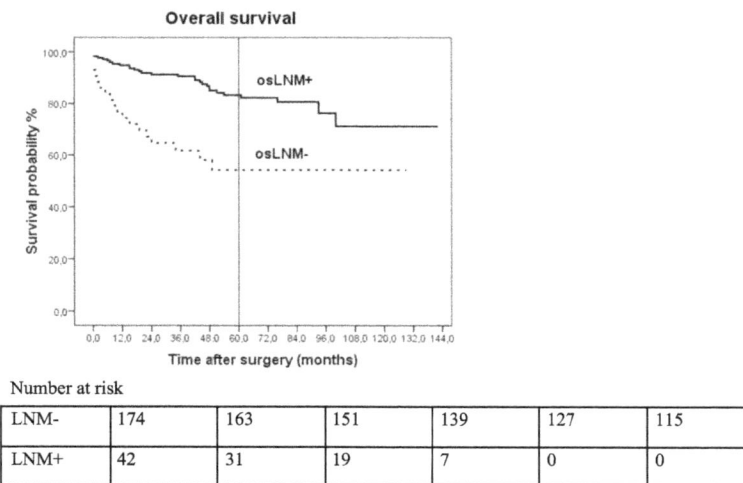

Fig. 1 Five-year overall survival rate of patients with EGC according to lymph node status

results also confirming lymphovascular invasion as a risk factor for LNM. Another risk factor which was studied in our data, submucosal tumor invasion, was mentioned in 3 of 6 previously published Western studies. Tumor differentiation was only mentioned as a risk factor for LMN in reports from Asian nations [15, 17, 19]. To our best knowledge, our study is the first report of Western countries which confirms tumor differentiation as an independent risk factor for LNM. Despite the discussed variation between Asian and Western regions, the use of EMR/ESD as a treatment option for ECG is increasing in the West [8]. Western guidelines such as the National Comprehensive Cancer Network (NCCN) guidelines for gastric cancer treatment and ESMO clinical practice guidelines recommend the endoscopic approach as an appropriate option for some cases of intramucosal gastric cancer. Indications for endoscopic treatment reported by these guidelines are very similar but display several discrepancies. While both guidelines note that tumor diameter should not exceed 2 cm, only the NCCN guidelines indicate lymphovascular invasion as a required criteria. On the other hand, the ESMO guidelines are more strict on the limits for differentiation grade. They suggest that only well differentiated tumors should be treated endoscopically. NCCN guidelines are more liberal by indicating that both well and moderately-well differentiated tumors can be treated by the endoscopic approach. Additionally, ESMO guidelines limit indications with ulceration criteria and NCCN guidelines do not. In our cohort of patients, 30 (13.7%) of 218 patients would have met the criteria for endoscopical treatment according to NCCN guidelines. 1 (3.13%) of these 30 patients had histologically confirmed LNM. Fewer patients fit ESMO criteria (13 of 218 patients) and none of them had LNM. While LNM risk is low or equal to zero for patients who match standard

endoscopical treatment criteria, implementation of expanded criteria in Western countries has been questioned. Furthermore, suspicions about different tumor behavior have increased after Ikoma et al. and Fukuhara et al. studies recently published that race is a risk factor for lymph node metastasis in gastric cancer [11, 12].

On the other hand, even non-curative endoscopic treatment could lead to satisfactory results. Hatta et al. recently published a large multi-center study, in which they evaluated and compared long term outcomes for patients who underwent non-curative endoscopic treatment of EGC followed by either radical surgery or only follow-up. The study revealed that patients who underwent radical surgery had significantly longer 3- and 5-year overall survival (OS) and disease-specific survival rates (DSS). However, the difference in DSS rates was rather small (99.4% vs. 98.7%) compared to the difference in OS rates (96.7% vs. 84.0%). Estimated rates of recurrence were significantly different, although both were low; 1.3% in the radical surgery group and 3.1% in the follow-up group. Nonetheless, positive results according to DSS and recurrence rates in the follow-up group should be interpreted carefully due to different clinico-pathological backgrounds between the two groups. Some risk factors for LNM (lymphatic invasion or deeper submucosal invasion) were significantly more frequent in the radical surgery group [20]. Furthermore, Nakamura et al. provided a direct correlation between lymphatic infiltration and worse survival [21]. Up to this date, evidence of a correlation between lymphatic invasion and worse survival results have been demonstrated only by studies performed in Asia, with Western studies confirming these findings. Haist et al. analyzed lymphatic invasion and survival result correlation in a Western cohort, however they did not display a significant effect

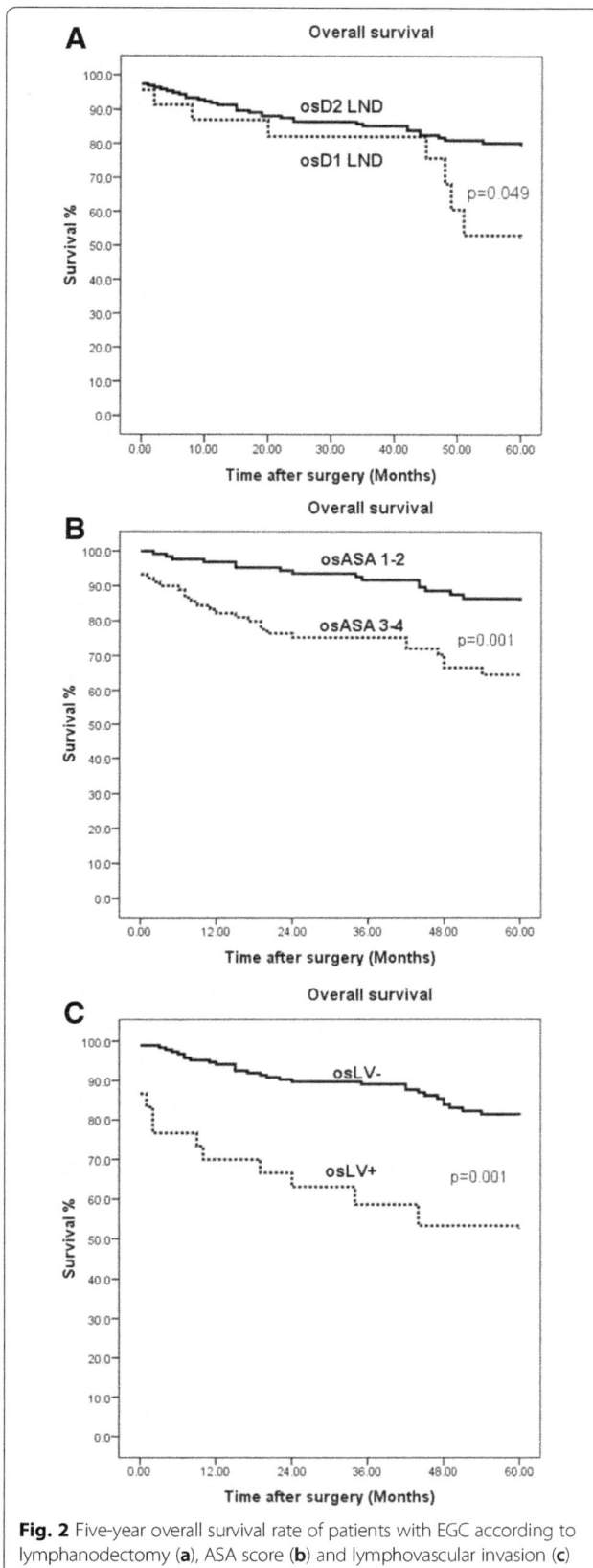

Fig. 2 Five-year overall survival rate of patients with EGC according to lymphanodectomy (**a**), ASA score (**b**) and lymphovascular invasion (**c**)

of lymphatic invasion on longtime survival results [22]. Consequently, our study became the first of such Western reports to present lymphovascular invasion as an independent prognostic factor associated with worse long-term survival results.

Several limitations of our study must be taken into consideration. First, it is a retrospective study originating from a single centre conducted over a long period of time. Second, surgical techniques used were not standardized. Even though the D2 lympahadenectomy remained institutionally standard over the entire study period and the number of examined lymph nodes was sufficient, the extent of resection and confirmation of lymph node removal was not clear in every case. Appropriate lymphadenectomy is important because the risk of lymph node metastasis could be underestimated in cases with incomplete lymphanodectomy. However, we believe that the quality of th obtained histological specimens was accurate and adequate, while the average number of removed lymph nodes was 19.89 ± 9.69. More than 15 lymph nodes were removed for 72% of the patients and only 9% of cases included less than ten dissected lymph nodes. Also, patients with insufficient lymphanodectomy were not excluded from our study to avoid discrepancies as we compared our study results to five other studies from Western countries, where patients with less than 15 examined lymph nodes were included [18, 20, 22–24]. Moreover if only patients with ≥15 resected LN would have been analyzed, the percentage of lymph node metastasis would not be much higher than in the whole series (T1a cancer - 5,1% vs 5,6%, T1b cancer 31,9% vs 36%). Therefore, the entire continuous series was used to avoid selection bias. Third, we were unable to use follow-up records, preventing us from estimating and evaluating recurrence rates, disease free survival and disease specific survival. Fourth, although our study was large enough when compared to other similar Western studies, the absolute number of patients with LNM was still relatively low. This reduces the statistical power of our analyses and the confidence of identifying correct risk factors for LNM.

Conclusion

In our study, LNM occurred in 19,7% of EGC cases. However, depending on varying criteria of several distinct guidelines, the rate of LNM meeting indications for an endoscopic resection was low or equal to zero. Additionally, this study identified submucosal tumor invasion, lympovascular invasion, and high grade tumor differentiation as risk factors for lymph node metastasis. Lymphatic invasion and submucosal tumor invasion were associated with worse 5-year overall survival results. Endoscopical treatment of EGC should be performed within the standard criteria. If risk factors for

Table 4 Lymph node metastasis in early gastric cancer – literature review and our results

Author	Country	Year	No. of patients	LNM+ in T1a cancer patients	LNM+ in T1b cancer patients	Risk factors for LNM
Studies from Asian countries						
Lim MS. et al. [14]	South Korea	2011	376	2.8%	18.4%	T1a: tumor size > 2 cm and lymphovascular invasion T1b: macroscopic type (elevated) and lymphovascular invasion
Ren G. el al. [25]	China	2013	202	9.0%	22.5%	Depth of invasion
Wang L. et al. [26]	China	2013	242	5.5%	20.0%	Depth of invasion, lymphovascular invasion.
Nakagawa M. et al. [27]	South Korea	2015	1042	Not available	Not available	Depth of invasion, tumor size, ulceration, age and positive nodal status by CT.
Wang Y. [16]	China	2015	198	6.0%	56.2%	Depth of invasion. Tumor size. Ulceration. histological type and venous invasion.
Park JH. et al. [28]	South Korea	2015	2270	2.8%	19.0%	Depth of invasion, tumor size >3 cm and lymphovascular invasion
Fang WL. et al. [29]	Taiwan	2015	391	4.9%	21.4%	T1a: Lauren's diffuse type and lymphatic invasion T1b: lymphatic invasion
Zhao LY. et al. [15]	China	2016	687	15.5%	35.9%	Depth of invasion. tumor size > 2 cm, ulceration, lymphovascular invasion, differentiation
Wang YW. et al. [30]	China	2016	230	8.5%	28.6%	Depth of invasion, tumor size ≥ 2 cm and P53 overexpression
Sekiguchi M. et al. [19]	Japan	2016	3131	4.2%	20.2%	Depth of invasion, tumor size ≥ 2 cm, ulceration, lymphovascular invasion, differentiation
Zheng Z. et al. [17]	China	2016	597	3.0%	18.3%	Depth of invasion, ulceration, lymphovascular invasion, age, differentiation.
Studies from Western countries						
Milhomem LM. et al. [31]	Brazil	2012	126	7.8%	22.6%	Depth of invasion, tumor size > 5 cm, ulceration and lymphatic invasion.
Bravo Neto GP. et al. [23]	Brazil	2014	26	16.7%	42.9%	Not available
Fukuhara S. et al. [10]	USA	2014	104	7.1%	35.4%	Lymphovascular invasion, non-Asian race and younger age.
Haist T. et al. [22]	Germany	2016	124	1.9%	22.5%	Depth of invasion, lymphovascular invasion.
Ahmad R. et al. [18]	USA	2016	67	4.3%	31.8%	Lymphovascular invasion and positive nodal status by endoscopic ultrasound.
Ronellenfitsch U. et al. [24]	Germany	2016	275	3.9%	18.2%	Depth of invasion, lymphovascular invasion, diffuse- and mixed-type according to Lauren.
Our study	Lithuania	2017	218	5.1%	31.9%	Depth of invasion, lymphovascular invasion and tumor differentiation grade
Indication for endoscopic treatment of EGC according to different guidelines						
ESMO-ESSO-ESTRO	Well-differentiated, lesion is ≤2 cm in diameter, confined to the mucosa and not ulcerated.					
NCCN	Well or moderately well differentiated, lesion is ≤2 cm in diameter, confined to the mucosa, does not exhibit lymphovascular invasion					

LNM are present in histological specimens, surgery with adequate lymphadenectomy should be followed. To successfully utilize the endoscopical approach in Western countries, criteria need to be expanded and applied to the appropriate population. For safe implementation, further research should be conducted by Western studies.

Acknowledgements

Not applicable.

Funding

This study was performed without funding.

Authors' contributions

RB and ES were guarantor of the integrity of the study. AB was responsible for literature research. DK, KM, IV and ML were responsible for data collection and statistical analysis. Manuscript was prepared by AB and IV, edited by RB and reviewed by ES and KS. All authors read and approved the final manuscript.

Competing interests

The authors declare that they have no competing interests.

Author details

[1]Department of Abdominal Surgery and Oncology, National Cancer Institute, Santariskiu str. 1, Vilnius 08660, Lithuania. [2]Faculty of Medicine, Vilnius University, Ciurlionio str. 21, Vilnius 03101, Lithuania. [3]School of Medicine, Georgetown University, Washington, D.C., USA. [4]Center of Abdominal surgery, Vilnius University Hospital Santaros Klinikos , Santariskiu str. 2, Washington 08661, USA.

References

1. Baušys A, Klimas D, Kilius A, Pauža K, Rudinskaite G, Samalavičius N, et al. Tumor differentiation is a risk factor for lymph node metastasis in patients with gastric cancer. Ann Oncol. 2015;26(suppl 4):iv28.
2. Roviello F, Rossi S, Marrelli D, Pedrazzani C, Corso G, Vindigni C, et al. Number of lymph node metastases and its prognostic significance in early gastric cancer: a multicenter Italian study. J Surg Oncol. 2006;94(4):275–80.
3. Nakahara K, Tsuruta O, Tateishi H, Arima N, Takeda J, Toyonaga A, et al. Extended indication criteria for endoscopic mucosal resection of early gastric cancer with special reference to lymph node metastasis– examination by multivariate analysis. Kurume Med J. 2004;51(1):9–14.
4. Hopkins S, Yang GY. FDG PET imaging in the staging and management of gastric cancer. J Gastrointest Oncol. 2011;2(1):39–44.
5. Hallinan JTPD, Venkatesh SK. Gastric carcinoma: imaging diagnosis, staging and assessment of treatment response. Cancer Imaging Off Publ Int Cancer Imaging Soc. 2013;13:212–27.
6. Hasbahceci M, Akcakaya A, Memmi N, Turkmen I, Cipe G, Yildiz P, et al. Diffusion MRI on lymph node staging of gastric adenocarcinoma. Quant Imaging Med Surg. 2015;5(3):392–400.
7. Soetikno R, Kaltenbach T, Yeh R, Gotoda T. Endoscopic mucosal resection for early cancers of the upper gastrointestinal tract. J Clin Oncol Off J Am Soc Clin Oncol. 2005;23(20):4490–8.
8. Gotoda T. Endoscopic resection of early gastric cancer. Gastric Cancer Off J Int Gastric Cancer Assoc Jpn Gastric Cancer Assoc. 2007;10(1):1–11.
9. Gotoda T, Yanagisawa A, Sasako M, Ono H, Nakanishi Y, Shimoda T, et al. Incidence of lymph node metastasis from early gastric cancer: estimation with a large number of cases at two large centers. Gastric Cancer Off J Int Gastric Cancer Assoc Jpn Gastric Cancer Assoc. 2000;3(4):219–25.
10. Yamaguchi N, Isomoto H, Fukuda E, Ikeda K, Nishiyama H, Akiyama M, et al. Clinical outcomes of endoscopic submucosal dissection for early gastric cancer by indication criteria. Digestion. 2009;80(3):173–81.
11. Fukuhara S, Yabe M, Montgomery MM, Itagaki S, Brower ST, Karpeh MS. Race/ethnicity is predictive of lymph node status in patients with early gastric cancer. J Gastrointest Surg Off J Soc Surg Aliment Tract. 2014;18(10):1744–51.
12. Ikoma N, Blum M, Chiang Y-J, Estrella JS, Roy-Chowdhuri S, Fournier K, et al. Race is a risk for lymph node metastasis in patients with gastric cancer. Ann Surg Oncol. 2017;24(4):960–5.
13. Suzuki H, Oda I, Abe S, Sekiguchi M, Nonaka S, Yoshinaga S, et al. Clinical outcomes of early gastric cancer patients after noncurative endoscopic

submucosal dissection in a large consecutive patient series. Gastric Cancer. 2016. [Epub ahead of print].
14. Lim MS, Lee H-W, Im H, Kim BS, Lee MY, Jeon JY, et al. Predictable factors for lymph node metastasis in early gastric cancer-analysis of single institutional experience. J Gastrointest Surg Off J Soc Surg Aliment Tract. 2011;15(10):1783–8.
15. Zhao L-Y, Yin Y, Li X, Zhu C-J, Wang Y-G, Chen X-L, et al. A nomogram composed of clinicopathologic features and preoperative serum tumor markers to predict lymph node metastasis in early gastric cancer patients. Oncotarget. 2016;7(37):59630–39.
16. Wang Y. The predictive factors for lymph node metastasis in early gastric cancer: a clinical study. Pak J Med Sci. 2015;31(6):1437–40.
17. Zheng Z, Zhang Y, Zhang L, Li Z, Wu X, Liu Y, et al. A nomogram for predicting the likelihood of lymph node metastasis in early gastric patients. BMC Cancer. 2015;16:92.
18. Ahmad R, Setia N, Schmidt BH, Hong TS, Wo JY, Kwak EL, et al. Predictors of lymph node metastasis in western early gastric cancer. J Gastrointest Surg Off J Soc Surg Aliment Tract. 2016;20(3):531–8.
19. Sekiguchi M, Oda I, Taniguchi H, Suzuki H, Morita S, Fukagawa T, et al. Risk stratification and predictive risk-scoring model for lymph node metastasis in early gastric cancer. J Gastroenterol. 2016;51(10):961–70.
20. Hatta W, Gotoda T, Oyama T, Kawata N, Takahashi A, Yoshifuku Y, et al. Is radical surgery necessary in all patients who do not meet the curative criteria for endoscopic submucosal dissection in early gastric cancer? A multi-center retrospective study in Japan. J Gastroenterol. 2017;52(2):175–84.
21. Nakamura Y, Yasuoka H, Tsujimoto M, et al. Importance of lymph vessels in gastric cancer: a prognostic indicator in general and a predictor for lymph node metastasis in early stage cancer. J Clin Pathol. 2006;59:77–82.
22. Haist T, Pritzer H, Pauthner M, Fisseler-Eckhoff A, Lorenz D. Prognostic risk factors of early gastric cancer-a western experience. Langenbecks Arch Surg Dtsch Ges Für Chir. 2016;401(5):667–76.
23. Bravo Neto GP, dos Santos EG, Victer FC, Carvalho CE de S. Lymph node metastasis in early gastric cancer. Rev Colégio Bras Cir 2014; 41(1):11–7.
24. Ronellenfitsch U, Lippert C, Grobholz R, Lang S, Post S, Kähler G, et al. Histology-based prediction of lymph node metastases in early gastric cancer as decision guidance for endoscopic resection. Oncotarget. 2016; 7(9):10676–83.
25. Ren G, Cai R, Zhang W-J, Ou J-M, Jin Y-N, Li W-H. Prediction of risk factors for lymph node metastasis in early gastric cancer. World J Gastroenterol. 2013;19(20):3096–107.
26. Wang L, Liang H, Wang X, Wu L, Ding X, Liu H. Mode of lymph node metastasis in early gastric cancer and risk factors. Zhonghua Wei Chang Wai Ke Za Zhi Chin J Gastrointest Surg. 2013;16(2):147–50.
27. Nakagawa M, Choi YY, An JY, Chung H, Seo SH, Shin HB, et al. Difficulty of predicting the presence of lymph node metastases in patients with clinical early stage gastric cancer: a case control study. BMC Cancer. 2015;15:943.
28. Park JH, Lee SH, Park JM, Park CS, Park KS, Kim ES, et al. Prediction of the indication criteria for endoscopic resection of early gastric cancer. World J Gastroenterol. 2015;21(39):11160–7.
29. Fang W-L, Huang K-H, Lan Y-T, Chen M-H, Chao Y, Lo S-S, et al. The risk factors of lymph node metastasis in early gastric cancer. Pathol Oncol Res POR. 2015;21(4):941–6.
30. Wang Y-W, Zhu M-L, Wang R-F, Xue W-J, Zhu X-R, Wang L-F, et al. Predictable factors for lymph node metastasis in early gastric cancer analysis of clinicopathologic factors and biological markers. Tumour Biol J Int Soc Oncodevelopmental Biol Med. 2016;37(7):8567–78.
31. Milhomem LM, Cardoso DMM, Mota ED, Fraga-Júnior AC, Martins E, da Mota OM. Frequency and predictive factors related to lymphatic metastasis in early gastric cancer. Arq Bras Cir Dig ABCD Braz Arch Dig Surg. 2012;25(4):235–9.

19

Excessive visceral fat area as a risk factor for early postoperative complications of total gastrectomy for gastric cancer: a retrospective cohort study

Masashi Takeuchi, Kenjiro Ishii*, Hiroaki Seki, Nobutaka Yasui, Michio Sakata, Akihiko Shimada and Hidetoshi Matsumoto

Abstract

Background: Obesity is a known risk factor for complications after digestive surgery. Body mass index (BMI) is commonly used as an index of obesity but does not always reflect the degree of obesity. Although some studies have shown that high visceral fat area (VFA) is associated with poor outcomes in digestive surgery, few have examined the relationship between VFA and total gastrectomy. In this study, we demonstrated that VFA is more useful than BMI in predicting complications after total gastrectomy.

Methods: Seventy-five patients who underwent total gastrectomy for gastric cancer were enrolled in this study; they were divided into two groups: a high-VFA group ($n = 26$, ≥ 100 cm^2) and a low-VFA group ($n = 49$, < 100 cm^2). We retrospectively evaluated the preoperative characteristics and surgical outcomes of all patients and examined postoperative complications within 30 days of surgery (including cardiac complications, pneumonia, ileus, anastomotic leakage, pancreatic fistula, incisional surgical site infection [SSI], abdominal abscess, and hemorrhage).

Results: The incidence of anastomotic leakage ($p = 0.03$) and incisional SSI ($p = 0.001$) were higher in the high-VFA group than in the low-VFA group. No significant differences were observed in the other factors. We used univariate analysis to identify risk factors for anastomotic leakage and incisional SSI. Age and VFA were risk factors for anastomotic leakage, and BMI and VFA were risk factors for incisional SSI. A multivariate analysis including these factors found that only VFA was a predictor of anastomotic leakage (hazard ratio [HR] 4.62; 95 % confidence interval [CI] 1.02–21.02; $p = 0.048$) and incisional SSI (HR 4.32; 95 % CI 1.18–15.80; $p = 0.027$].

Conclusions: High VFA is more useful than BMI in predicting anastomotic leakage and SSI after total gastrectomy. Therefore, we should consider the VFA value during surgery

Keywords: Excessive visceral fat area, Total gastrectomy, Gastric cancer, Anastomotic leakage, Incisional SSI

Background

Total gastrectomy for gastric cancer is one of the highly invasive surgeries in gastroenterology, and is associated with high morbidity and mortality. A recent study reported a 30-day morbidity rate of 36 % and mortality rate of 4.7 % after total gastrectomy [1], with common postoperative complications being respiratory complications (16 %), sepsis (15 %), organ/space infection (9 %), and surgical site infection (SSI) (8 %). Other known severe complications are pancreatic fistula and anastomotic insufficiency. As these are difficult to manage, careful management of postoperative complications in total gastrectomy is necessary.

Obesity is a known risk factor for postoperative complications in digestive surgery [2]. Although body mass index (BMI) is commonly used as an index of obesity, it does not always reflect the degree of obesity [3]. It has also been reported that Asians have a higher percentage of body fat than Caucasians at the same BMI level [4, 5].

* Correspondence: tomukuru-zu@hotmail.co.jp
Department of Surgery, Keiyu Hospital, 3-7-3 Minatomirai, Nishi-ku, Yokohama-shi, Kanagawa 220-8521, Japan

Recent studies have shown that high visceral fat area (VFA) is associated with poor outcomes in digestive surgery [6, 7]. However, there have been few studies on the relationship between VFA and total gastrectomy.

In the present study, we demonstrated that VFA is more useful than BMI in predicting postoperative complications in total gastrectomy.

Methods

Patients

Seventy-five patients who underwent total gastrectomy for gastric cancer at the Keiyu Hospital, Kanagawa, Japan between June 2009 and February 2015. There was no limitation with regards to age, and patients' ECOG performance status scores ranged from 0 to 2. Patients who underwent total gastrectomy with combined resection of other organs and those who had surgery following neoadjuvant chemotherapy were also included in the sample.

Patients' preoperative examinations included upper gastrointestinal endoscopy, abdominal computed tomography (CT) scan, and laboratory tests. Gastric cancer diagnoses were based on pathologic findings [8].

Lymph node dissection and gastric reconstruction were determined according to the Japanese classification of gastric carcinoma [8]. Patients with clinical T2, T3, T4a, T4b, or N+ underwent D2 dissection; those with clinical T1a or a part of T1b with N0 underwent D1 or D1+ dissection. All patients underwent Roux-en-Y reconstruction. We resected the transverse colon or pancreas tail simultaneously if there was direct tumor invasion of both organs.

We retrospectively evaluated patients' preoperative characteristics from hospital records, including age, sex, history of diabetes mellitus, cardiac history, pulmonary history, and history of chronic kidney disease. We also assessed intraoperative findings, such as gastrectomy with splenectomy, gastrectomy with jejunostomy, number of retrieved lymph nodes, operating time, amount of blood loss, and pathologic stage. Pathologic findings were defined by the Japanese classification of gastric carcinoma. We obtained BMI data and American Society of Anesthesiologists (ASA) scores from patients' anesthesia records. Three patients who had surgery following neoadjuvant chemotherapy were included. Three patients received neoadjuvant chemotherapy preoperatively. S-1 was administered to one patient, and two patients received S-1 + cisplatin.

We collected data on postoperative complications within 30 days of surgery. This included cardiac complications, pneumonia, ileus, anastomotic leakage, pancreatic fistula, incisional SSI, abdominal abscess, and hemorrhage. Anastomotic leakage was diagnosed on the basis of CT scan findings or the characteristics of abdominal drains. Pancreatic fistula was diagnosed if the amylase content of the drain around the pancreas after postoperative day 3 was greater than three times the upper limit of its normal serum value [9]. The diagnosis of incisional SSI was based on the definition of the United States Centers for Disease Control and Prevention Guidelines for the prevention of SSIs [10]. We used the Clavien–Dindo classification for complications and identified complication cases as those having a Clavien–Dindo classification greater than grade 2, with the exception of incisional SSI cases. Incisional SSI was only investigated as postoperative SSI. The treatment for incisional SSI is open drainage of wound infections; this treatment represents a grade 1 Clavien–Dindo classification. Therefore, we selected patients with a Clavien–Dindo classification greater than grade 1 for incisional SSI.

We excluded one patient who underwent laparoscopic gastrectomy. Patients with esophagogastric junction cancer, those who underwent emergency surgery due to gastric perforation, and one patient who underwent additional total gastrectomy after a positive surgical margin post-distal gastrectomy were also excluded. This study was approved by the Keiyu hospital ethics committee (approval number:H27-No31).

Evaluation of fat area

We measured VFA and subcutaneous fat area (SFA) at the umbilical level on available CT scan images (LightSpeed VCT 64 slice CT, GE Yokogawa Medical Systems). CT was performed 4 weeks preoperatively. To calculate VFA, we first traced the outline of the intraperitoneal tissue [11, 12]. Thereafter, using this outlined region, we determined a histogram of the CT numbers ranging from -150 HU to -50 HU [13]. SFA was calculated in a similar manner by using a manually traced contour of the subcutaneous region. Japanese criteria for obesity disease have been provided by the Japan Society for Study of Obesity [3]. These criteria were adopted by the Japanese Ministry of Health, Labour and Welfare and set the cut-off value of visceral obesity as 100 cm2. As only Japanese individuals were included in our study, we used a cut-off value of 100 cm2 for VFA. Patients were divided into two groups: a high-VFA group ($n = 26$, ≥ 100 cm^2) and a low-VFA group ($n = 49$, <100 cm^2).

Statistical analysis

Statistical analyses were performed using Stata/SE 12.1 for Mac (StataCorp, TX, USA). Categorical variables were analyzed with chi-square tests for univariate analysis, and continuous variables were analyzed with the Mann–Whitney U test. A p value < 0.05 was considered significant. Variables with p values < 0.05 in the univariate analysis were subsequently entered into a logistic regression model for multivariate analysis.

Table 1 Comparison of the baseline characteristics of patients who underwent total gastrectomy ($n = 75$)

	High-VFA ($n = 26$)	Low-VFA ($n = 49$)	p value
Sex (men/women)	22/4	35/14	0.20
Age (mean ± SD)	70.8 ± 9.7	70.7 ± 10.2	0.71
ASA (I/II/III)	7/15/4	6/36/7	0.25
BMI (kg/m^2) in mean ± SD	25.1 ± 3.0 (20.0–32.2)	20.8 ± 2.6 (14.7–25.4)	<0.0001
VFA (cm^2) (mean ± SD)	146.9 ± 38.2 (101.8–240.9)	54.3 ± 27.1 (5.9–99.9)	<0.0001
SFA (cm^2) (mean ± SD)	157.1 ± 54.8 (77.3–292.3)	86.1 ± 54.9 (5.1–200.5)	<0.0001
Total fat area (cm^2) (mean ± SD)	304.0 ± 74.7 (194.7–481.2)	140.5 ± 72.0 (14.3–286.0)	<0.0001
Diabetes mellitus	7	7	0.18
Cardiac history	5	8	0.75
Pulmonary history	1	3	0.68
Chronic kidney disease	4	0	0.005
Pathologic T (1a/1b/2/3/4a/4b)	1/7/7/4/7/0	2/6/9/20/10/2	0.19
Pathologic N (0/1/2/3)	12/4/3/7	17/6/13/13	0.48
Pathologic M (0/1)	26/1	44/5	0.33
Pathologic stage (I/II/III/IV)	11/6/8/1	14/10/20/5	0.51
Neoadjuvant chemotherapy	0	3	0.198
Residual gastrectomy	0	6	0.06
Splenectomy	8	10	0.32
Resection of pancreatic tail	1	2	0.24
Partial resection of colon	1	1	0.64

SD standard deviation; *ASA* American Society of Anesthesiologists; *BMI* body mass index; *SFA* subcutaneous fat area; *VFA* visceral fat area; *T* tumor status; *N* nodal status; *M* metastasis status

Results

Comparison of baseline characteristics

We compared the baseline characteristics of the two groups (Table 1). The groups were similar in terms of mean age (high VFA group: 70.8 ± 9.7 years vs. low VFA group: 70.7 ± 10.2 years; $p = 0.71$), ASA scores, disease stage, and underlying diseases. The groups differed significantly on BMI ($p < 0.0001$), VFA ($p < 0.0001$), SFA ($p < 0.0001$), total fat area ($p < 0.0001$), and history of chronic kidney disease ($p = 0.005$).

Table 2 Comparison of outcomes and complications after total gastrectomy ($n = 75$)

	High-VFA ($n = 26$)	Low-VFA ($n = 49$)	p value
Number of retrieved lymph nodes (mean ± SD)	42.7 ± 18.7	43.0 ± 24.2	0.81
Operating time (min) in mean ± SD	225.9 ± 92.0	200.9 ± 58.3	0.08
Blood loss (ml) in mean ± SD	467.9 ± 600.2	318.5 ± 407.1	0.32
Postoperative hospital stay (day) in mean ± SD	22.8 ± 15.7	18.8 ± 9.6	0.70
Postoperative complications			
Cardiac	0	3	0.20
Pneumonia	4	4	0.33
Incisional SSI	12	6	0.001
Ileus	2	0	0.05
Anastomotic leakage	6	3	0.03
Pancreatic fistula	2	1	0.23
Abdominal abscess	4	3	0.19
Postoperative hemorrhage	1	2	0.96
Other	4	5	0.53

SD standard deviation; *SSI* surgical site infection; *VFA* visceral fat area

Table 3 Univariate analyses of factors associated with anastomotic leakage following total gastrectomy

Risk factors	anastomotic leakage (+)	anastomotic leakage (−)	Univariate analysis	Logistic regression analysis	
				Hazard ratio (95 % CI)	p value
Sex					
Men	9	48	0.072		
Women	0	18			
Age (mean ± SD)	64.6 ± 7.5	71.6 ± 10.0	0.017	0.94 (0.87–1.01)	0.057
ASA					
I	2	11	0.891		
II	6	45			
III	1	10			
BMI (≥25/<25 kg/m^2)	4/5	12/54	0.071		
VFA (≥100/<100 cm^2)	6/3	20/46	0.032	4.6 (1.05–20.25)	0.044
SFA (cm^2) (mean ± SD)	126.5 ± 56.5	108.6 ± 65.3	0.434		
Diabetes mellitus	2	12	0.77		
Cardiac history	2	11	0.695		
Pulmonary history	0	4	0.444		
Chronic kidney disease	1	3	0.419		
Pathologic Stage					
I	1	24	0.269		
II	3	13			
III	5	23			
IV	0	6			
Neoadjuvant chemotherapy	0	3	0.514		
Residual gastrectomy	0	6	0.346		
Splenectomy	2	16	0.894		
Resection of pancreatic tail	1	2	0.246		
Partial resection of colon	0	2	0.597		
Number of retrieved lymph nodes (mean ± SD)	38.4 ± 22.3	43.5 ± 22.4	0.487		
Operating time (min) (mean ± SD)	254.8 ± 118.8	207.3 ± 59.0	0.23		
Blood loss (ml) (mean ± SD)	572.5 ± 663.7	351.4 ± 460.2	0.428		

CI confidence interval; *SD* standard deviation

Comparison of surgical outcomes and postoperative complications

Compared with the low-VFA group, the high VFA group had a higher incidence of anastomotic leakage ($p = 0.03$) and incisional SSI ($p = 0.001$). No significant differences were observed for the other factors (Table 2).

Risk factors for anastomotic leakage and incisional SSI

We used univariate analysis to determine the risk factors for anastomotic leakage and incisional SSI from variables, such as background and surgical outcomes. Age and VFA were risk factors for anastomotic leakage, and BMI and VFA were risk factors for incisional SSI. In the multivariate analysis that included these factors, only

Table 4 Multivariate analysis of factors associated with anastomotic leakage after total gastrectomy

Risk factors	anastomotic leakage (+)	anastomotic leakage (−)	β	SE	Hazard ratio (95 % CI)	p value
Age (≥70/<70 years)	2/7	35/31	−0.20	0.22	0.25 (0.05–1.36)	0.108
VFA (≥100/<100 cm^2)	6/3	20/46	0.25	3.57	4.62 (1.02–21.02)	0.048

CI, confidence interval; β, standard regression coefficient; SE, standard error

Table 5 Univariate analyses of factors associated with incisional SSI following total gastrectomy

Risk factors	Incisional SSI (+)	Incisional SSI (−)	Univariate analysis	Logistic regression analysis Hazard ratio (95 % CI)	p value
Sex					
Men	15	42	0.403		
Women	3	15			
Age (years)	71.2 ± 9.4	70.6 ± 10.2	0.98		
ASA					
I	1	12	0.318		
II	14	37			
III	3	8			
BMI (≥25/<25 kg/m^2)	8/10	8/49	0.006	4.9 (1.49–16.15)	0.009
VFA (≥100/<100 cm^2)	12/6	14/43	0.001	6.14 (1.94–19.41)	0.002
SFA (cm^2) (mean ± SD)	136.9 ± 73.3	102.5 ± 59.5	0.104		
Diabetes mellitus	3	11	0.803		
Cardiac history	5	8	0.144		
Pulmonary history	1	3	0.921		
Chronic kidney disease	2	2	0.186		
Pathologic Stage					
I	6	19	0.527		
II	4	12			
III	8	20			
IV	0	6			
Neoadjuvant chemotherapy	1	2	0.699		
Residual gastrectomy	0	6	0.151		
Splenectomy	3	15	0.403		
Resection of pancreatic tail	1	2	0.699		
Partial resection of colon	1	1	0.383		
Number of retrieved lymph nodes (mean ± SD)	39.7 ± 18.2	43.9 ± 23.5	0.85		
Operating time (min) (mean ± SD)	225.1 ± 64.2	208.6 ± 69.6	0.278		
Blood loss (ml) (mean ± SD)	368.2 ± 369.9	377.4 ± 517.7	0.985		

SSI surgical site infection; *CI* confidence interval; *SD* standard deviation

VFA was identified as a predictor of anastomotic leakage (hazard ratio [HR] 4.62; 95 % confidence interval [CI] 1.02–21.02; $p = 0.048$] (Tables 3 and 4) and incisional SSI (HR 4.32; 95 % CI 1.18–15.80; $p = 0.027$) (Tables 5 and 6).

Discussion

We reached two conclusions based on the results of our study: 1) high VFA is a more useful risk factor than high BMI in predicting anastomotic leakage after total gastrectomy, and 2) compared with high SFA, high VFA resulted in more incisional SSIs.

There have been some studies on the relationship between VFA and complications following digestive surgery [14, 15]. A few studies have reported that VFA was a more useful index than BMI in predicting postoperative complications in gastrectomy. Sugisawa et al. indicated that excessive visceral fat was an independent risk factor for pancreas-related infection and anastomotic leakage after gastrectomy [16]. Tokunaga et al. investigated

Table 6 Multivariate analysis of factors associated with incisional SSI after total gastrectomy

Risk factors	Incisional SSI (+)	Incisional SSI (−)	β	SE	Hazard ratio (95 % CI)	p value
BMI (≥25/<25 kg/m^2)	8/10	8/49	0.31	1.60	2.28 (0.57–9.04)	0.241
VFA (≥100/<100 cm^2)	12/6	14/43	0.38	2.86	4.32 (1.18–15.80)	0.027

CI confidence interval; *β* standard regression coefficient; *SE* standard error

the relationship between fat area and early surgical outcomes after gastrectomy [17] and concluded that excessive visceral fat was likely to result in intra-abdominal infections, such as anastomotic leakage, pancreas-related infection, and intra-abdominal abscess. Tanaka et al. evaluated risk factors (including VFA) for postoperative complications after total gastrectomy [18] and found that the VFA value was a better indicator of pancreatic fistula compared with BMI. Our study showed that VFA was useful in predicting anastomotic leakage. Previous studies did not consider background characteristics (e.g., cardiovascular diseases) that are usually associated with patients with obesity; these background factors may have contributed to the incidence of anastomotic leakage due to insufficient microcirculation [19, 20] and may have confounded their results. Therefore, in our study, we considered baseline characteristics, such as cardiac history or diabetes mellitus, which may affect the incidence of anastomotic leakage.

Kim et al. showed that male sex, preoperative/intraoperative transfusion, cardiovascular disease, and disease location on the upper third of the stomach were predictive of postoperative anastomotic leakage after gastrectomy [19]. Although some factors, such as splenectomy or malnutrition, were identified as risk factors for anastomotic leakage [21, 22], excessive tension on the anastomosis site was also reported to be a risk factor [16, 23].

In our study, high VFA resulted in more incisional SSIs compared with high SFA. Mike et al. evaluated the incidence of incisional SSI and identified the predictors after digestive surgery [24]. They identified four risk factors for incisional SSI after stoma reversal: history of fascial dehiscence, colostomy, Caucasian origin, and thick subcutaneous fat. In the present study, incisional SSI was observed in 18 patients, seven (39 %) of whom had anastomotic leakage. Therefore, anastomotic leakage was a confounding factor. Moreover, there are large confidence intervals for VFA in multivariate analysis, because our single-center study had a small number of patients. We thought that it was not appropriate to investigate the patients in more previous periods for increasing the number of patients, because patients who underwent a surgery of different quality might also be included.

This study had several limitations. First, it was a retrospective, single-center study limited to Asian population. Our hospital also has extensive experience and a high workload in gastric cancer surgery due to higher local incidence; thus, our outcomes may not be applicable to other centers in other countries. Second, to calculate VFA, the outlines of intraperitoneal tissue were traced manually; this may have led to measurement errors, compared with automatic tracing.

Conclusions

High VFA is more useful than BMI in predicting anastomotic leakage and SSI after total gastrectomy. Therefore, we should consider the VFA value during surgery.

Funding
None.

Authors' contributions
MT and KI designed the study, acquired the data, performed the analysis and interpretation of data, and drafted and revised the manuscript, HS, NY, MS, AS and HM helped to acquire the data. All authors read and approved the final manuscript.

Competing interests
The authors declare that they have no conflicts of interest.

References
1. Bartlett EK, Roses RE, Kelz RR, Drebin JA, Fraker DL, Karakousis GC. Morbidity and mortality after total gastrectomy for gastric malignancy using the American College of Surgeons National Surgical Quality Improvement Program database. Surgery. 2014;156:298–304.
2. Wakefield H, Vaughan-Sarrazin M, Cullen JJ. Influence of obesity on complications and costs after intestinal surgery. Am J Surg. 2012;204:434–40.
3. Oda E. New criteria for "obesity disease" in Japan. Circ J. 2006;70:150.
4. Kadowaki T, Sekikawa A, Murata K, Maegawa H, Takamiya T, Okamura T, et al. Japanese men have larger areas of visceral adipose tissue than Caucasian men in the same levels of waist circumference in a population-based study. Int J Obes. 2006;30:1163–5.
5. Deurenberg P, Deurenberg-Yap M, Guricci S. Asians are different from Caucasians and from each other in their body mass index/body fat per cent relationship. Obes Rev. 2002;3:141–6.
6. Watanabe J, Tatsumi K, Ota M, Suwa Y, Suzuki S, Watanabe A, et al. The impact of visceral obesity on surgical outcomes of laparoscopic surgery for colon cancer. Int J Colorectal Dis. 2014;29:343–51.
7. Moon H-G, Ju Y-T, Jeong C-Y, Jung E-J, Lee Y-J, Hong S-C, et al. Visceral obesity may affect oncologic outcome in patients with colorectal cancer. Ann Surg Oncol. 2008;15:1918–22.
8. Sano T, Kodera Y. Japanese classification of gastric carcinoma: 3rd English edition. Gastric Cancer. 2011;14:101–12.
9. Bassi C, Dervenis C, Butturini G, Fingerhut A, Yeo C, Izbicki J, et al. Postoperative pancreatic fistula: an international study group (ISGPF) definition. Surgery. 2005;138:8–13.
10. Mangram AJ, Horan TC, Pearson ML, Silver LC, Jarvis WR. Guideline for prevention of surgical site infection, 1999. Centers for Disease Control and Prevention (CDC) Hospital Infection Control Practices Advisory Committee. Am J Infect Control. 1999;27:97–132. quiz 133–4;discussion 96.
11. Yoshizumi T, Nakamura T, Yamane M, Islam AH, Menju M, Yamasaki K, et al. Abdominal fat: standardized technique for measurement at CT. Radiology. 1999;211:283–6.
12. Ryo M. Clinical significance of visceral adiposity assessed by computed tomography: a Japanese perspective. World J Radiol. 2014;6:409.
13. Roriz AKC, Passos LCS, de Oliveira CC, Eickemberg M, Moreira PDA, Sampaio LR. Evaluation of the accuracy of anthropometric clinical indicators of visceral Fat in adults and elderly. PLoS One. 2014;9:e103499.
14. Seki Y, Ohue M, Sekimoto M, Takiguchi S, Takemasa I, Ikeda M, et al. Evaluation of the technical difficulty performing laparoscopic resection of a rectosigmoid carcinoma: Visceral fat reflects technical difficulty more accurately than body mass index. Surg Endosc Other Interv Tech. 2007;21:929–34.
15. Tsujinaka S, Konishi F, Kawamura YJ, Saito M, Tajima N, Tanaka O, et al. Visceral obesity predicts surgical outcomes after laparoscopic colectomy for sigmoid colon cancer. Dis Colon Rectum. 2008;51:1757–65.
16. Sugisawa N, Tokunaga M, Tanizawa Y, Bando E, Kawamura T, Terashima M. Intra-abdominal infectious complications following gastrectomy in patients with excessive visceral fat. Gastric Cancer. 2012;15:206–12.

17. Tokunaga M, Hiki N, Fukunaga T, Ogura T, Miyata S, Yamaguchi T. Effect of individual fat areas on early surgical outcomes after open gastrectomy for gastric cancer. Br J Surg. 2009;96:496–500.

18. Tanaka K, Miyashiro I, Yano M, Kishi K, Motoori M, Seki Y, et al. Accumulation of excess visceral fat is a risk factor for pancreatic fistula formation after total gastrectomy. Ann Surg Oncol. 2009;16:1520–5.

19. Kim S, Son S, Park Y, Ahn S, Park DJ, Kim H. Risk factors for anastomotic leakage: a retrospective cohort study in a Single Gastric Surgical Unit. J Gastric Cancer. 2015;15:167–75.

20. Jeong S-H, Ahn HS, Yoo M-W, Cho J-J, Lee H-J, Kim H-H, et al. Increased morbidity rates in patients with heart disease or chronic liver disease following radical gastric surgery. J Surg Oncol. 2010;101:200–4.

21. Kodera Y, Yamamura Y, Shimizu Y, Torii A, Hirai T, Yasui K, et al. Lack of benefit of combined pancreaticosplenectomy in D2 resection for proximal-third gastric carcinoma. World J Surg. 1997;21:622–8.

22. Marano L, Porfidia R, Pezzella M, Grassia M, Petrillo M, Esposito G, et al. Clinical and immunological impact of early postoperative enteral immunonutrition after total gastrectomy in gastric cancer patients: a prospective randomized study. Ann Surg Oncol. 2013;20:3912–8.

23. Kang KC, Cho GS, Han SU, Kim W, Kim HH, Kim MC, et al. Comparison of Billroth I and Billroth II reconstructions after laparoscopy-assisted distal gastrectomy: A retrospective analysis of large-scale multicenter results from Korea. Surg Endosc Other Interv Tech. 2011;25:1953–61.

24. Liang MK, Li LT, Avellaneda A, Moffett JM, Hicks SC, Awad SS. Outcomes and predictors of incisional surgical site infection in stoma reversal. JAMA Surg. 2013;148:183–9.

20

Short-term outcomes of laparoscopic local resection for gastric submucosal tumors: a single-center experience of 266 patients

Ke Chen, Yu Pan, Shu-ting Zhai, Jun-hai Pan, Wei-hua Yu, Ding-wei Chen, Jia-fei Yan and Xian-fa Wang[*]

Abstract

Background: Laparoscopic resections for submucosal tumors (SMTs) of the stomach have been developed rapidly over the past decade. Several types of laparoscopic methods for gastric SMTs have been created. We assessed the short-term outcomes of two commonly used types of laparoscopic local resection (LLR) for gastric SMTs and reported our findings.

Methods: We retrospectively analyzed the clinicopathological results of 266 patients with gastric SMTs whom underwent LLR between January 2006 and September 2016. 228 of these underwent laparoscopic exogastric wedge resection (LEWR), the remaining 38 patients with the tumors near the esophagogastric junction (EGJ) or antrum underwent laparoscopic transgastric resection (LTR).

Results: All the patients underwent laparoscopic resections successfully. The mean operation times of LEWR and LTR were 90.2 ± 37.2 min and 101.7 ± 38.5 min respectively. The postoperative length of hospital stays for LEWR and LTR were 5.1 ± 2.1 days and 5.3 ± 1.7 days respectively. There was a low complication rate (4.4%) and zero mortality in our series.

Conclusion: ELWR is technically feasible therapy of gastric SMTs. LTR is secure and effective for gastric intraluminal SMTs located near the EGJ or antrum.

Keywords: Laparoscopy, Gastrectomy, Submucosal tumors, Complications

Background

Submucosal tumors (SMTs) of the stomach are defined as tumors located beneath the gastric mucosa and include gastrointestinal stromal tumors (GISTs), schwannomas, leiomyomas, malignant lymphomas, lymphangiomas, lipomas, hemangiomas, heterotopic pancreas, *et al.* [1]. We can always perceive gastric SMTs accidently, which make up 2% of whole gastric neoplasms [2]. A broad clinical spectrum was shown from benign to malignant. It seems tough to deal with diagnosis of the tumors before the operation and evaluation of the extent of latent malignancy. Moreover, even a benign tumor can cause a variety of complications such obstruction and bleeding. Therefore, surgical excision of the lesions remains the first choice.

Achieving a disease-free margin to complete the partial excision of the tumor is favored and lymphadenectomy is not usually needed, because nearly 80% of gastric SMTs are GISTs, whose periodicity of lymph node metastasis is low [3, 4].

Laparoscopic resection, which has been regarded as the most appropriate treatment, not only offers minimal normal tissue loss and maintains gastrointestinal continuity, but is also characterized by minimally invasive to the patient. Exogastric laparoscopic wedge resection (ELWR) is the most prevailing laparoscopic local resection (LLR). However, as to neoplasms located at cardia, especially near the esophagogastric junction (EGJ), or lay to antrum, LEWR increases the risk of generating stenosis or deformity in the gastric inlet or outlet [5]. Based on our extensive laparoscopic gastrectomy (LG) [6–10], we developed laparoscopic transgastric resection (LTR) for tumors located at cardia or antrum

* Correspondence: srrshwxf@163.com
Department of Gastrointestinal Surgery, Sir Run Run Shaw Hospital, School of Medicine, Zhejiang University, 3 East Qingchun Road, Hangzhou 310016, Zhejiang Province, China

to avoid a total, proximal or distal gastrectomy. We herein give notice to our results from these two types of laparoscopic resection methods and also an assessment of the postoperative surgical outcomes to evaluate the feasibility and safety of those procedures.

Methods

Patients

At the Department of General Surgery, Sir Run Run Shaw Hospital, 266 patients suffered LLR for probable gastric SMTs. In order to assess the site, dimension, and development mode of the tumor, all of patients experienced preoperative process, including gastroscopy, endoscopic ultrasound (EUS), and abdominal computed tomography (CT). Some patients with enormous tumors were diagnosed before the operation, whose tumors may have intruded on neighboring organs, including various organs because of metastatic disease, or suffered an emergency surgery due to acute upper gastrointestinal bleeding. These people were not taken account into the research. Written consent was obtained from every patient prior to enrollment in the study, which was confirmed by the Zhejiang University's Ethics Committee.

Data collection

People analyzed retrospectively and kept track of demographic message, surgical procedures, pathologic message, clinical presentation, and the process for these patients after operation. Pathologic features of GIST patients were studied, including tumor size, location, mitotic rate and Fletcher classification [11]. On the basis of the Risk Assessment Classification presented by Fletcher and colleagues, the GISTs were quadripartite. [10] (National Institutes of Health [NIH] consensus criteria). A skilled pathologist counted mitotic figures for total specimen in 50 high-power fields (HPFs), which were chosen at random. We also analyzed surgical outcomes involved with the loss of blood, the time of operation, and complications after operation et al.

Surgical procedure

The former described approach was utilized for site and trocar place [6]. We built five trocars in a V-shape setting. In order to eliminate tumor spread and transfer, we operate an entire laparoscopic abdominal examination before the resection. Gastroscopy was taken advantage to assess tumor positioning during the operation if necessary. Tumor positions were first made clear by laparoscopic handing when using LEWR. Before excision, we always mobilize the tumor as follows: Tumor in anterior wall of the gastric body was excised directly using ultrasonic coagulating shears or endoscopic linear staples (Fig. 1). It will be effortless to redeploy the tumor by taking advantage of ultrasonic coagulating shears, where the greater omentum incision was originated from the middle-inferior pole of the spleen to the greater

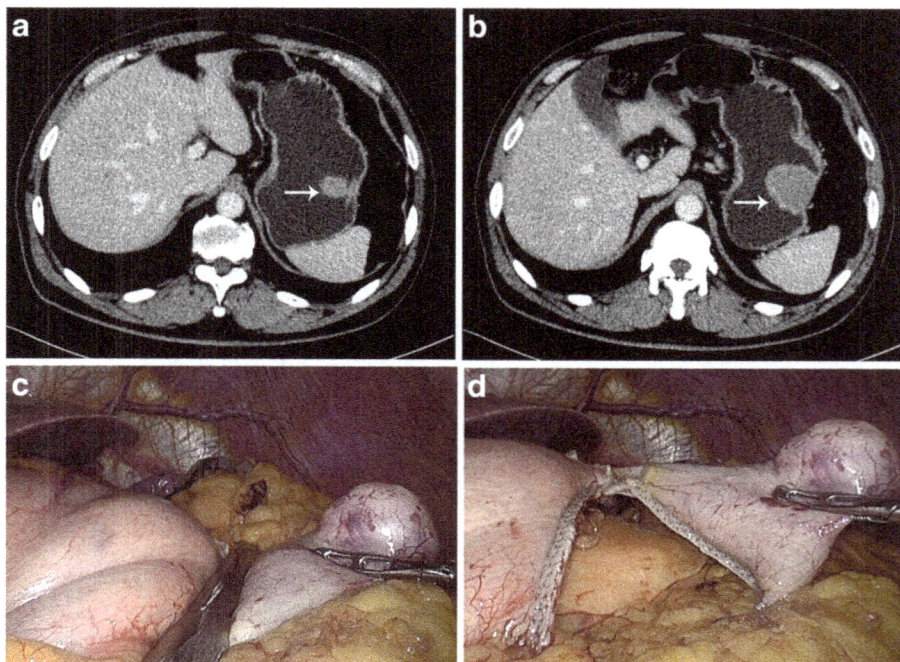

Fig. 1 Resection of tumor in anterior wall of gastric body. (**a**) Image of the tumor from abdominal CT scan. (*white arrow*). (**b**) Image of the tumor from abdominal CT scan. (*white arrow*). (**c**) Resect the wall included the gastric SMTs using linear stapler. (**d**) Fire the anastomat and complete the resection

outer winding of the vessel of the gastric omentum. Moreover, in order to redeploy the tumor, the hepato-gastric ligament was anatomized. They anatomized the gastrocolic and gastrosplenic ligaments, and then held up the stomach to make the tumor clear for tumors which were lay on the posterior wall (Figs. 2 and 3). In order to redeploy the fundus and make the tumor clear, they also anatomized gastrocolic and gastrosplenic ligament as well as left gastroepiploic vessels and short gastric vessels for tumors which were in fundus. Utilizing ultrasonic coagulating shears or endoscopic staples with at lowest 1–2 cm surgical margin, we resected the tumor. Based on the measurement of the tumor, each

excision needed 2 to 3 staples. If the tumor was relatively large, we recommend resecting the tumor using ultrasonic coagulating shears. In order to hold the corners, several sutures were utilized as long stay sutures, and the endoscopic linear staplers played the role of concluding the start. The defect from the stapler line was reinforced using laparoscopic manual sutures to avoid bleeding or leakage (Fig. 4).

We used LTR for tumors located at cardia, near EGJ or the antrum, especially those with intraluminal growth, to avoid deformity or stenosis in the gastric inlet or outlet. If the tumor was located in the cardia, the process was originated from distributing the gastrocolic ligament

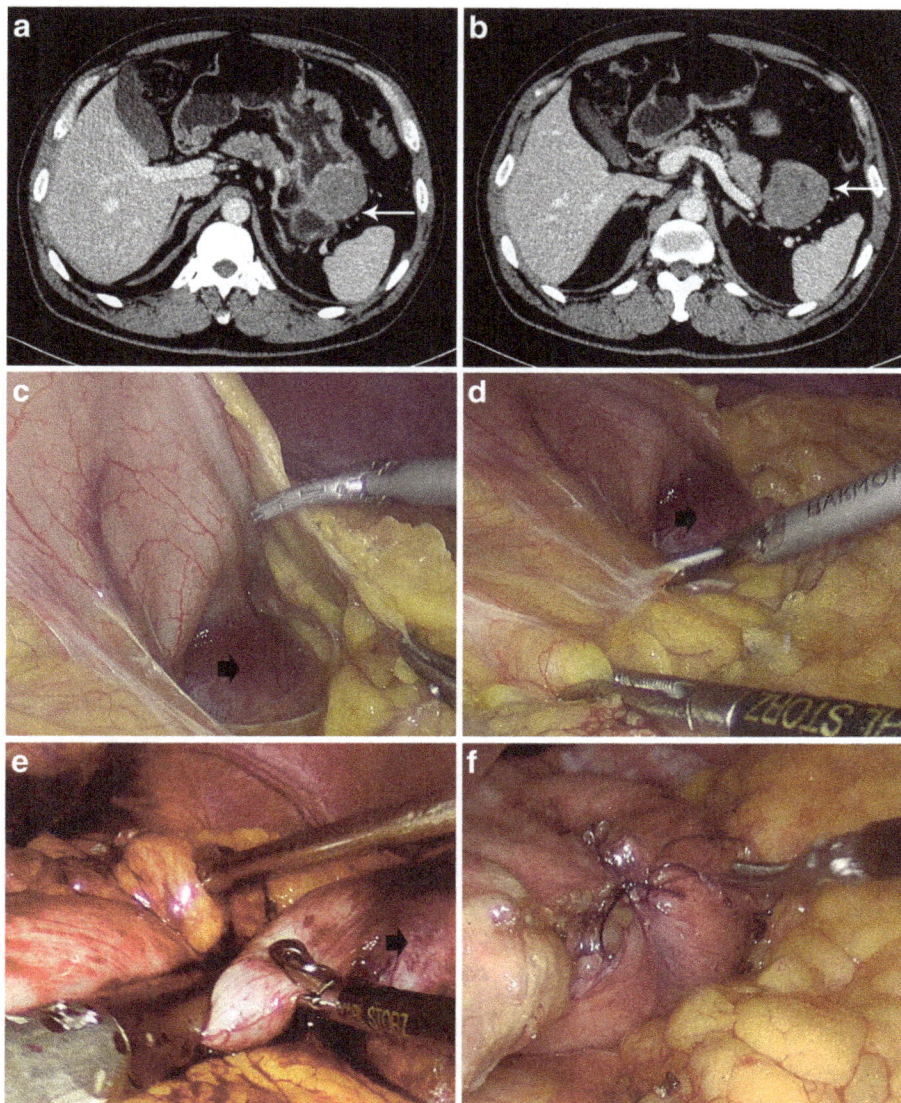

Fig. 2 Resection of tumor in posterior wall of gastric body. (**a**) Image of the tumor from abdominal CT scan. (*white arrow*). (**b**) Image of the tumor from abdominal CT scan. (*white arrow*). (**c**) Open the greater omentum to splenic hilum. (*black arrow*). (**d**) Dissect the pancreatic stomach plica to expose the tumor. (*black arrow*). (**e**) Resect the wall included the gastric SMTs using linear stapler. (**f**) Complete the resection

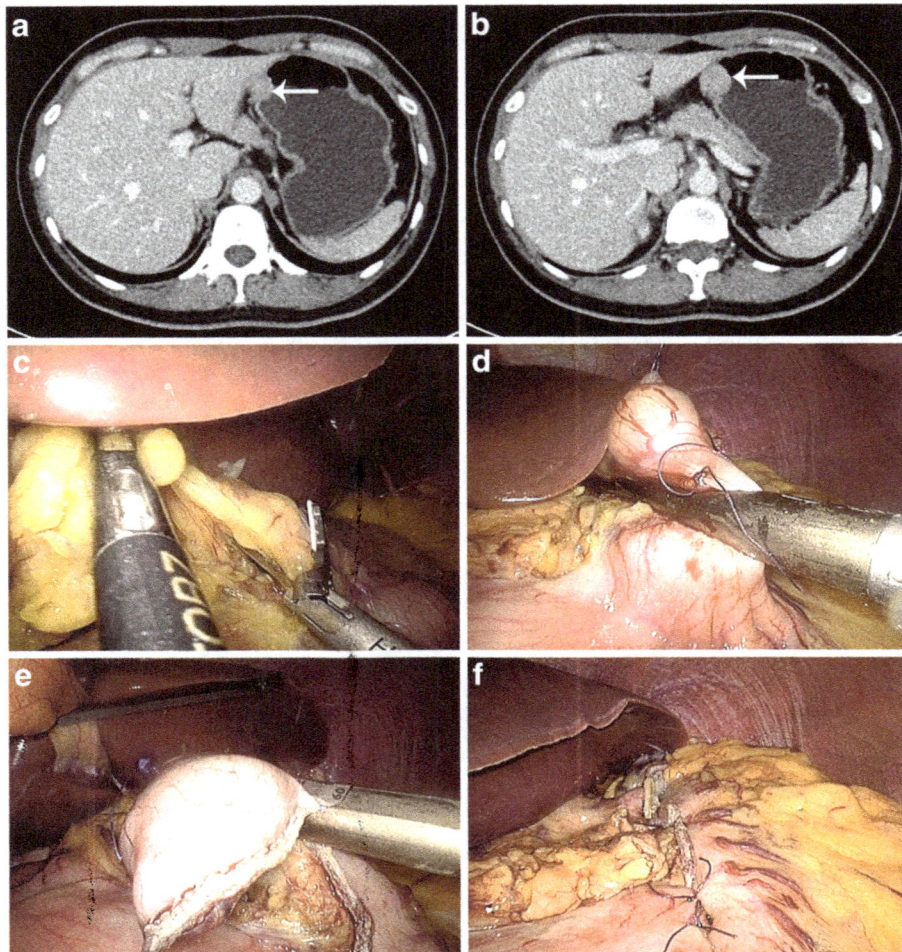

Fig. 3 Resection of tumor in lesser curvature. (**a**) Image of the tumor from abdominal CT scan. (*white arrow*). (**b**) Image of the tumor from abdominal CT scan. (*white arrow*). (**c**) Explore the hepatogastric ligament. (**d**) Resect the wall included the gastric SMTs using linear stapler. (**e**) Complete the resection using another stapler. (**f**) Reinforce the resection using several sutures

up to the spleen or the duodenum degree. In order to come near the EGJ, the hepatogastric or hepatoduodenal ligament was opened. We used ultrasonic coagulating shears to make a perpendicular gastrotomy cut on the anterior wall of the stomach at the possible site of the tumor after redeployment of the EGJ. It was effortless to observe the SMTs marked with the titanium clip and the mucosa directly from the opening (Fig. 5a). Using a stay suture, we upturned the full-thickness gastric wall from this gastrotomy in the lesion area (Fig. 5b). In order to excising transgastricly, we used several endoscopic linear staples to excise the tumor with the entire layer of gastric wall (Fig. 5c.d). Then, the utilizing of endoscopic linear staples longitudinally or laparoscopic manual sutures brought an end to the gastrotomy. The tumor was retrieved from the umbilical wound and placed in a specimen bag.

If the imageological examinations or intraoperative findings showed the tumor was near the pylorus.

Resection commenced with dissection of the appropriate section of the greater omentum with ultrasonic coagulating shears. The short gastric vessels near the tumor were then transected to a height dependent on the level of transection. The right gastric artery was divided and cut. The left lobe of the liver was retracted upward, while the stomach was stretched downward to expose the lesser omentum. At this stage, dissection was continued at the side with the least curvature of the stomach. After mobilization of the pylorus, the excision was similar to those near EGJ.

Results

Patient characteristics

The clinical characteristics of the 266 patients whom underwent laparoscopic surgical resection of gastric SMTs are summarized in Table 1. The 266 patients included 91 males and 175 females. The mean age was

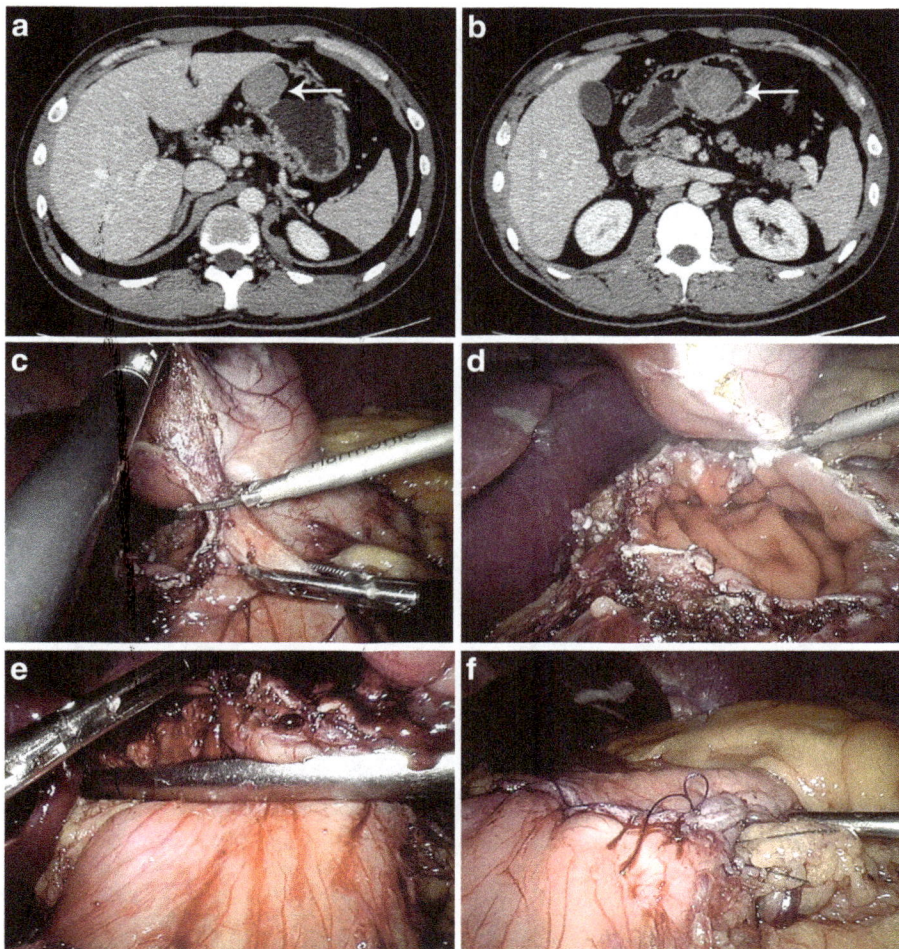

Fig. 4 Resection of tumor using ultrasonic coagulating shears. (**a**) Image of the tumor from abdominal CT scan. (*white arrow*). (**b**) Image of the tumor from abdominal CT scan. (*white arrow*). (**c**) Resect along the tumor using ultrasonic coagulating shears. (**d**) Resect the tumor. (**e**) Close the opening using endoscopic linear staplers. (**f**) Reinforce the resection using several sutures

57.8 years (range 22 to 81 years). The mean body mass index (BMI) was 23.4 kg/m^2 (range: 13.6 to 31.3). Of these patients, 228 underwent LEWR and 38 patients underwent LTR. According to the pathological reports, 229 patients were diagnosed with GIST. The remaining patients were diagnosed with submucosal tumors other than GIST, such as schwannomas (15 patients), ectopic pancreas (4 patients), leiomyoma (14 patients), lipomas (2 patients) and plasmacytoma (2 patients).

Pathologic features of GIST patients

As shown in Table 2, among the patients with GISTs, 203 suffered from LEWR and 26 suffered from LTR. The mean tumor size of LEWR group was 3.6 ± 2.5 cm, and that of LTR group was 2.1 ± 1.3 cm. On the basis of pathological reports, 202 patients were reported to have a mitotic rate of < 5 per 50HPF, 18 patients were reported to have a mitotic rate of 5 ~

10 per 50HPF and 8 patients were reported to have a mitotic rate of > 10 per 50HPF. Adopting the standard of Fletcher classification, our patients were assigned to four groups: very low risk (68 patients), low risk (111 patients), intermediate risk (36 patients) and high risk (14 patients).

Surgical and postoperative outcomes

As shown in Table 3, the mean operation time of LTR was 101.7 ± 38.5 min and was 90.2 ± 37.2 min in LEWR group. The mean blood loss of LEWR and LTR were 50.4 ± 51.6 mL and 42.2 ± 30.2 mL respectively. The postoperative hospital stay of LEWR and LTR were 5.1 ± 2.1 days and 5.3 ± 1.7 days respectively. In the LEWR group, 1 patient suffered from intraluminal bleeding, 4 patients suffered from delayed gastric emptying and 2 patients suffered from pulmonary infections. This group had a complication

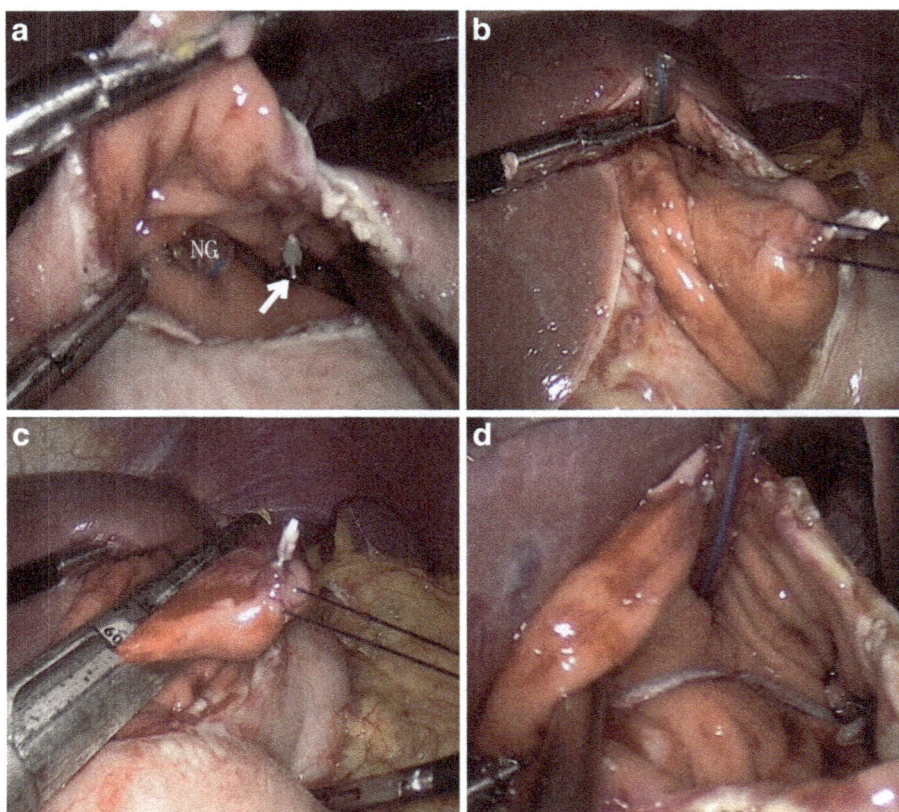

Fig. 5 laparoscopic transgastric resection of gastric SMTs located near the EGJ. (**a**) A gastrotomy was performed at the anterior wall of the proximal stomach and the SMTs marked with the titanium clip and mucosa of EGJ were directly observed from the openings. (arrow: SMTs marked with the titanium clip; NG: nasogastric tube). (**b**) Evert the tumor from the gastrotomy by a stay suture. (**c**) Stapled resection of the tumor. (**d**) Complete the transgastric resection

Table 1 Clinical characteristics

Variable	LEWR (n = 228)	LTR (n = 38)
Gender (male/female)	78/150	13/25
Age (years)	58.7 ± 11.8	52.4 ± 10.3
BMI (kg/m2)	23.4 ± 3.6	23.5 ± 2.7
ASA classification (I/II/III)	113/108/7	19/15/4
Comorbidities (yes)	104	16
Hypertension	77	9
Diabetes mellitus	23	7
Cardiovascular	13	2
Pulmonary	6	3
Pathology		
GIST	203	26
Schwannoma	12	3
Ectopic pancreas	3	1
Leiomyoma	7	7
Lipomas	1	1
Plasmacytoma	2	0

Abbreviation: *BMI* body mass index, *ASA* American Society of Anesthesiologists
Data are means ± standard deviations or number

rate of 3.07%. Two patients (7.14%) developed intraluminal bleeding and one patient developed a pulmonary infection in the LTR group. There were no incidences of conversion to open surgery during the operation. All patients with complications were cured with a conservation treatment. There was no perioperative mortality in our series.

Table 2 Pathologic features of GIST patients

Variable	LEWR (n = 203)	LTR (n = 26)
Tumor size (cm)	3.6 ± 2.5	2.1 ± 1.3
Mitotic rate (per 50 HPF)		
<5	180	22
5 ~ 10	15	3
>10	8	0
Fletcher classification		
Very low risk	55	13
Low risk	100	11
Intermediate risk	34	2
High risk	14	0

Table 3 Surgical outcomes of 266 patients

Variable	LEWR ($n = 228$)	LTR ($n = 38$)
Operation time (min)	90.2 ± 37.2	101.7 ± 38.5
Blood loss (mL)	50.4 ± 51.6	42.2 ± 30.2
First flatus (day)	2.4 ± 1.1	2.2 ± 0.9
Oral intake (days)	3.2 ± 1.1	3.0 ± 1.0
Postoperative hospital stay (days)	5.1 ± 2.1	5.3 ± 1.7
Postoperative complications		
Intraluminal bleeding	1	2
Delayed gastric emptying	4	
Abdominal abscess		
Pulmonary infection	2	1

Discussion

Gastric SMTs are potentially life-threatening tumors. Although the majority of SMTs are benign, some have the potential to become malignant. GISTs make up a large portion of SMTs. It has been reported that the pathogenesis of GIST is closely related to mutations at c-Kit proto-oncogene, and GISTs that do not have c-Kit mutations might be correlated with gain-of-function mutations of platelet-derived growth factor-a (PDGFRa) [12]. Secondary to these findings, imatinib mesylate (Gleevec®) therapy, which can inhibit the intracellular kinase activities of CD117 and PDGFRa, has been manifested to increase the overall tumor control rate of GIST by 85%. It has been report that Gleevec® is the standard treatment for unresectable or metastatic GIST in many countries [13]. However, resection remains the first option for primary GIST. On the one hand, it can establish the diagnosis; on the other hand, it may be curative. SMTs that are not obviously benign should be excised as assumed GISTs. Patients with a diagnosis for GISTs are mainly treated by laparoscopic local resection [14].

Lukaszczyk and colleagues reported in 1992 the use of laparoscopy for gastric GIST resection in a patient [15]. Since then, there have been multiple small series using the laparoscopic approach for these kinds of tumors. In this study, LLR was successfully performed within an acceptable operation time. It is lowest of the average blood loss and morbidity rate, and mortality hardly happened. All patients started oral feeding earlier, the average oral intake day is 3.2 days (range: 2 to 6 days) after the operation. Hospital stays were also short and acceptable. Pathologic examination of the surgical specimens showed that all surgical margins were microscopically tumor free (R0 resection). Although there are no randomized studies comparing laparoscopic versus open approach in the management of gastric SMTs, several retrospective studies have shown the advantages of the laparoscopic approach in treating gastric SMTs, with similar disease free survival, mortality and oncologic

outcomes comparable with the open approach [16–24]. It is not only the technical potential of laparoscopic excision, but also its effectiveness facilitated by the data.

LLR can be distributed into ELWR or LTR according to the development mode, tumor measurement, and site. ELWR is the most ordinary method and the first thought for gastric SMTs. We can use the laparoscopic vision or the haptic retroaction of the laparoscopic tools to locate lesions straightly for the tumors which were located in the anterior wall along the greater curvature of the stomach. Considering the remarkable superfluity and mobility of the stomach in these sites, a laparoscopically stapled gastric wedge excision often is always greatly potential. With a project for a stapled wedge excision, it is easy to come near laparoscopically for tumors in this site. In order to avoid cardiac stricture for tumors located in the fundus, the left gastroepiploic artery should be transected. The gastrophrenic ligament and gastrosplenic ligament should be dissected for mobility of the stomach and then making sure there is enough distance between the cutting line and the left side of the cardia when applying the second staple. Otherwise it would cause stricture due to the Endo-GIA position being too close to the cardia. Because the stomach where tumors along the lesser curvature are short of redundancy, and the lesser curvature is restricted in length, so it is tough to treat laparoscopically. To make the posterior wall of the stomach clear, we are supposed to do dissection to part the stomach from the greater omentum. Then, the lesser curvature was everted and the tumor was removed. The vagus nerve branch (Latarjet nerves) and blood vessels in the lesser omentum should be protected.

For the reason that ELWR has the chance of stenosis or deformity conducing to excessive excision of the normal gastric wall, it is difficult to apply to tumors which are located close to the gastric inlet or outlet [5]. In our series, there seemed to be 65 cases with tumors which were located close to the esophagogastric junction or the pylorus which were thought improper to undergo ELWR by laparoscopic stapling. We had better utilize ultrasonic coagulating shears with the excision margin paralleling the round edge of the tumor to reduce the fine tissue loss and to hold back luminal narrowing to operate manual excision, on condition that the tumor has exogastric development and is located on the anterior wall. Then, the laparoscopic intracorporeal handsewn method was used to close the incision. It is advisable to use the laparoscopic transgastric method for the excision of an intraluminal tumor which is located at the posterior wall of the stomach, which offered straight observation of the lesion and inner stomach, and brings greater command of the surgical margin. [25, 26]. The outcomes of our retrospective research proved that the process was secure and effective. Two cases had postoperative gastric intraluminal bleeding, but this was cured with a conservation treatment. In our experience, the exact site of tumors is crux of this method, which is using endoscopic before the operation, marking with titanium clips, intact redeployment of the EGJ or pylorus before excision, and step cutting transversely along the foundation of the tumor. However, restrictions related to attached bleeding venture and intraperitioneal contanmination by seeping gatric juices are common.[26, 27]. The endoscopic linear staple resection line of the stomach wall is weak and leakage and bleeding occur easily. Therefore, intracorporeal hand-sewn was used in our center to reinforce this area. Intraperitioneal contamination with gastric juice seemed to be a dominating problem of this technique, as the gastric cavity requires opening temporarily. Hence, it is necessary to operate abundant decompression of the stomach before gastrotomy and comprehensive irrigation of the operating area after closing the gastrotomy for preventing abdominal or wound infection.

There is another technique designed to resect tumors located near the EGJ or pylorus is laparoscopic intragastric resection [26]. This technique involves a difficult procedure to set up the view before resection. By blowing up a balloon sticked on the trocars, the gastric wall is supposed to be attached to the abdominal wall after inserting several trocars into the gastric lumen through the gastric wall. This method not only offers an abundant operative area, but also generates less deformity of the EGJ compared with an extragastric approach. However, the need of specific ballon-type ports and the trouble originated from inserting the ports into stomach restricted its feasibility. In addition, if a tumor is larger than 4 cm, the intragastric resection is inapposite, because it is difficult to retract the large specimen orally. We did not use this method in our center.

If a relatively large tumor is located at EGJ and antrum, the surgeons must consider the problems incurred by LLR that include the possibility of stenosis and deforming the gastric inlet or outlet. For tumors located at antrum or large tumors in the lower stomach close to antrum, we recommended laparoscopic distal gastrectomy (LDG). For tumors at EGJ or large tumors in the middle or upper body we recommend laparoscopic total gastrectomy (LTG) instead of laparoscopy proximal gastrectomy (LPG) due to the relatively lower rate of reflux esophagitis. Another tip, observation by flexible endoscope during the resection of the GIST is recommended to avoid gastric inlet or outlet narrowing. During endoscope examination, we looped the pylorus with a silk band to stop gas from entering the intestine, which would interfere with vision and subsequent manipulation.

Several limitations of this study warrant mention and require special attentions in the interpretation. First,

because it was a retrospective study performed at a single institution, case selection was inevitably affected by bias. Second, the uneven surgical skills of the different surgeons might result in flaws of the study. Third, it's a one-arm study and long-term outcomes were not evaluated because of the short observation period. Therefore, randomized controlled trials or prospective comparative studies with long-term follow-up are necessary to adequately evaluate the status of LLR for gastric SMTs.

Conclusion
In conclusion, for the reason that the process provides reasonable morbidity and well-pleasing short-term outcomes, it seems that ELWR is technically practicable for the therapy of gastric SMTs. For gastric intraluminal SMTs which are located close to the EGJ or pylorus, LTR is easy, secure, and efficient. When LLR are inappropriate for bulky tumors located at EGJ or antrum, LDG or LTG could be used to avoid stenosis.

Abbreviations
CT: Computed tomography; EGJ: Esophagogastric junction; EUS: Endoscopic ultrasound; GISTs: Gastrointestinal stromal tumors; HPFs: High-power fields; LDG: Laparoscopic distal gastrectomy; LEWR: Laparoscopic exogastric wedge resection; LG: Laparoscopic gastrectomy; LLR: Laparoscopic local resection; LPG: Laparoscopy proximal gastrectomy; LTG: laparoscopic total gastrectomy; LTR: Laparoscopic transgastric resection; NIH: National Institutes of Health; SMTs: Gastric submucosal tumors

Acknowledgements
The authors thank Hendi Maher from Australia for editing the English language.

Funding
This study was supported by the Nature Science Foundation of Zhejiang Province (No.LY12H16026) and the Chinese Medical Technology Foundation of Zhejiang Province (No.2012ZA087).

Authors' contributions
KC designed the study; XFW, KC and STZ performed the operation; KC and YP wrote the manuscript. JHP, WHY and JFY collected data; WXF proofread and revised the manuscript; all authors have approved the version to be published.

Competing interests
The authors declare that they have no competing interests.

References
1. Guo J, Liu Z, Sun S, Wang S, Ge N, Liu X, Wang G, Liu W. Endosonography-assisted diagnosis and therapy of gastrointestinal submucosal tumors. Endoscopic Ultrasound. 2013;2:125–33.
2. Cheng HL, Lee WJ, Lai IR, Yuan RH, Yu SC. Laparoscopic wedge resection of benign gastric tumor. Hepatogastroenterology. 1999;46:2100–4.
3. Ryu KJ, Jung SR, Choi JS, Jang YJ, Kim JH, Park SS, Park BJ, Park SH, Kim SJ, Mok YJ, Kim CS. Laparoscopic resection of small gastric submucosal tumors. Surg Endosc. 2011;25:271–7.
4. Pidhorecky I, Cheney RT, Kraybill WG, Gibbs JF. Gastrointestinal stromal tumors: current diagnosis, biologic behavior, and management. Ann Surg Oncol. 2000;7:705–12.
5. Tagaya N, Mikami H, Kubota K. Laparoscopic resection of gastrointestinal mesenchymal tumors located in the upper stomach. Surg Endosc. 2004;18: 1469–74.

Short-term outcomes of laparoscopic local resection for gastric submucosal...

135

6. Chen K, Xu X, Mou Y, Pan Y, Zhang R, Zhou Y, Wu D, Huang C. Totally laparoscopic distal gastrectomy with D_2 lymphadenectomy and Billroth II gastrojejunostomy for gastric cancer: short- and medium-term results of 139 consecutive cases from a single institution. Int J Med Sci. 2013;10:1462–70.

7. Chen K, Mou YP, Xu XW, Pan Y, Zhou YC, Cai JQ, Huang CJ. Comparison of short-term surgical outcomes between totally laparoscopic and laparoscopic-assisted distal gastrectomy for gastric cancer: a 10-y single-center experience with meta-analysis. J Surg Res. 2015;194:367–74.

8. Chen K, Mou YP, Xu XW, Cai JQ, Wu D, Pan Y, Zhang RC. Short-term surgical and long-term survival outcomes after laparoscopic distal gastrectomy with D_2 lymphadenectomy for gastric cancer. BMC Gastroenterol. 2014;14:41.

9. Chen K, Pan Y, Cai JQ, Xu XW, Wu D, Yan JF, Chen RG, He Y, Mou YP. Intracorporeal esophagojejunostomy after totally laparoscopic total gastrectomy: A single-center 7-year experience. World J Gastroenterol. 2016;22:3432–40.

10. Chen K, Wu D, Pan Y, Cai JQ, Yan JF, Chen DW, Maher H, Mou YP. Totally laparoscopic gastrectomy using intracorporeally stapler or hand-sewn anastomosis for gastric cancer: a single-center experience of 478 consecutive cases and outcomes. World J Surg Oncol. 2016;14:115.

11. Fletcher CD, Berman JJ, Corless C, Gorstein F, Lasota J, Longley BJ, Miettinen M, O'Leary TJ, Remotti H, Rubin BP, Shmookler B, Sobin LH, Weiss SW. Diagnosis of gastrointestinal stromal tumors: A consensus approach. Hum Pathol. 2002;33:459–65.

12. Hirota S, Isozaki K, Moriyama Y, Hashimoto K, Nishida T, Ishiguro S, Kawano K, Hanada M, Kurata A, Takeda M, Muhammad Tunio G, Matsuzawa Y, Kanakura Y, Shinomura Y, Kitamura Y. Gain-of-function mutations of c-kit in human gastrointestinal stromal tumors. Science. 1998;279:577–80.

13. Group LR. Gleevec for GIST. Available at: https://liferaftgroup.org/gleevec/. November 2012.

14. Joensuu H, Fletcher C, Dimitrijevic S, Silberman S, Roberts P, Demetri G. Management of malignant gastrointestinal stromal tumours. Lancet Oncol. 2002;3:655–64.

15. Lukaszczyk JJ, Preletz RJ. Laparoscopic resection of benign stromal tumor of the stomach. J Laparoendosc Surg. 1992;2:331–4.

16. Catena F, Di Battista M, Fusaroli P, Ansaloni L, Di Scioscio V, Santini D, Pantaleo M, Biasco G, Caletti G, Pinna A. Laparoscopic treatment of gastric GIST: report of 21 cases and literature's review. J Gastrointest Surg. 2008;12:561–8.

17. Silberhumer GR, Hufschmid M, Wrba F, Gyoeri G, Schoppmann S, Tribl B, Wenzl E, Prager G, Laengle F, Zacherl J. Surgery for gastrointestinal stromal tumors of the stomach. J Gastrointest Surg. 2009;13:1213–9.

18. Goh BK, Chow PK, Chok AY, Chan WH, Chung YF, Ong HS, Wong WK. Impact of the introduction of laparoscopic wedge resection as a surgical option for suspected small/medium-sized gastrointestinal stromal tumors of the stomach on perioperative and oncologic outcomes. World J Surg. 2010;34:1847–52.

19. Karakousis GC, Singer S, Zheng J, Gonen M, Coit D, DeMatteo RP, Strong VE. Laparoscopic versus open gastric resections for primary gastrointestinal stromal tumors (GISTs): a size-matched comparison. Ann Surg Oncol. 2011;18:1599–605.

20. De Vogelaere K, Hoorens A, Haentjens P, Delvaux G. Laparoscopic versus open resection of gastrointestinal stromal tumors of the stomach. Surg Endosc. 2013;27:1546–54.

21. Melstrom LG, Phillips JD, Bentrem DJ, Wayne JD. Laparoscopic versus open resection of gastric gastrointestinal stromal tumors. Am J Clin Oncol. 2012;35:451–4.

22. Lee HH, Hur H, Jung H, Park CH, Jeon HM, Song KY. Laparoscopic wedge resection for gastric submucosal tumors: a size-location matched case-control study. J Am Coll Surg. 2011;212:195–9.

23. Pucci MJ, Berger AC, Lim PW, Chojnacki KA, Rosato EL, Palazzo F. Laparoscopic approaches to gastric gastrointestinal stromal tumors: an institutional review of 57 cases. Surg Endosc. 2012;26:3509–14.

24. Chen K, Zhou YC, Mou YP, Xu XW, Jin WW, Ajoodhea H. Systematic review and meta-analysis of safety and efficacy of laparoscopic resection for gastrointestinal stromal tumors of the stomach. Surg Endosc. 2015;29:355–67.

25. Basso N, Silecchia G, Pizzuto G, Surgo D, Picconi T, Materia A. Laparoscopic excision of posterior gastric wall leiomyoma. Surg Laparosc Endosc. 1996;6:65–7.

26. Tagaya N, Mikami H, Kogure H, Kubota K, Hosoya Y, Nagai H. Laparoscopic intragastric stapled resection of gastric submucosal tumors located near the esophagogastric junction. Surg Endosc. 2002;16:177–9.

27. Motson RW, Fisher PW, Dawson JW. Laparoscopic resection of a benign intragastric stromal tumour. Br J Surg. 1995;82:1670.

21

Nodal skip metastasis in thoracic esophageal squamous cell carcinoma: a cohort study

Francesco Cavallin[1*], Rita Alfieri[1], Marco Scarpa[1], Matteo Cagol[1], Alberto Ruol[2], Matteo Fassan[3], Massimo Rugge[3], Ermanno Ancona[1] and Carlo Castoro[1]

Abstract

Background: Nodal skip metastasis is a prognostic factor in some sites of malignancies, but its role in esophageal cancer is still unclear. The present study aimed to investigate occurrence and effect of nodal skip metastases in thoracic esophageal squamous cell carcinoma.

Methods: All 578 patients undergoing esophagectomy for thoracic esophageal squamous cell carcinoma at the Center for Esophageal Diseases located in Padova between January 1992 and December 2010 were retrospectively evaluated. Selection criteria were R0 resection, pathological M0 stage and pathological lymph node involvement. Patients receiving neoadjuvant therapy were excluded.

Results: The selection identified 88 patients with lymph node involvement confirmed by pathological evaluation. Sixteen patients (18.2%) had nodal skip metastasis. Adjusting for the number of lymph node metastases, patient with nodal skip metastasis had similar 5-year overall survival (14% vs. 13%, $p = 0.93$) and 5-year disease free survival (14% vs. 9%, $p = 0.48$) compared to patients with both peritumoral and distant lymph node metastases. The risk difference of nodal skip metastasis was: −24.1% (95% C.I. -43.1% to −5.2%) in patients with more than one lymph node metastasis compared to those with one lymph node metastasis; −2.3% (95% C.I. -29.8% to 25.2%) in middle thoracic esophagus and −23.0% (95% C.I. -47.8% to 1.8%) in lower thoracic esophagus compared to upper thoracic esophagus; 18.1% (95% C.I. 3.2% to 33.0%) in clinical N0 stage vs. clinical N+ stage.

Conclusions: Nodal skip metastasis is a common pattern of metastatic lymph involvement in thoracic esophageal squamous cell carcinoma. However, neither overall survival nor disease free survival are associated with nodal skip metastasis occurrence.

Keywords: Esophageal cancer, Nodal skip metastasis, Metastasis, Lymph node involvement, Esophagectomy

Background

Esophageal cancer is a very aggressive malignancy, with poor prognosis in resected patients. Although the incidence of esophageal adenocarcinoma (EAC) has been increasing in Western Countries [1], esophageal squamous cell carcinoma (ESCC) is still the predominant esophageal malignancy in Eastern Countries, like Japan and China [2, 3].

The most important factor affecting the prognosis of ESCC patients is lymph node (LN) involvement, which

is included in the American Joint Committee of Cancer (AJCC) TNM classification [4]. The role of lymph node metastases (LNMs) on prognosis has been widely investigated, from the simple involvement to the number of involved nodes [5–7]. The ratio of LNMs on harvested nodes has also been evaluated to take into account the variability of lymph node dissection, but its role is still unclear [8]. The 7th edition of the AJCC staging system took into account all these results on LN involvement and it increased the classes of N-stage according to the number of LNMs [4]. Apart from the number, the localization of LNMs could also play a role in ESCC prognosis. Since the esophagus is an organ that passes

---
* Correspondence: cescocava@libero.it
[1]Esophageal and Digestive Tract Surgical Unit, Regional Centre for Esophageal Disease, Veneto Institute of Oncology IOV IRCCS, Padova, Italy
Full list of author information is available at the end of the article

through three main anatomic regions (neck, chest, abdomen), the prognosis of patients with the same number of positive LNs might be different due to localization of LNMs in one or more anatomic regions [9].

Nodal skip metastasis (NSM) is a particular pattern of LNMs, which involves the LNs distant from the tumor site but not the peritumoral LNs. This pattern has been evaluated to be relevant in other kinds of malignancies [10, 11] but its role in esophageal cancer patients is still controversial [12]. The aim of this study was to investigate the factors predicting NSM and to assess its effect on survival and recurrence in thoracic ESCC.

Methods
Study design
The present study aimed to investigate the factors predicting NSM and to assess its effect on survival and recurrence in thoracic ESCC. All 578 patients undergoing esophagectomy for thoracic ESCC at the Center for Esophageal Diseases located in Padova between January 1, 1992 and December 31, 2010 were retrospectively evaluated for inclusion in this study using a prospectively collected database. Inclusion criteria were pathological lymph node involvement, R0 resection and absence of distant metastasis (M0) on final specimen. Patients receiving neoadjuvant therapy were excluded according to literature [12] because neoadjuvant therapy modifies frequency and distribution of LNMs [13]. Patients included in the study did not receive neoadjuvant therapy due to clinical N0 stage, contraindications to chemo-radio therapy (i.e. previous radio therapy or hematopoietic comorbidities) or patient's refusal. The study was conducted according to Helsinki Declaration principles of 1975, as revised in 1983, and patients gave their consent to have their data collected for scientific purposes. This retrospective study was notified to the Ethical Committee of Veneto Oncology Institute IOV IRCCS who did not find any ethical problems (2014–06-16-Note4).

Preoperative evaluation
In all patients, preoperative evaluation was performed, including barium tests; esophageal endoscopy; computed tomography (CT) of the neck, chest, and abdomen; and bronchoscopy. Endosonography (EUS) of the esophagus and positron emission tomography scan have been part of routine esophageal cancer staging since 2000 and 2005, respectively. Indication for surgery was determined by an experienced multidisciplinary team composed of a dedicated upper gastrointestinal surgeon, a medical oncologist and radiation oncologist.

Pathology
Histopathological examination of all resected specimens consisted in evaluation of: tumor stage, residual tumor,

grading, and number of lymph nodes involved. The specimens were fixed in 5% formaldehyde and set in paraffin. The lymph nodes were counted and assessed by a pathologist. A series of sections from each node were selected and stained with hematoxylin and eosin (H&E) as well as with periodic acid-Schiff (PAS). All dissected lymph nodes were microscopically analyzed for metastatic disease [13].

Tumor location and lymph node classification
The seventh edition of AJCC cancer staging system was used to determine TNM stage and to classify thoracic ESCC in upper, middle and lower thoracic esophagus [4]. LNMs were assigned to five groups [12]. Laterocervical and supraclavicular nodes were assigned to cervical group. Upper and lower paratracheal nodes and upper paraesophageal nodes were assigned to upper mediastinal group, while middle paraesophageal and subcarinal nodes to middle mediastinal group, and lower paraesophageal and inferior pulmonary vein nodes to lower mediastinal group. Paracardial, perigastric and celiac nodes were assigned to abdominal group [4]. LNMs were then classified as peritumoral or distant according to the location of the tumor (Fig. 1). NSM was defined as presence of distant LNMs without presence of peritumoral LNMs. Patients with peritumoral LNMs (with or without presence of distant LNMs) were included in non-NSM group.

Surgery and post-surgical follow up
The surgical treatment consisted in open radical transthoracic esophagectomy with cervical or mediastinal anastomosis. Briefly, esophagectomy was performed using an Ivor-Lewis procedure, via laparotomy and right thoracotomy, for tumors of the mid-lower esophagus and gastric cardia. A three-stage McKeown's procedure, with an additional left cervical incision, was performed in tumors in the upper third of the esophagus. At least 6–8 cm of healthy esophagus was resected above the proximal edge of the tumor to avoid neoplastic involvement of the resection margins. In this group of patients, en bloc lymph node dissection was performed, including the paraesophageal, sub carinal, posterior mediastinal and paracardial lymph nodes, as well as those located along the lesser gastric curvature, the origin of the left gastric artery, the celiac trunk, the common hepatic artery and the splenic artery. Cervical nodal dissection (three-field dissection) was performed in case of suspected LNMs at preoperative evaluation. The alimentary tract was reconstructed using the gastric pull-up technique; if the stomach was unavailable, either a jejunal loop or the left colon was used. Follow-up visits were scheduled every 3 months in the first year after surgery, every 6 months during the next 2 years and every 12 months thereafter. An upper gastrointestinal endoscopy was performed regularly 1 year after surgery, or earlier based on the clinical findings, with

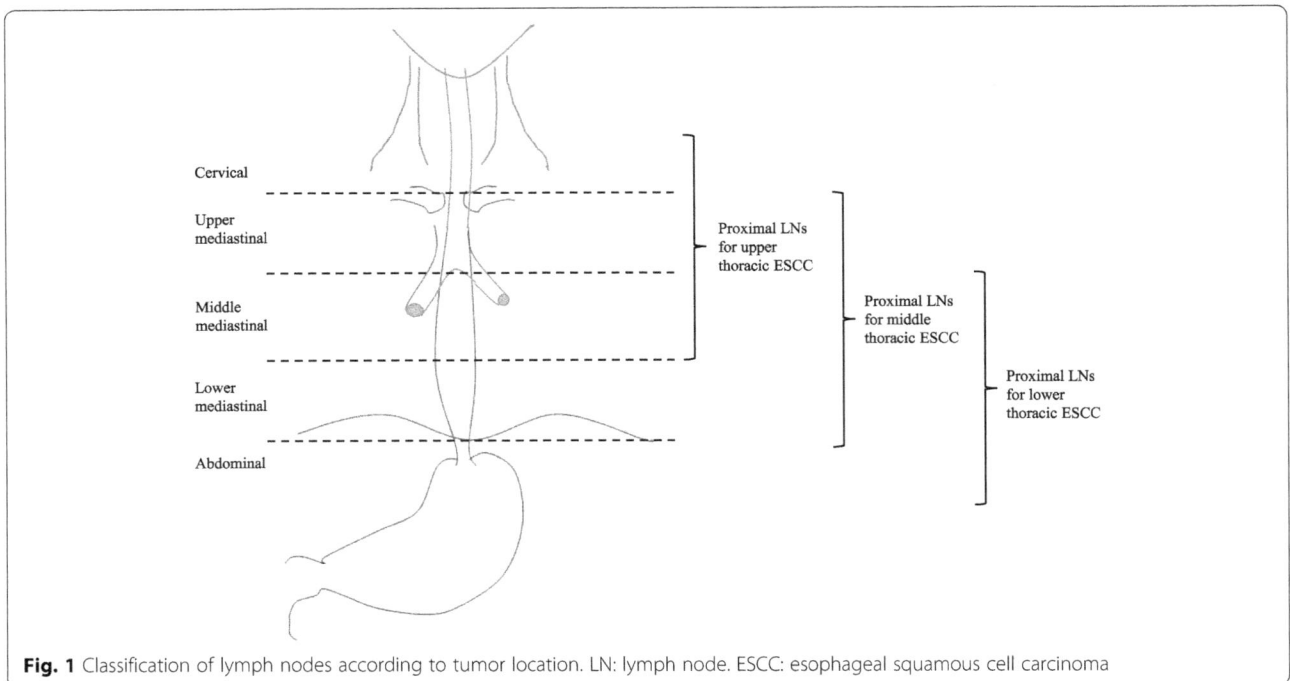

Fig. 1 Classification of lymph nodes according to tumor location. LN: lymph node. ESCC: esophageal squamous cell carcinoma

direct evaluation of the remaining esophagus, anastomosis and of the esophageal replacement conduct. Functional results were assessed based on clinical and endoscopical findings.

Statistical analysis

Continuous data were expressed as median and interquartile range (IQR). Categorical data were compared between patients with NSM and those without NSM using Fisher's exact test and continuous data using Mann-Whitney test. Multivariable analysis of risk factors for NSM was not performed due to the small number of patient with NSM. Overall survival (OS) and disease-free survival (DFS) estimates were calculated for patients with NSM and those without NSM using Cox regression models, adjusting for the number of LNM. In addition, we reviewed the short-term follow-up of pN0 patients, who were excluded from the main analysis. The occurrence of LNM at cervical, mediastinal or abdominal LNs within 6 months from surgery identified the patients who were wrongly considered pN0 due to 2-field lymphadenectomy and might have been benefit from a complete lymphadenectomy. All tests were two-sided and a p-value less than 0.05 was considered significant. Statistical analysis was performed using SAS 9.1 (SAS Institute Inc., Cary, NC, USA).

Results

Patients

Eighty-eight patients were included in the final sample according to selection criteria (Fig. 2). These 88 patients did not receive neoadjuvant therapy due to clinical N0 stage (50 patients), contraindications to chemo-radio therapy (12 patients) or patient's refusal (26 patients). The majority were males (71, 80.7%) and the median age was 62 years (IQR 57–70). The median harvested lymph nodes was 17 (IQR 12–25). Patient characteristics are shown in Table 1.

Nodal skip metastasis

Sixteen patients (18.2%) showed NSM and 72 (81.8%) had both peritumoral and distant LNMs. The number of harvested lymph nodes was similar in the two groups (median 18 in NSM vs. 17 in non-NSM patients, $p = 0.72$; Table 2), but patients with NSM had lower number of metastatic lymph nodes than those without NSM (median 1 vs. 2, $p = 0.01$; Table 2). The risk difference of NSM was –24.1% (95% C.I. -43.1% to –5.2%) in patients with more than one LNM compared to those with one LNM. The rate of NSM was different according to tumor location ($p = 0.02$; Table 2) and clinical N stage ($p = 0.04$; Table 2). Compared to upper thoracic esophagus, the risk difference of NSM was –2.3% (95% C.I. -29.8% to 25.2%) in middle thoracic esophagus and –23.0% (95% C.I. -47.8% to 1.8%) in lower thoracic esophagus. The risk difference of NSM was 18.1% (95% C.I. 3.2% to 33.0%) in clinical N0 stage vs. clinical N+ stage.

Survival

Median follow-up was 23 months (IQR 14–41). Three patients died of postoperative complications (two cardio-pulmonary and one sepsis). The 5-year OS was similar

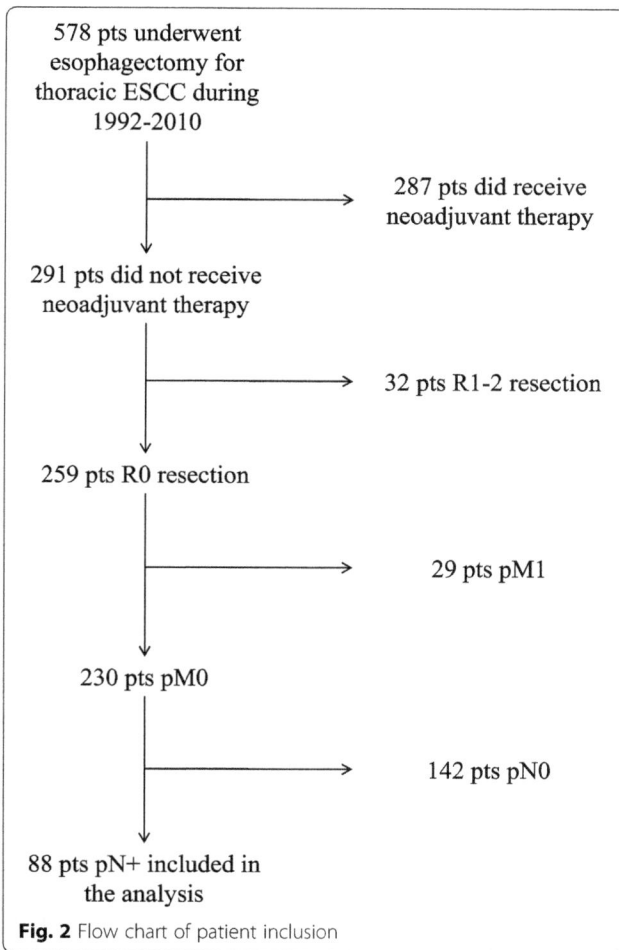

578 pts underwent esophagectomy for thoracic ESCC during 1992-2010

287 pts did receive neoadjuvant therapy

291 pts did not receive neoadjuvant therapy

32 pts R1-2 resection

259 pts R0 resection

29 pts pM1

230 pts pM0

142 pts pN0

88 pts pN+ included in the analysis

Fig. 2 Flow chart of patient inclusion

Table 1 Clinical and pathological characteristics

Number	88
Age (years)[a]	62 (57–70)
Sex Male: Female	71:17
Advanced liver disease	18 (20.5)
Pulmonary disease	17 (19.3)
Tumor location:	
Upper thoracic esophagus	14 (15.9)
Middle thoracic esophagus	38 (43.2)
Lower thoracic esophagus	36 (40.9)
Tumor differentiation:	
Well	16 (18.2)
Moderately	57 (64.8)
Poor	15 (17.0)
Tumor length (mm)[a]	50 (40–70)
Pathologic T stage	
T1	11 (12.5)
T2	10 (11.4)
T3	58 (65.9)
T4	9 (10.2)
Harvested lymph nodes[a]	17 (12–25)
Lymph node metastasis:	
Peritumoral or Peritumoral and distant (non-NSM)	72 (81.8)
Only distant (NSM)	16 (18.2)
Adjuvant therapy: yes	28 (31.8)

Data expressed as n (%) or [a]median(IQR). NSM: nodal skip metastasis

in patients with NSM and in those without NSM (14% vs. 13% respectively; p = 0.93; Fig. 3a), adjusting for the number of LNM. The 5-year DFS was similar in patients with NSM and in those without NSM (14% vs. 9% respectively; p = 0.48; Fig. 2b), adjusting for the number of LNM.

Recurrence pattern in NSM patients

Recurrence was detected in 10 out of 16 NSM patients. One patient had upper esophageal ESCC with abdominal NSM and the recurrence site was locoregional. One patient had upper esophageal ESCC with abdominal NSM and the recurrence site was both locoregional and distant (pulmonary LN). Four patients had middle esophageal ESCC with abdominal lymph node involvement and the recurrence site was locoregional. Three patients had middle esophageal ESCC with abdominal lymph node involvement and the recurrence site was distant. One patient had middle esophageal ESCC with abdominal lymph node involvement and the recurrence site was both locoregional and distant (pulmonary LN and abdominal LN).

Sub-analysis of pN0 patients

Among the 142 pN0 patients who were excluded from the main analysis (Fig. 1), 3 patients (2.1%) had LNM at cervical, mediastinal or abdominal LNs within 6 months from surgery. One patient out of 41 (2.4%) with upper thoracic ESCC had a cervical LNM (i.e. would have been included in the non-NSM group) and died after CTRT treatment at 10 months from surgery. Two patients out of 67 (3%) with middle thoracic ESCC had a cervical LNM (i.e. would have been included in the NSM group) and died after palliative resection and CTRT at 13 and 19 months, respectively. None of pN0 patients with lower thoracic ESCC had LNM at cervical, mediastinal or abdominal LNs within 6 months from surgery. Adding these 3 patients to the 88 patients of the main analysis, the rate of NSM would have increased from 18.2% (16 out of 88) to 19.8% (18 out of 91).

Discussion

NSM is not an uncommon form of metastatic spread to lymph nodes and has been found to be of clinical importance in some sites of malignancies, i.e. non-small cell lung cancer or thyroid cancer [10, 11]. The presence

Table 2 Factors associated with nodal skip metastasis

	Non-NSM	NSM	p-value
Number	72	16	-
Age (years)[a]	63 (57–70)	59 (54–69)	0.64
Sex Male: Female	59:13	12:4	0.50
Advanced liver disease	15 (20.8)	3 (18.8)	0.99
Pulmonary disease	14 (19.4)	3 (18.8)	0.99
Tumor location:			0.02
Upper thoracic esophagus	10 (13.9)	4 (25.0)	
Middle thoracic esophagus	28 (38.9)	10 (62.5)	
Lower thoracic esophagus	34 (47.2)	2 (12.5)	
Tumor differentiation:			0.21
Well	11 (15.3)	5 (31.3)	
Moderate	47 (65.3)	10 (62.5)	
Poor	14 (19.4)	1 (6.2)	
Tumor length (mm)[a]	50 (40–70)	50 (35–50)	0.22
Preoperative clinical N stage:			0.04
cN+	35 (48.6)	3 (18.8)	
cN0	37 (51.4)	13 (81.2)	
Pathologic T stage:			0.99
pT1-pT2	17 (23.6)	4 (25.0)	
pT3-pT4	55 (76.4)	12 (75.0)	
Harvested lymph nodes[a]	17 (12–25)	18 (13–23)	0.72
Metastatic lymph nodes[a]	1 (1–3)	2 (1–5)	0.01

Data expressed as n (%) or [a]median(IQR), *NSM* nodal skip metastasis

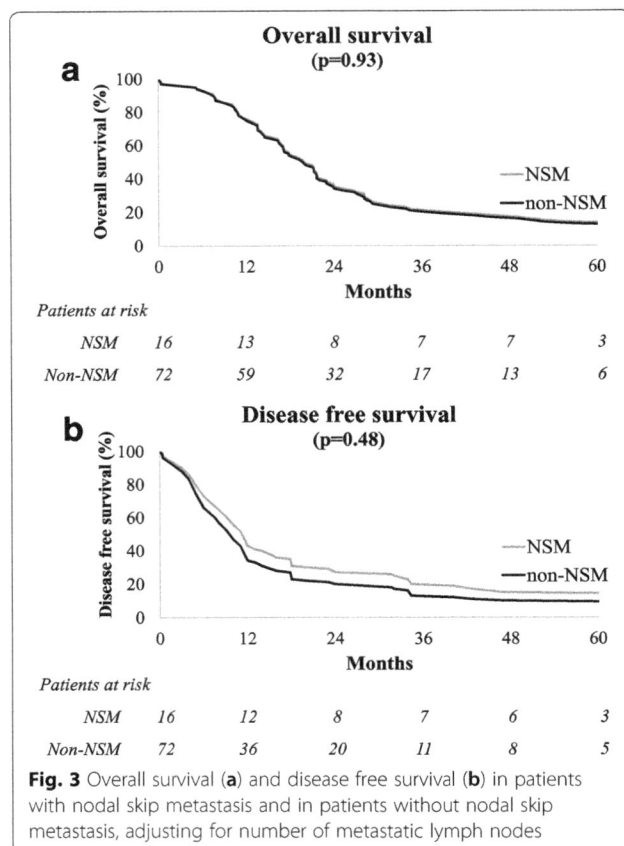

Fig. 3 Overall survival (**a**) and disease free survival (**b**) in patients with nodal skip metastasis and in patients without nodal skip metastasis, adjusting for number of metastatic lymph nodes

of NSM has also been evaluated in esophageal cancer but its prognostic role is still unclear and requires further investigation [12, 14–18]. Recent studies on this topic are summarized in Table 3. The rate of NSM in esophageal cancer varied widely across the studies (from 20.3% to 76.3%, Table 3), increasing the uncertainty about this type of metastatic spread. Such variability could be explained by the different criteria of lymph node classification criteria that were used by the authors. Briefly, NSM has been defined as a) metastatic involvement of distant LNs with peritumoral LNs free of tumor infiltration [12, 16, 18,], b) cervical and/or abdominal involvement but no mediastinal metastasis [14, 15, 19], or c) metastatic infiltration of N2 through N4 lymph nodes but not of N1 nodes according to the Japanese staging system of the Japanese Society for Esophageal Disease [15, 17]. The first definition (metastatic involvement of distant LNs with peritumoral LNs free of tumor infiltration) was used in the present study because we believed it would afford a stricter definition of skip lymph nodes. It is noteworthy that Wu et al. [15] used different lymph node classification criteria to evaluate the same sample and reported very different rates of NSM (24.2% and 69.7%). In addition, the different node dissection (both

2-field and 3-field node dissections have been reported) [19] and the inclusion of both EAC and ESCC patients in 2 studies could have contributed to the variability of the reported rate of NSM (Table 3).

Predictors of NSM in esophageal cancer has been investigated in three previous studies [12, 17, 18] that reported tumor location as the main factor associated to NSM (Table 3). In our series, the number of NSM patients did not allow any meaningful multivariable analysis of risk factors for NSM. However, univariate analysis suggested a higher NSM occurrence in upper and middle thoracic esophagus. In literature, tumors located in the middle thoracic esophagus were identified as risk factor for NSM, despite slight differences among the studies regarding the comparison of tumor sites (Table 3). The association between NSM and middle thoracic esophageal tumors could be explained by its anatomic location (which allows both upper and lower spread directions) and by the definition itself of NSM (cervical and abdominal lymph nodes are possible NSMs), which increase the likelihood of finding NSMs in tumors located in middle thoracic esophagus [20–22].

In our series, patients with NSM showed similar overall survival and disease free survival compared to those with peritumoral LNM, adjusting for the number of

Table 3 Main findings of recent literature: all patients had thoracic esophageal cancer and were treated with esophagectomy without neoadjuvant therapy

First author and year	Country	Histotype	Node dissection	N pts. with LNM	NSM rate	Predictors of NSM	Effect of NSM on OS	Effect of NSM on DFS
Zhu, 2013 [a][13]	China	ESCC	3-field	207	28%	Tumor location (middle esophagus)	Similar prognosis	Not evaluated
Li, 2013 [b][14]	China	Superficial ESCC	2-field/3-field	49	40.8%	Not evaluated	Not evaluated	Not evaluated
Wu, 2012 [b][c][15]	China	Middle thoracic ESCC	2-field/3-field	33	24.2% to 69.7% [d]	Not evaluated	Similar prognosis	Not evaluated
Xu, 2011 [a][16]	China	ESCC	Not reported	38	76.3%	Not evaluated	Similar prognosis	Not evaluated
Prenzel, 2010 [c][17]	Germany	EAC/ESCC	2-field	128	20.3%	Tumor location (middle/upper esophagus) and T1 stage	Better prognosis	Not evaluated
Chen, 2009 [a][18]	China	ESCC	3-field	1081	73.6%	Tumor location (middle/lower esophagus)	Not evaluated	Not evaluated

LNM lymph node metastasis, *NSM* nodal skip metastasis, *OS* overall survival, *DFS* disease free survival, *ESCC* esophageal squamous cell carcinoma, *EAC* esophageal adenocarcinoma. [a]NSM defined as metastatic involvement of distant LNs with peritumoral LNs free of tumor infiltration. [b]NSM defined as cervical and/or abdominal involvement but no mediastinal metastasis. [c]NSM defined as metastatic infiltration of N2 through N4 lymph nodes but not of N1 nodes according to the Japanese staging system of the Japanese Society for Esophageal Disease. [d]According to the different definitions evaluated in the study

LNMs. Similar findings on overall survival in ESCC patients were shown by 3 previous Chinese studies [12, 15, 16] while Prenzel et al. [17] reported a favorable prognosis associated with the presence of NSM in a heterogeneous group of both ESCC and EAC patients. It was surprising that NSM (distant metastases in absence of local metastases) did not affect overall survival. Our hypothesis is that patient immune response to cancer cells cleared the peritumoral metastases while some surviving clones proceeded to further nodal stations. Therefore, NSM might represent a final escape step of ESCC progression [23]. In addition, previous data on favorable prognosis of NSM in ESCC might have been biased by the lower number of LNMs in NSM patients. We think that these considerations might be extended to disease free survival, but the literature did not provide useful data on the association between NSM and disease free survival in ESCC.

Our series included over 50% clinical N0 stages, thus the role of radical lymphadenectomy is further enhanced, even in case of apparent N0 stage at clinical evaluation. Moreover, NSM was less likely identified than local LN involvement during preoperative evaluation (cN0 rate 81.2% vs. 51.4%). These findings support the potential usefulness of innovative techniques such as sentinel node assessment in order to intraoperatively identify the pattern of LN involvement [24].

The present study has some limitations. First, it is a retrospective study on a single-institution series. Second, the number of patients may have prevented some findings from being extrapolated. Third, the quality of lymphadenectomy could have affected the results. However, all esophagectomies were performed by the same surgical team; – thus the warranted homogeneity of the

surgical approach - and the number of harvested nodes were acceptable. In fact, 2-field lymphadenectomy failed to identify LNM in only 3 patients (2.1%) who had cervical nodal metastasis and had been staged N0 at pathologic evaluation upon final specimen.

Conclusions

NSM is a common pattern of metastatic LN involvement in thoracic ESCC, but it does not affect the prognosis. The heterogeneity of the studies on NSM in literature requires further evaluation in order to investigate this lymph node metastatic spread.

Abbreviations
CT: Computed tomography; DFS: Disease free survival; EAC: Esophageal adenocarcinoma; ESCC: Esophageal squamous cell carcinoma; EUS: Endosonography; IQR: Interquartile range; LN: Lymph node; LNM: Lymph node metastasis; NSM: Nodal skip metastasis; OS: Overall survival

Acknowledgments
The authors are grateful to Ms. Christina Drace (Language Revision Service, Veneto Institute of Oncology IOV IRCCS, Padova, Italy) for the English revision of the manuscript. Ms. Christina Drace is a native English speaker.

Funding
None.

Authors' contributions
FC, MS and CC designed the study; MC, RA, AR, MF, MR and EA collected the data; FC and MS analyzed the data; FC, MS and CC wrote the manuscript; MC, RA, AR, MF, MR and EA critically revised the manuscript for important intellectual content; all authors read and approved the final manuscript.

Competing interests
The authors declare that they have no competing interests.

Author details
[1]Esophageal and Digestive Tract Surgical Unit, Regional Centre for
Esophageal Disease, Veneto Institute of Oncology IOV IRCCS, Padova, Italy.
[2]3rd Surgical Clinic, Azienda Ospedaliera di Padova, Padova, Italy.
[3]Department of Medicine (DIMED), Surgical Pathology & CytopathologyUnit,
University of Padova, Padova, Italy.

References

1. Torre LA, Bray F, Siegel RL, Ferlay J, Lortet-Tieulent J, Jemal A. Global cancer statistics, 2012. CA Cancer J Clin. 2015;65:87–108.

2. Domper Arnal MJ, Ferrández Arenas Á, Lanas AÁ. Esophageal cancer: risk factors, screening and endoscopic treatment in western and eastern countries. World J Gastroenterol. 2015;21:7933–43.

3. Tran GD, Sun XD, Abnet CC, Fan JH, Dawsey SM, Dong ZW, Mark SD, Qiao YL, Taylor PR. Prospective study of risk factors for esophageal and gastric cancers in the Linxian general population trial cohort in China. Int J Cancer. 2005;113:456–63.

4. Edge SB, Byrd DR, Compton CC, Fritz AG, Greene FL, Trotti A. AJCC cancer staging manual. 7th ed. New York: Springer; 2009.

5. Kayani B, Zacharakis E, Ahmed K, Hanna GB. Lymph node metastases and prognosis in oesophageal carcinoma - a systematic review. Eur J Surg Oncol. 2011;37:747–53.

6. Akutsu Y, Shuto K, Kono T, Uesato M, Hoshino I, Shiratori T, Isozaki Y, Akanuma N, Uno T, Matsubara H. The number of pathologic lymph nodes involved is still a significant prognostic factor even after neoadjuvant chemoradiotherapy in esophageal squamous cell carcinoma. J Surg Oncol. 2012;15(105):756–60.

7. Zheng YZ, Zhao W, Hu Y, Ding-Lin XX, Wen J, Yang H, Liu QW, Luo KJ, Huang QY, Chen JY, Fu JH. Aggressive surgical resection does not improve survival in operable esophageal squamous cell carcinoma with N2-3 status. World J Gastroenterol. 2015;21:8644–52.

8. Mariette C, Piessen G, Briez N, Triboulet JP. The number of metastatic lymph nodes and the ratio between metastatic and examined lymph nodes are independent prognostic factors in esophageal cancer regardless of neoadjuvant chemoradiation or lymphadenectomy extent. Ann Surg. 2008;247:365–71.

9. Zheng WH, Zhu SM, Zhao A, Mao WM. The prognostic impact of lymph node involvement in large scale operable node-positive esophageal Squamous cell carcinoma patients: a 10-year experience. PLoS One. 2015;10:e0133076.

10. Prenzel KL, Mönig SP, Sinning JM, Baldus SE, Gutschow CA, Grass G, Schneider PM, Hölscher AH. Role of skip metastasis to mediastinal lymph nodes in non-small cell lung cancer. J Surg Oncol. 2003;82:256–60.

11. Machens A, Holzhausen HJ, Dralle H. Skip metastases in thyroid cancer leaping the central lymph node compartment. Arch Surg. 2004;139:43–5.

12. Zhu Z, Yu W, Li H, Zhao K, Zhao W, Zhang Y, Sun M, Wei Q, Chen H, Xiang J, Fu X. Nodal skip metastasis is not a predictor of survival in thoracic esophageal squamous cell carcinoma. Ann Surg Oncol. 2013;20:3052–8.

13. Castoro C, Scarpa M, Cagol M, Ruol A, Cavallin F, Alfieri R, Zanchettin G, Rugge M, Ancona E. Nodal metastasis from locally advanced esophageal cancer: how neoadjuvant therapy modifies their frequency and distribution. Ann Surg Oncol. 2011;18:3743–54.

14. Li B, Chen H, Xiang J, Zhang Y, Kong Y, Garfield DH, Li H. Prevalence of lymph node metastases in superficial esophageal squamous cell carcinoma. J Thorac Cardiovasc Surg. 2013;146:1198–203.

15. Wu J, Chen QX, Zhou XM, Mao WM, Krasna MJ, Teng LS. Prognostic significance of solitary lymph node metastasis in patients with squamous cell carcinoma of middle thoracic esophagus. World J Surg Oncol. 2012;10:210.

16. Xu QR, Zhuge XP, Zhang HL, Ping YM, Chen LQ. The N-classification for esophageal cancer staging: should it be based on number, distance, or extent of the lymph node metastasis? World J Surg. 2011;35:1303–10.

17. Prenzel KL, Bollschweiler E, Schröder W, Mönig SP, Drebber U, Vallboehmer D, Hölscher AH. Prognostic relevance of skip metastases in esophageal cancer. Ann Thorac Surg. 2010;90:1662–7.

18. Chen J, Liu S, Pan J, Zheng X, Zhu K, Zhu J, Xiao J, Ying M. The pattern and prevalence of lymphatic spread in thoracic oesophageal squamous cell carcinoma. Eur J Cardiothorac Surg. 2009;36:480–6.

19. Li H, Zhang Y, Cai H, Xiang J. Pattern of lymph node metastases in patients with squamous cell carcinoma of the thoracic esophagus who underwent three-field lymphadenectomy. Eur Surg Res. 2007;39:1–6.

20. Tachibana M, Kinugasa S, Hirahara N, Yoshimura H. Lymph node classification of esophageal squamous cell carcinoma and adenocarcinoma. Eur J Cardiothorac Surg. 2008;34:427–31.

21. Skandalakis JE, Ellis H. Embryologic and anatomic basis of esophageal surgery. Surg Clin North Am. 2000;80:85–155.

22. Hosch SB, Stoecklein NH, Pichlmeier U, Rehders A, Scheunemann P, Niendorf A, Knoefel WT, Izbicki JR. Esophageal cancer: the mode of lymphatic tumor cell spread and its prognosticsignificance. J Clin Oncol. 2001;19:1970–5.

23. Dunn GP, Bruce AT, Ikeda H, Old LJ, Schreiber RD. Cancer immunoediting: from immunosurveillance to tumor escape. Nat Immunol. 2002;3:991–998.

24. Filip B, Scarpa M, Cavallin F, Alfieri R, Cagol M, Castoro C. Minimally invasive surgery for esophageal cancer: a review on sentinel node concept. Surg Endosc. 2014;28:1238–49.

22

BariSurg trial: Sleeve gastrectomy versus Roux-en-Y gastric bypass in obese patients with BMI 35–60 kg/m² – a multi-centre randomized patient and observer blind non-inferiority trial

Lars Fischer[1*†], Anna-Laura Wekerle[1†], Thomas Bruckner[2], Inga Wegener[3], Markus K. Diener[1,3], Moritz V. Frankenberg[4], Daniel Gärtner[5], Michael R. Schön[5], Matthias C. Raggi[6], Emre Tanay[6], Rainer Brydniak[7], Norbert Runkel[7], Corinna Attenberger[8], Min-Seop Son[9], Andreas Türler[9], Rudolf Weiner[10], Markus W. Büchler[1] and Beat P. Müller-Stich[1]

Abstract

Background: Roux-en-Ygastric bypass (RYGB) and sleeve gastrectomy (SG) rank among the most frequently applied bariatric procedures worldwide due to their positive risk/benefit correlation. A systematic review revealed a similar excess weight loss (EWL) 2 years postoperatively between SG and RYGB. However, there is a lack of randomized controlled multi-centre trials comparing SG and RYGB, not only concerning EWL, but also in terms of remission of obesity-related co-morbidities, gastroesophageal reflux disease (GERD) and quality of life (QoL) in the mid- and long-term.

Methods: The BariSurg trial was designed as a multi-centre, randomized controlled patient and observer blind trial. The trial protocol was approved by the corresponding ethics committees of the centres. To demonstrate EWL non-inferiority of SG compared to RYGB, power calculation was performed according to a non-inferiority study design. Morbidity, mortality, remission of obesity-related co-morbidities, GERD course and QoL are major secondary endpoints. 248 patients between 18 and 70 years, with a body mass index (BMI) between 35–60 kg/m² and indication for bariatric surgery according to the most recent German S3-guidelines will be randomized. The primary and secondary endpoints will be assessed prior to surgery and afterwards at discharge and at the time points 3–6, 12, 24, 36, 48 and 60 months postoperatively.

Discussion: With its five year follow-up, the BariSurg-trial will provide further evidence based data concerning the impact of SG and RYGB on EWL, remission of obesity-related co-morbidities, the course of GERD and QoL.

Keywords: Sleeve gastrectomy, Roux-en-Ygastric bypass, Randomized controlled trial, Patient and observer blind trial, Long-term excess weight loss, Obesity related co-morbidity, Gastroesophageal reflux disease, Quality of life, Morbidity, Mortality

* Correspondence: lars.fischer@med.uni-heidelberg.de
†Equal contributors
[1]Department of General, Visceral and Transplantation Surgery, University of Heidelberg, Im Neuenheimer Feld 110, 69120 Heidelberg, Germany
Full list of author information is available at the end of the article

Background

Rationale of the trial

The effect of bariatric surgery on obesity and related co-morbidities such as type 2 diabetes mellitus (T2DM) or hypertension is no longer doubted [1–3]. Reliable data showing improved overall patient survival and a reduced cancer incidence, especially in females, following bariatric surgery are available [4]. Additionally, bariatric surgery can now be performed safely and with acceptable morbidity and mortality [5, 6]. The procedures performed in the field of bariatric surgery are still evolving and include rather simple procedures such as gastric banding and more advanced techniques, such as biliopancreatic diversion or ileal transposition. Looking from a more general point of view, Roux-en-Y gastric bypass (RYGB) and sleeve gastrectomy (SG) are the most commonly performed procedures worldwide and in Germany, a finding that is likely due to their positive risk/benefit correlation [6]. However, RYGB is still considered superior to SG [7, 8]. This belief, however, is mostly based on historical considerations, as RYGB was one of the first bariatric procedures ever performed [9]. Because of recent evidence including systematic reviews and randomized controlled trials, SG has become more and more accepted as a stand-alone bariatric surgery procedure [9–17]. The systematic review data revealed, among other things, that excess weight loss (EWL) after SG was not significantly different from EWL following RYGB, 24 months after surgery [13]. This finding is consistent with that of Peterli et al., who also observed no significant differences in 12 month post-op EWL between SG and RYGB [9]. Another randomized controlled trial (RCT) from Finland, comparing SG and RYGB, revealed a significantly reduced operative time and complication rates in favour of the SG group [12]. As a result, the German statistic on obesity surgery for 2011 revealed for the first time, that more SG resections than RYBGs were performed [13, 18, 19]. Nevertheless, SG is still regarded with some scepticism due to the lack of valid long-term results and RCTs. Major criticism includes not only the effect of SG on EWL, but also on the course of obesity-related co-morbidities, on gastro-esophageal reflux disease (GERD), and on quality of life (QoL) [20–23]. Furthermore, it seems that SG is correlated with rather specific complications such as fistulas and/or stenosis. The incidence of these complications is reported with the range 0 % to 17.5 % [19]. However, SG has a rather fast learning curve and can be performed within a short operative time. In addition, SG is considered less technically challenging than RYGB, due to the lack of anastomosis. Based on these unresolved controversies, further RCTs comparing SG and RYGB are urgently needed. The available RCT's show that the clinical efficacy regarding EWL and T2DM remission between both procedures are comparable [14, 15, 24]. This goes along with similar morbidity rates even though it seems that the morbidity rate of RYGB in these RCTs is higher [12, 15].

Objective

The primary endpoint of the BariSurg RCT, to compare EWL rates 2 years after SG and RYGB, was chosen based upon systematic review findings [13]. BariSurg will be a multi-centre, randomized controlled, patient and observer blind trial. Major secondary endpoints will be morbidity, mortality, re-operation rate, remission of obesity-related co-morbidities, the occurrence and course of GERD, QoL, the course of the dumping syndrome, and the EWL rate 60 months after surgery.

Trial locations

The BariSurg RCT will be conducted at seven bariatric centres: the University of Heidelberg, Städtisches Klinikum Karlsruhe, Agaplesion Bethesda Krankenhaus Stuttgart, Schwarzwald-BaarKlinikum (Villingen-Schwenningen), Caritas-Krankenhaus St. Josef (Regensburg), Johanniter Krankenhaus (Bonn) and Sana Klinikum Offenbach GmbH (Offenbach).

Methods/Design

Trial design

The BariSurg trial is a multi-centre, randomized controlled, patient and observer blind trial.

Sample size

A total of 248 patients will be randomized, with 124 patients assigned to each treatment arm. A dropout rate of approximately 20 % is considered realistic and has been accounted for the total number of randomized patients.

Patient selection criteria

Patients between 18 and 70 years old with a BMI between 35 and 60 kg/m^2 with indication for bariatric surgery according to the most recent German S3 guidelines will be eligible. Patients with a BMI of 35–40 kg/m^2 need to have at least one obesity-related co-morbidities such as T2DM or hypertension (see Table 1).

Recruitment and timelines

Patients will be recruited by the above mentioned seven participating centres. The recruitment period is estimated at 18 months. The time from enrollment of the first patient to study completion of the last, will be approximately 78 months, and the proposed duration of the entire trial is 90 months.

Table 1 Inclusion and exclusion criteria

Inclusion criteria	Exclusion criteria
BMI 40-60 kg/m^2	Lack of informed consent
BMI 35–40 kg/m^2 with at least one obesity-related co-morbidity	Expected lack of compliance
Age 18–70 years	Previous bariatric surgery
	Pregnancy

Randomization

Patients fulfilling all inclusion without meeting any exclusion criteria and after receiving their informed consent, randomization will be performed intraoperatively via an internet-based randomization tool (http://www.randomizer.at). Randomization is performed by block randomization and will be stratified for each centre until the enrolment goal of 248 patients has been reached.

Interventions

Patients will be asked to complete standard preoperative diagnostics including esophagogastroduodenoscopy (EGD), endocrine assessment and psychosomatics, and will also fill out four questionnaires (Short-Form-36 Health Survey (SF-36) [25], Gastrointestinal Quality of Life Index (GIQLI) [26], the Dumping questionnaire (Sigstad score) and Gastrointestinal Symptom Rating Score (GSRS) [27, 28]). Two weeks before surgery, patients will be asked to reduce their weight by following a low calorie liquid diet [29]. Preoperatively, a single-shot antibiotic prophylaxis will be given. For the surgical procedure, the patient will be placed in the supine position 45° (reverse Trendelenburg).

Roux-en-Y-gastric bypass

After the gastroesophageal junction is identified, the stomach is transsected with a linear stapler 6 cm below the junction. A pouch with a 4–6 cm height and 14–16 mm width is created using a 42 French tube. A 70 cm biliopancreatic limb is defined and an end-to-side gastroenterostomy will be performed using either a 30 mm linear or 25 mm circular stapling technique. The common channel (side-to-side jejunojejunostomy) will be stapled after another 150 cm antecolic limb. To identify a leak of the proximal anastomosis methylene blue is applied through a nasogastric tube [30]. All patients will be discharged with the recommendation of oral intake of multivitamin tablets twice daily. During the follow up examination vitamin levels will be assessed regularly. In case of vitamin deficiency substitution of vitamins will be performed.

Sleeve gastrectomy

The gastroepiploic vessels are divided 6 cm prepyloric along the great curvature, until the angle of His and the left crus of the diaphragm are visible. Along with a 42 French bougie, the stomach is then resected using linear stapler devices. At the angle of His the stapler line is sutured. The sleeve is checked for leakage using methylene blue. All patients will be discharged with the recommendation of oral intake of multivitamin tablets twice daily.

Study visits

Study documentation and visits of patients will be performed by both surgeons and study nurses. Since the trial is designed as observer and patient blind RCT, information about the surgical procedure will not be reported during the follow-up examinations. There will be 9 study visits during the BariSurg RCT (see Fig. 1). During the first postoperative year, study visits will be performed at discharge, 3–6 months and 12 months postoperatively. Then visits will be performed annually. Every postoperative study visit includes data collection of weight, morbidity, mortality, course of obesity-related co-morbidities (including laboratory parameters and current medication), analysis of nutritional supplementation, occurrence of GERD and analysis of dumping syndrome using the Sigstad score. In addition to the above mentioned information, extended study visits will yearly assess general laboratory parameters, EGD results and the questionnaires (SF-36, GIQLI, GSRS, see Fig. 1).

Risk-benefit ratio

SG is associated with a morbidity rate between 0–17.5 % and a mortality rate between 0–1.2 % [13]. The most frequently occurring postoperative complications are insufficiencies/fistulas at the staple line, leakage, stenosis of the sleeve and dilatation of the sleeve [5]. RYGB has a morbidity rate of 2-10 % and a mortality of 0.5-0.8 % [7, 12, 15]. Frequently observed complications include anastomotic insufficiency, especially with regard to the gastrojejunostomy, and dumping syndrome. Dumping syndrome is observed in 42 % after RYGB and up to 29 % after SG [31–33]. Therefore patients will be assessed for dumping syndrome. If the diagnosis dumping syndrome is confirmed patients will get the optimal treatment for dumping syndrome [28]. For both bariatric procedures, nutritional supplementation might be necessary for the remainder of the patient's life.

Outcome

The summary of the primary and the secondary endpoints depicts different points of view concerning the efficacy and safety of bariatric procedures. In doing so, medical issues as well as patient assessment can be analyzed.

Primary endpoint

The primary endpoint is defined as EWL at 24 months after surgery (RYGB or SG). Power calculation was made according to the systematic review of Fischer et al. [13].

| Population | - Patients with a BMI between 35-60 kg/m²
- Patients with a BMI between 35-40 kg/m² must have at least one obesity-related co-morbidity such as T2DM, hypertension, joint pain, sleep apnoea
- Age 18-70 years |

Screening	Inclusion/exclusion criteria
	Eligible Not eligible
	Informed consent/Enrollment
	Assessment of X and O

Start of intervention	Randomisation
	Roux-en-Y gastric bypass	Sleeve gastrectomy
Discharge	Assessment of O	Assessment of O
Follow-up 3-6 months	Assessment of O	Assessment of O
Follow-up 12 months	Assessment of O	Assessment of O
Follow-up 24 months	Assessment of X and O	Assessment of X and O
Follow-up 36 months	Assessment of O	Assessment of O
Follow-up 48 months	Assessment of O	Assessment of O
Follow-up 60 months	Assessment of X and O	Assessment of X and O

Postoperative outcome:
X: regular laboratory parameters, EGD, questionnaires (SF-36, GIQLI, GSRS)
O: EWL, morbidity, mortality, obesity-related co-morbidities, nutritional supplementation, medication, occurence of GERD, dumping syndrome (Sigstad score)

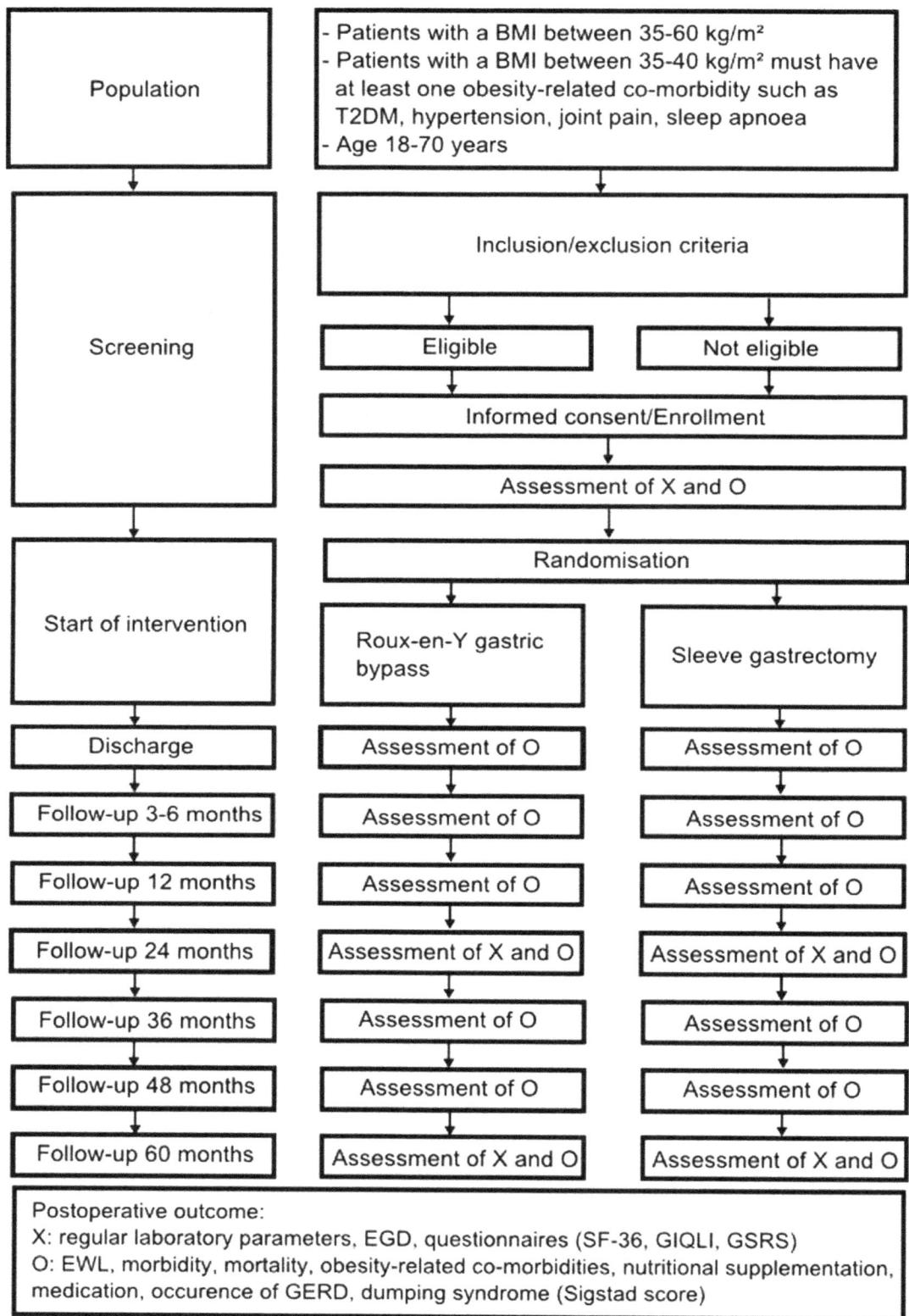

Fig. 1 Flow chart of BariSurg trial, showing the timeline and the course for trial participants. Abbreviations: BMI: body mass index, T2DM: type 2 diabetes mellitus, EWL: excess weight loss, EGD: esophagogastroduodenoscopy, SF-36: Short-Form-36 Health Survey, GIQLI: gastrointestinal quality of life index, GSRS: gastrointestinal symptom rate score, EWL: excess weight loss, GERD: gastroesphageal reflux disease

Secondary endpoints

Long-term EWL at 60 months after surgery, morbidity, mortality, course of obesity-related co-morbidities (T2DM, hypertension, joint pain, sleep apnoea, dyslipidemia), vitamin status, incidence and/or course of GERD and QoL (as defined by the SF 36) and dumping syndrome (as defined by the Sigstad score) will form the secondary endpoints. The course of obesity-related co-morbidities is assessed by laboratory examinations and current medication use. T2DM remission will be measured by HbA1c, fasting glucose and medication use. Hypertension will be monitored by medication and blood pressure measurements. The course of joint pain and dyslipidemia are assessed by pain and respectively lipid metabolism medication. The course of sleep apnoea is analysed by patients' application of CPAP-mask. Nutritional substitution will be assessed using a questionnaire which was developed in the bariatric centre of the University of Heidelberg. GERD incidence and course of GERD will be assessed with EGD and by using GSRS and GIQLI as standardized questionnaires. To evaluate QoL, the validated SF-36 questionnaire will be used. The Dumping score will be evaluated by using the validated Sigstad score. Secondary endpoints will be evaluated preoperatively, at discharge, 3-6, 12, 24, 36, 48 and 60 months postoperatively. Questionnaires will be filled out 12, 24 and 60 months after surgery. The EGD will be performed 12 and 60 months postoperatively.

Data management

Trial-relevant data will be documented in the case report form (CRF). The original CRFs will remain at the investigating centre and copies will be sent to the primary investigating centre, i.e. University Heidelberg. Data extraction and analysis will be made by the contract research organization, R&P Ryschlick and Partner GmBH (Burscheid, Germany). Data will be analyzed for completeness, validity and plausibility. The investigator will be consulted in case of uncertainty of the data.

Safety evaluation and reporting of adverse events

Patients will receive regular medical treatment, including any necessary emergency treatment, throughout the duration of the trial. Serious adverse events (SAE) are defined as the need for re-operation, prolonged hospitalization, life-threatening situations, readmission for any reason, and death. The principal investigator must be informed about all occurring SAEs within 24 hours of knowledge of the event. All SAEs must be reported to the principle investigator.

Unblinding

Blinding of patients has been done many times even in surgery [34–36]. Besides randomization, blinding of patients (and observers) reduces bias. Subsequently, internal and external validity will be increased. The fact that this study will be a patient and observer blinded study made a thoroughly ethical and clinical evaluation necessary. Based on the given evidence there is reliable data available that both procedures are similar in their clinical efficacy regarding excess weight loss, diabetes remission and complication rates [13–15]. Taking aside historical considerations and looking only at the RCT regarding RYGB and SG one can truly suggest to patients that both procedures are equally effective and safe.

During the BariSurg trial, all patients get extensive oral and written information about both procedures with all relevant pros and cons. Patients are informed that they will not know which procedure will be performed. Randomization will be performed intraoperatively after confirming that both procedures can be performed safely. All relevant documents including operation report and discharge letter state that the patient was enrolled in a randomized controlled patient and observer blind clinical trial comparing RYGB and SG and that the patient does not know about the procedure. These documents also include an emergency number which patients or physicians can call any time (24 hours, 365 days service) in case unblinding is necessary. Thus, blinding patients during the BariSurg trial is reasonable both from a clinical point of view as well as from ethical considerations.

Statistical methods
Sample size

According to a systematic review by Fischer et al. the mean EWL two years after SG and RYGB was 56.1 % and 68.3 % respectively, with a common standard deviation of 22.5 % [13]. Based on these results, the null hypothesis is that there exits inferiority of SG compared to RYGB in EWL 24 months after surgery. Based on the assumption that a difference in EWL of 10 % or more is clinically relevant, the margin to consider EWL as similar is set to 9 %. The power calculation for a non-inferiority trial with a one-sided t-test (alpha = 0.025 % and beta = 20 %) and a standard deviation of 22.5 % revealed that 99 patients per intervention group need to be randomized. Since a high dropout rate of 20 % is expected, a further 25 patients per intervention group should be randomized. Hence a total of 124 patients for each group will be recruited (overall 248 patients).

Analysis of primary endpoint

The primary endpoint is percent of EWL 24 months after surgery. To formalize the statistical approach, the following notations will be used: $\mu RYGB/\mu SG$, population mean of primary endpoint in RYGB/SG group. The following one-sided non-inferiority test problem is defined as

H0: μRYGB - μSG > = delta vs.

H1: μRYGB - μSG < delta

(For definition and specification of delta, see sample size calculation). This hypothesis will be tested using a one-sided t-test applied to each protocol population (see below). A low number of missing values for the primary endpoint is expected. If any values are missing, they will be replaced by methods of multiple imputation.

Secondary analyses

Concerning secondary endpoints, exploratory data analysis will be performed and appropriate summary measures for the empirical distribution, as well as descriptive two-sided p-values, will be calculated. Homogeneity of the treatment groups will be described by comparing the baseline values. Each patient's allocation to the different analysis populations [full analysis set (FAS) according to the intention-to-treat (ITT) principle, per protocol (PP) analysis set, safety analysis set] will be defined prior to analysis and documented in the analysis plan prior to database closure. During the data review, deviations from the protocol will be assessed as 'minor' or 'major'. Major deviations from the protocol will lead to the patient's exclusion from the PP analysis set. In addition to the evaluation of PP, an ITT analysis will be performed as a sensitivity analysis.

Safety measures

Safety analysis includes frequency of SAEs and complications. Homogeneity of the study arms will be described by comparing demographic data with baseline values.

Withdrawals and stopping guidelines

Patient withdrawal from the trial is possible at any time and without explanation. The trial will be ended in cases of insufficient patient recruitment and a high rate of SAEs due to SG or RYGB.

Data safety monitoring board

Reports of SAEs will be collected by an independent data and safety monitoring board (DSMB). Furthermore, the DSMB will inform the trial management about relevant imbalances between the two groups.

Trial organization and administration

Ethical considerations

SG and RYGB are frequently performed, standard techniques in bariatric surgery. The overall complication rate in SG and in RYGB described by Birkmeyer et al. is 5.9 % and 10.3 % respectively. A mortality of 0 % in SG and 0.3-0.9 % in RYGB was observed [12, 15, 37]. All participating centres perform both techniques frequently. In this manner morbidity and mortality rate can be expected like above

mentioned. Furthermore, all participating centres received positive approvals of the according ethic committees (i.e. the University of Heidelberg from the Heidelberg ethics committee (S500/2012), Johanniter Hospital (Bonn) (2015179/2014), Städtisches Klinikum Karlsruhe, Schwarzwald-Baar-Klinikum (Villingen-Schwenningen), Agaplesion Bethesda Krankenhaus Stuttgart from the ethics committee of the State Board of Physicians of Baden-Württemberg which is responsible for the mentioned hospitals (B-F-2014-059)). The Caritas-Krankenhaus St. Josef (Regensburg) requested formal information of the ethics committee of the Bavarian State Board of Physicians to be legally considered a positive ethic vote.)

Good clinical practice

The BariSurg trial will be conducted according to national and international trial standards (ICH-GCP, Declaration of Helsinki 2008).

Registration

This trial is registered in the German Clinical Trials Register (DRKS00004766).

Discussion

The positive effects of bariatric surgery on weight loss and obesity-related co-morbidities are no longer doubted. In addition, these procedures can also be performed safely with low mortality and morbidity [5, 12, 38]. The range of available bariatric procedures is tremendous [7, 17, 39–45]. Almost every year, a "new" procedure is focussed upon within the scientific community [18, 19]. However, there are only few RCTs comparing the two most commonly performed bariatric procedures, i.e. RYGB and SG with regard to actual weight loss and/or improvement of obesity-related co-morbidities in the mid- and long-term [12, 15]. It is therefore impossible to advocate any particular, bariatric surgical method, because one still does not know which patient benefits most from which procedure. A systematic review revealed that the EWL after 24 months is not statistically different between RYGB and SG [41]. In addition, the same publication demonstrated the poor data quality among publications dealing with SG. The urgent questions concerning comparisons between SG and the current gold standard of RYGB with respect to long-term EWL, course of obesity-related co-morbidities, course of GERD and QoL, are still not answered. In the last 2 years, however, a small number of RCTs were started with the goal of examining some of these issues [12, 14, 15, 17, 39]. To our knowledge, the BariSurg trial will be the first multi-centre, randomized controlled patient and observer blind clinical trial with a sufficient sample size analyzing hard clinical endpoints such as mid- and long-term EWL, morbidity and mortality. In addition BariSurg will also answer some of the urgent questions associated with SG, such as course of obesity-related co-morbidities, dumping syndrome and GERD. Thus, BariSurg will contribute to class 1B evidence, which enable future class 1A evidence in form of meta-analyses. The remission of obesity-related co-morbidities, such as T2DM, following bariatric procedures is already known [1–3, 40]. In particular, the RYGB has been considered as a potential therapy for T2DM, even in patients with a BMI of less than 35 kg/m^2 [41, 42]. However, SG also has a significant impact on T2DM remission [24, 43, 46]. Prior RCTs have suggested similar outcomes after RYGB and SG with regard to glucose metabolism [15, 44, 47]. The incidence of GERD seems to be more frequent after SG whereas RYGB is considered a therapeutic option in patients with GERD [15, 45, 48]. Nevertheless, the course of GERD after SG is controversial and definite evidence supporting either side does not exist [23, 49, 50]. The current discussion among bariatric surgeons is almost unidirectional and focused on "hard" clinical facts such as weight loss, T2DM remission, and the course of other obesity-related co-morbidities. "Soft" clinical facts such as QoL have gained importance. At the present, there is few literature about patients' expectation concerning surgical intervention. Data from the Michigan Bariatric Surgery Collaborative on a total of 8.847 patients showed an increased qoL after SG and RYGB [51]. However long-term results of QoL after RYGB and SG are not available. The combined evaluation within this trial of the primary endpoint of EWL after 24 months plus the course of EWL, obesity-related co-morbidities, GERD, morbidity and mortality over 5 years, will lead to further insights of the pros and cons of both procedures. Additionally, the setting of this multi-centre, randomized trial enables a maximum reduction of bias and increases internal and external validity [52].

Trial status
Recruitment started in November 2013.

Abbreviations
RYGB: Roux-en-Y gastric bypass; SG: Sleeve gastrectomy; BMI: Body mass index; GERD: Gastroesophageal reflux disease; EWL: Excess weight loss; T2DM: Type 2 diabetes mellitus; QoL: Quality of life; GIQLI: Gastrointestinal quality of life index; GSRS: Gastrointestinal symptom related score; SF-36: Short-Form-36 Health Survey.

Competing interests
The authors hereby declare that they have no competing interests.

Authors' contributions
All authors contributed to the design of the present study and revised the manuscript critically. All authors read and approved the final manuscript.

Acknowledgements
We would like to thank Inga Rossion, Colette Dörr-Harim and R & P Ryschlick and Partner GmBH for their support.

Author details
[1]Department of General, Visceral and Transplantation Surgery, University of Heidelberg, Im Neuenheimer Feld 110, 69120 Heidelberg, Germany. [2]Institute of Medical Biometry and Informatics, University of Heidelberg, Im Neuenheimer Feld 305, 69120 Heidelberg, Germany. [3]Study Centre of the German Surgical Society (SDGC), University of Heidelberg, Im Neuenheimer Feld 110, 69120 Heidelberg, Germany. [4]Salem Hospital, Zeppelinstraße 11 – 33, 69121 Heidelberg, Germany. [5]Department of General and Visceral Surgery, Städtisches Krankenhaus Karlsruhe, Moltkestraße 90, 76133 Karlsruhe, Germany. [6]Department of General and Visceral Surgery, Agaplesion Bethesda Krankenhaus Stuttgart, Hohenheimer Straße 21, 70184 Stuttgart, Germany. [7]Department of General and Visceral Surgery, Schwarzwald- Baar Klinikum, Klinikstraße 11, 78052 Villingen-Schwenningen, Germany. [8]Department of Surgery, Caritas-Krankenhaus St. Josef, Landshuter Straße 65, 93053 Regensburg, Germany. [9]Department of General and Visceral Surgery, Johanniter Krankenhaus, Johanniter GmbH, Johanniterstraße 3, 53113 Bonn, Germany. [10]Department of Bariatric Surgery and Metabolic Surgery, Sana Klinikum Offenbach GmbH, Starkenburgring 66, 63069 Offenbach, Germany.

References
1. Buchwald H, Estok R, Fahrbach K, Banel D, Jensen MD, Pories WJ, et al. Weight and Type 2 Diabetes after Bariatric Surgery: Systematic Review and Meta-analysis. Am J Med. 2009;122:248–256.e5.
2. Sjöström L, Lindroos A-K, Peltonen M, Torgerson J, Bouchard C, Carlsson B, et al. Lifestyle, Diabetes, and Cardiovascular Risk Factors 10 Years after Bariatric Surgery. N Engl J Med. 2004;351:2683–93.
3. Scopinaro N, Adami GF, Papadia FS, Camerini G, Carlini F, Fried M, et al. Effects of biliopancreatic diversion on type 2 diabetes in patients with BMI 25 to 35. Ann Surg. 2011;253:699–703.
4. Sjöström L, Gummesson A, Sjöström CD, Narbro K, Peltonen M, Wedel H, et al. Effects of bariatric surgery on cancer incidence in obese patients in Sweden (Swedish Obese Subjects Study): a prospective, controlled intervention trial. Lancet Oncol. 2009;10:653–62.
5. Herron D, Roohipour R. Complications of Roux-en-Y gastric bypass and sleeve gastrectomy. Abdom Imaging. 2012;37:712–8.
6. Franco JVA, Ruiz PA, Palermo M, Gagner M. A review of studies comparing three laparoscopic procedures in bariatric surgery: sleeve gastrectomy, Roux-en-Y gastric bypass and adjustable gastric banding. Obes Surg. 2011;21:1458–68.
7. Buchwald H, Avidor Y, Braunwald E, Jensen MD, Pories W, Fahrbach K, et al. Bariatric surgery: a systematic review and meta-analysis. JAMA J Am Med Assoc. 2004;292:1724–37.
8. Buchwald H, Oien DM. Metabolic/bariatric surgery worldwide 2011. Obes Surg. 2013;23:427–36.
9. Peterli R, Steinert RE, Woelnerhanssen B, Peters T, Christoffel-Courtin C, Gass M, et al. Metabolic and hormonal changes after laparoscopic Roux-en-Y gastric bypass and sleeve gastrectomy: a randomized, prospective trial. Obes Surg. 2012;22:740–8.
10. Leyba JL, Aulestia SN, Llopis SN. Laparoscopic Roux-en-Y gastric bypass versus laparoscopic sleeve gastrectomy for the treatment of morbid obesity. A prospective study of 117 patients. Obes Surg. 2011;21:212–6.
11. Zachariah SK, Chang P-C, Ooi ASE, Hsin M-C, Kin Wat JY, Huang CK. Laparoscopic sleeve gastrectomy for morbid obesity: 5 years experience from an Asian center of excellence. Obes Surg. 2013;23:939–46.
12. Helmiö M, Victorzon M, Ovaska J, Leivonen M, Juuti A, Jaser N, et al. SLEEVEPASS: a randomized prospective multicenter study comparing laparoscopic sleeve gastrectomy and gastric bypass in the treatment of morbid obesity: preliminary results. Surg Endosc. 2012;26:2521–6.
13. Fischer L, Hildebrandt C, Bruckner T, Kenngott H, Linke GR, Gehrig T, et al. Excessive weight loss after sleeve gastrectomy: a systematic review. Obes Surg. 2012;22:721–31.
14. Lee W-J, Chong K, Ser K-H, Lee Y-C, Chen S-C, Chen J-C, et al. Gastric bypass vs sleeve gastrectomy for type 2 diabetes mellitus: a randomized controlled trial. Arch Surg Chic Ill 1960. 2011;146:143–8.

15. Peterli R, Borbély Y, Kern B, Gass M, Peters T, Thurnheer M, et al. Early Results of the Swiss Multicentre Bypass Or Sleeve Study (SM-BOSS): A Prospective Randomized Trial Comparing Laparoscopic Sleeve Gastrectomy and Roux-en-Y Gastric Bypass. Ann Surg. 2013;258(5):690–4.

16. Leyba JL, Llopis SN, Aulestia SN. Laparoscopic Roux-en-Y gastric bypass versus laparoscopic sleeve gastrectomy for the treatment of morbid obesity. A prospective study with 5 years of follow-up. Obes Surg. 2014;24:2094–8.

17. Kehagias I, Karamanakos SN, Argentou M, Kalfarentzos F. Randomized clinical trial of laparoscopic Roux-en-Y gastric bypass versus laparoscopic sleeve gastrectomy for the management of patients with BMI < 50 kg/m2. Obes Surg. 2011;21:1650–6.

18. O'Brien PE, McPhail T, Chaston TB, Dixon JB. Systematic review of medium-term weight loss after bariatric operations. Obes Surg. 2006;16:1032–40.

19. Brethauer SA, Hammel JP, Schauer PR. Systematic review of sleeve gastrectomy as staging and primary bariatric procedure. Surg Obes Relat Dis Off J Am Soc Bariatr Surg. 2009;5:469–75.

20. Himpens J, Dobbeleir J, Peeters G. Long-term results of laparoscopic sleeve gastrectomy for obesity. Ann Surg. 2010;252:319–24.

21. Weiner RA, Weiner S, Pomhoff I, Jacobi C, Makarewicz W, Weigand G. Laparoscopic sleeve gastrectomy–influence of sleeve size and resected gastric volume. Obes Surg. 2007;17:1297–305.

22. Bohdjalian A, Langer FB, Shakeri-Leidenmühler S, Gfrerer L, Ludvik B, Zacherl J, et al. Sleeve Gastrectomy as Sole and Definitive Bariatric Procedure: 5-Year Results for Weight Loss and Ghrelin. Obes Surg. 2010;20:535–40.

23. Zhang N, Maffei A, Cerabona T, Pahuja A, Omana J, Kaul A. Reduction in obesity-related comorbidities: is gastric bypass better than sleeve gastrectomy? Surg Endosc. 2013;27:1273–80.

24. Schauer PR, Kashyap SR, Wolski K, Brethauer SA, Kirwan JP, Pothier CE, et al. Bariatric Surgery versus Intensive Medical Therapy in Obese Patients with Diabetes. N Engl J Med. 2012;366:1567–76.

25. Bullinger M. German translation and psychometric testing of the SF-36 Health Survey: preliminary results from the IQOLA Project. International Quality of Life Assessment. Soc Sci Med 1982. 1995;41:1359–66.

26. Eypasch E, Williams JI, Wood-Dauphinee S, Ure BM, Schmülling C, Neugebauer E, et al. Gastrointestinal Quality of Life Index: development, validation and application of a new instrument. Br J Surg. 1995;82:216–22.

27. Kulich KR, Malfertheiner P, Madisch A, Labenz J, Bayerdörffer E, Miehlke S, et al. Psychometric validation of the German translation of the Gastrointestinal Symptom Rating Scale (GSRS) and Quality of Life in Reflux and Dyspepsia (QOLRAD) questionnaire in patients with reflux disease. Health Qual Life Outcomes. 2003;1:62.

28. Sigstad H. A Clinical Diagnostic Index in the Diagnosis of the Dumping Syndrome. Acta Med Scand. 1970;188:479–86.

29. Colles SL, Dixon JB, Marks P, Strauss BJ, O'Brien PE. Preoperative weight loss with a very-low-energy diet: quantitation of changes in liver and abdominal fat by serial imaging. Am J Clin Nutr. 2006;84:304–11.

30. Kenngott HG, Clemens G, Gondan M, Senft J, Diener MK, Rudofsky G, et al. DiaSurg 2 trial–surgical vs. medical treatment of insulin-dependent type 2 diabetes mellitus in patients with a body mass index between 26 and 35 kg/m2: study protocol of a randomized controlled multicenter trial–DRKS00004550. Trials. 2013;14:183.

31. Banerjee A, Ding Y, Mikami DJ, Needleman BJ. The role of dumping syndrome in weight loss after gastric bypass surgery. Surg Endosc. 2013;27:1573–8.

32. Papamargaritis D, Koukoulis G, Sioka E, Zachari E, Bargiota A, Zacharoulis D, et al. Dumping symptoms and incidence of hypoglycaemia after provocation test at 6 and 12 months after laparoscopic sleeve gastrectomy. Obes Surg. 2012;22:1600–6.

33. Tzovaras G, Papamargaritis D, Sioka E, Zachari E, Baloyiannis I, Zacharoulis D, et al. Symptoms suggestive of dumping syndrome after provocation in patients after laparoscopic sleeve gastrectomy. Obes Surg. 2012;22:23–8.

34. Sihvonen R, Paavola M, Malmivaara A, Itälä A, Joukainen A, Nurmi H, et al. Arthroscopic partial meniscectomy versus sham surgery for a degenerative meniscal tear. N Engl J Med. 2013;369:2515–24.

35. Nieuwenhuizen J, Eker HH, Timmermans L, Hop WC, Kleinrensink G-J, Jeekel J, et al. A double blind randomized controlled trial comparing primary suture closure with mesh augmented closure to reduce incisional hernia incidence. BMC Surg. 2013;13:48.

36. Boelens OB, van Assen T, Houterman S, Scheltinga MR, Roumen RM. A double-blind, randomized, controlled trial on surgery for chronic abdominal pain due to anterior cutaneous nerve entrapment syndrome. Ann Surg. 2013;257:845–9.

37. Birkmeyer NJO, Dimick JB, Share D, Hawasli A, English WJ, Genaw J, et al. Hospital complication rates with bariatric surgery in Michigan. JAMA J Am Med Assoc. 2010;304:435–42.

38. Zacharoulis D, Sioka E, Papamargaritis D, Lazoura O, Rountas C, Zachari E, et al. Influence of the learning curve on safety and efficiency of laparoscopic sleeve gastrectomy. Obes Surg. 2012;22:411–5.

39. Paluszkiewicz R, Kalinowski P, Wróblewski T, Bartoszewicz Z, Białobrzeska-Paluszkiewicz J, Ziarkiewicz-Wróblewska B, et al. Prospective randomized clinical trial of laparoscopic sleeve gastrectomy versus open Roux-en-Y gastric bypass for the management of patients with morbid obesity. Wideochirurgia Inne Tech Mało Inwazyjne Videosurgery Miniinvasive Tech Kwart Pod Patronatem Sekc Wideochirurgii TChP Oraz Sekc Chir Bariatrycznej TChP. 2012;7:225–32.

40. Mingrone G, Panunzi S, De Gaetano A, Guidone C, Iaconelli A, Leccesi L, et al. Bariatric surgery versus conventional medical therapy for type 2 diabetes. N Engl J Med. 2012;366:1577–85.

41. Müller-Stich BP, Fischer L, Kenngott HG, Gondan M, Senft J, Clemens G, et al. Gastric bypass leads to improvement of diabetic neuropathy independent of glucose normalization-results of a Prospective Cohort Study (DiaSurg 1 Study). Ann Surg. 2013;258(5):760–5.

42. Maggard-Gibbons M, Maglione M, Livhits M, Ewing B, Maher AR, Hu J, et al. Bariatric surgery for weight loss and glycemic control in nonmorbidly obese adults with diabetes: a systematic review. JAMA J Am Med Assoc. 2013;309:2250–61.

43. Vidal J, Ibarzabal A, Romero F, Delgado S, Momblán D, Flores L, et al. Type 2 diabetes mellitus and the metabolic syndrome following sleeve gastrectomy in severely obese subjects. Obes Surg. 2008;18:1077–82.

44. Ramón JM, Salvans S, Crous X, Puig S, Goday A, Benaiges D, et al. Effect of Roux-en-Y gastric bypass vs sleeve gastrectomy on glucose and gut hormones: a prospective randomised trial. J Gastrointest Surg Off J Soc Surg Aliment Tract. 2012;16:1116–22.

45. Patterson EJ, Davis DG, Khajanchee Y, Swanström LL. Comparison of objective outcomes following laparoscopic Nissen fundoplication versus laparoscopic gastric bypass in the morbidly obese with heartburn. Surg Endosc Interv Tech. 2003;17:1561–5.

46. Schauer PR, Bhatt DL, Kirwan JP, Wolski K, Brethauer SA, Navaneethan SD, et al. Bariatric surgery versus intensive medical therapy for diabetes–3-year outcomes. N Engl J Med. 2014;370:2002–13.

47. Jiménez A, Casamitjana R, Flores L, Viaplana J, Corcelles R, Lacy A, et al. Long-term effects of sleeve gastrectomy and Roux-en-Y gastric bypass surgery on type 2 diabetes mellitus in morbidly obese subjects. Ann Surg. 2012;256:1023–9.

48. Prachand VN, Alverdy JC. Gastroesophageal reflux disease and severe obesity: Fundoplication or bariatric surgery? World J Gastroenterol WJG. 2010;16:3757–61.

49. Petersen WV, Meile T, Küper MA, Zdichavsky M, Königsrainer A, Schneider JH. Functional importance of laparoscopic sleeve gastrectomy for the lower esophageal sphincter in patients with morbid obesity. Obes Surg. 2012;22:360–6.

50. Elazary R, Phillips EH, Cunneen S, Burch MA. Comments on "Increase in gastroesophageal reflux disease symptoms and erosive esophagitis 1 year after laparoscopic sleeve gastrectomy among obese adults" (doi:10.1007/s00464-012-2593-9). Surg Endosc. 2013;27:3935–6.

51. Carlin AM, Zeni TM, English WJ, Hawasli AA, Genaw JA, Krause KR, et al. The comparative effectiveness of sleeve gastrectomy, gastric bypass, and adjustable gastric banding procedures for the treatment of morbid obesity. Ann Surg. 2013;257:791–7.

52. Fischer L, Knaebel HP, Golcher H, Bruckner T, Diener MK, Bachmann J, et al. To whom do the results of the multicenter, randomized, controlled INSECT trial (ISRCTN 24023541) apply?–assessment of external validity. BMC Surg. 2012;12:2.

23

Short-term surgical outcomes of laparoscopy-assisted versus totally laparoscopic Billroth-II gastrectomy for gastric cancer: a matched-cohort study

Ji-Hyun Kim, Kyong-Hwa Jun[*] and Hyung-Min Chin

Abstract

Background: To evaluate feasibility and benefits of intracorporeal anastomosis, we compared short-term surgical outcomes between laparoscopy-assisted distal gastrectomy (LADG) and totally laparoscopic distal gastrectomy (TLDG) with Billroth-II (B-II) anastomosis for gastric cancer.

Methods: Sixty patients underwent attempted B-II TLDG from 2011 through 2013. Patients who underwent B-II LADG prior to 2011 were matched to TLDG cases for demographics, comorbidities, tumor characteristics, and TNM stage. Perioperative and short-term surgical outcomes were compared between the two groups.

Results: Clinicopathological characteristics of both groups were comparable. The B-II TLDG group had a shorter hospital stay (9.4 vs. 12.0 days, $P = 0.038$) and average incision size was smaller (3.5 vs. 5.4 cm, $P = 0.030$) than in the B-II LADG group. Anastomotic leakage was not recorded in either group, and there were no differences in the rates of perioperative complications and in inflammatory parameters between the two groups.

Conclusions: This study suggests that B-II TLDG is feasible, compared to B-II LADG, and that it has several advantages over LADG, including a smaller incision, a shorter hospital stay, and more convenience during surgery. However, prospective randomized controlled studies are still needed to confirm that B-II TLDG can be used as a standard procedure for LDG.

Keywords: Gastric cancer, Billroth-II anastomosis, Laparoscopic gastrectomy, Surgical outcome

Background

The frequency of early detection of gastric cancer has increased due to recent advances in diagnostic techniques and widespread screening. Laparoscopy-assisted distal gastrectomy (LADG) for early gastric cancer is widely accepted because many clinical studies demonstrated its minimal invasiveness and comparable outcomes to those of open distal gastrectomy (ODG) [1, 2]. Moreover, several recent randomized controlled trials reported that LADG results in less estimated blood loss, fewer postoperative complications, and a shorter hospital stay than ODG [3, 4].

In LADG, lymph node dissection is performed laparoscopically. Subsequent resection and reconstruction of the stomach are performed extracorporeally, through a minilaparotomy. Most surgeons prefer LADG to totally laparoscopic distal gastrectomy (TLDG) because of the technical difficulties of intracorporeal anastomosis and concern over complications associated with anastomosis [5]. However, extracorporeal anastomosis in a narrow space with restricted vision is often problematic, particularly in obese patients with a thick abdominal wall and in those with a small remnant stomach. TLDG enables better visualization during anastomosis compared with LADG, overcoming those difficulties.

Goh et al. [6] first reported intracorporeal Billroth-II (B-II) gastrojejunostomy using laparoscopic linear staplers in 1992. Since then, advances in laparoscopic technique

* Correspondence: dkkwkh@catholic.ac.kr
Department of Surgery, St. Vincent's Hospital, College of Medicine, The Catholic University of Korea, Seoul, Republic of Korea

and instruments have made possible various totally laparoscopic anastomoses. Recent clinical studies of Billroth-I (B-I) gastroduodenostomy or Roux-en Y (R-Y) esophagojejunostomy have demonstrated that TLDG is safer, more technically feasible, and less invasive than LADG [7–9]. Meanwhile, the benefits of intracorporeal B-II anastomosis are often assumed and remain unproven. Only a few studies have reported the surgical outcomes of B-II TLDG [10, 11]. We therefore conducted this study to expand our experience and to perform a comparative analysis. B-II LADG patients were individually matched to B-II TLDG patients for demographics, tumor characteristics, and TNM stage, to assess the potential benefits of B-II TLDG.

Methods
Patients and matching process
The study was approved by the Institutional Review Board of St. Vincent's Hospital (No. VC14RISI0107). Laparoscopic distal subtotal gastrectomy was restricted to patients whose tumors were clinical stage I. Sixty patients underwent B-II TLDG from 2011 through 2013. B-I or R-Y anastomoses were not included in this study. Matched-pair control patients were selected from 318 patients who underwent B-II LADG prior to the use of intracorporeal anastomosis (2008–2011). Candidates for controls were matched to TLDG cases for age, gender, comorbidities, body mass index (BMI), size and number of tumors, location of tumors, and TNM stage. First, tumor number and size were matched. After this first step of selection, the location of tumors and TNM stage were matched, and the LADG candidate who was best matched to each individual TLDG patient for demographics and comorbidities was selected. Peri- and postoperative outcomes were compared between the TLDG group ($n = 60$) and the matched-pair LADG group ($n = 60$).

Surgical procedure
The operations were performed by two surgeons (HM and KH), who had each performed more than 300 laparoscopic procedures, including 60 laparoscopy-assisted gastrectomies, before this study. Under general anesthesia, patients were placed in the supine position with their legs apart and five trocars were used. Pneumoperitoneum was established using a Veress needle. One initial 11-mm trocar for the laparoscope was inserted below the umbilicus and four additional trocars were placed in the upper abdomen. In principle, laparoscopic lymph node dissection was performed in the same manner as the conventional open gastrectomy. All of the patients underwent at least D1+ or D2 lymph node dissection as described in the Japanese Classification of Gastric Carcinoma [12]. All of the dissecting procedures were performed using laparoscopic coagulation shears. Separation of the greater omentum from the

transverse colon and dissection of the lymph nodes along the left gastroepiploic vessels (No. 4sb) was performed. Dissection was continued toward the pylorus, including the infrapyloric nodes (No. 6) and division of the right gastroepiploic vessels (No. 4d). The hepatoduodenal ligament was dissected and the suprapyloric nodes (No. 5) and the nodes along the common hepatic artery (No. 8) were dissected. Using a 60-mm Endo-GIA stapler (Covidien, Mansfield, MA), the duodenum was divided at a point 1 cm distal to the pylorus. Dissection of the nodes along the proper hepatic artery (No. 12a) and the proximal splenic artery (No. 11p) was performed when dissection of the D2 lymph node was necessary. After dissection of the nodes along the left gastric artery (No. 7) and celiac artery (No. 9), skeletonization of the lesser curvature of the gastroesophageal junction, with dissection of the right paracardial nodes (No.1) and the nodes along the lesser curvature (No. 3) was performed.

In LADG, epigastric incision was extended longitudinally to 4–5 cm in length and a wound protector was placed. The mobilized stomach was pulled out via the minilaparotomy. After resection of the distal part of the stomach using linear staplers, the proximal jejunum, 15–20 cm distal from Treitz's ligament, was pulled out and gastrojejunostomy was performed using hand-sewn running sutures.

In TLDG, the stomach was divided using linear staplers, followed by removal of the resected specimen through the extended U-shaped skin incision below the umbilicus using a large plastic bag. The surgeon then checked the location of the tumor and the proximal cut margin on the removed specimen. If needed, additional gastric resection could be performed for oncological safety. However, there were no cases requiring additional resection among the patients enrolled in this study. Laparoscopic intracorporeal antecolic gastrojejunostomy and closure of the entry hole were performed using linear staplers.

Postoperative data
Data related to patients' clinicopathological characteristics, surgical procedures, and postoperative outcomes were collected retrospectively. In all of the cases, the disease was pathologically staged according to the 7th edition of the Union for International Cancer Control (UICC) TNM Cancer Staging Manual [13]. Clinicopathological characteristics of patients included age, sex, BMI, comorbidity, TNM stage, retrieved lymph nodes, tumor size, and tumor location. Surgical outcome parameters included the operative time, estimated blood loss, retrieved number of lymph nodes, intraoperative complications, incision size, time to first flatus, time to first soft diet, and duration of postoperative hospital stay. Postoperative complications were defined and graded according to the Claviend-Dindo

surgical complication grading system [14]. Laboratory parameters, including white blood cell (WBC) count, neutrophil count, and CRP level at 1 and 4 days after surgery, were analyzed to compare the postoperative inflammatory response between the two groups. These data were compared between the two groups.

Statistical analysis

Continuous data are presented as means ± SD and categorical data are presented as proportions. Statistical analyses were performed using Student's t- test, the chi-squared test or Fisher's exact probability test. A P value < 0.05 was considered statistically significant. All of the statistical analyses were performed using the Statistical Package for the Social Science (SPSS) version 20.0 for Windows (SPSS, Inc., Chicago IL).

Results

Patients' demographics

Patient demographics (age, sex, BMI, and comorbidities), tumor characteristics (tumor size, number, and location), and TNM stage were comparable between TLDG and matched-pair LADG groups (Table 1). Because patients in the LADG group were selected from an earlier time period (before 2011) than the TLDG group (2011–2013), the median follow-up time was shorter in the TLDG group (median 23 months vs. 36.2 months, $P = 0.045$). By the criteria of the 7th edition of the UICC TNM Cancer Staging Manual, almost all of the patients (96.7%) were in stage I.

Surgical outcomes

Intraoperative surgical outcomes are shown in Table 2. Operative time was not significantly different between the groups (205.0 vs. 197.3 min, $P = 0.381$). For estimated blood loss, there was not statistically significant difference between two groups (100.5 vs. 117.2 mL, $P = 0.056$). There were no significant differences in time to flatus or start of soft diet. However, hospital stay and incision size in the TLDG group were significantly reduced compared to the LADG group. In obese patients (BMI ≥25 kg/m^2), operation time was not statistically significant between two groups (218.2 ± 12.1 vs 201.7 ± 17.5 $P = 0.054$). There were no differences between the two groups in postoperative complications or in hospital stay (Table 3).

Postoperative complications

Both TLDG and LADG had a complication rate of 8.3% (Table 4). Ileus with a paralytic obstruction pattern was observed on abdominal X-ray in two patients in the TLDG group and one patient in the LADG group. There was neither anastomotic leakage nor stricture in both groups. One patient in both groups suffered from duodenal stump leakage, which was managed conservatively. Anastomotic

Table 1 Demographics of patients undergoing gastrectomy

	LADG ($n = 60$)	TLDG ($n = 60$)	P value
Age (yr)	60.9 ± 11.4	60.5 ± 12.1	0.889
Sex			
Male	40 (66.7)	40 (66.7)	1.000
Female	20 (33.3)	20 (33.3)	
BMI (kg/m^2)	24.7 ± 2.8	24.1 ± 3.7	0.705
Comorbidity			
Diabetes	8 (13.3)	10 (16.7)	0.728
Cardiac	11 (18.3)	8 (13.3)	
Pulmonary	5 (8.3)	7 (11.7)	
Liver disease	3 (5.0)	2 (3.3)	
Cerebral infarction	0 (0)	1 (1.7)	
Tumor size	2.5 ± 1.4	2.8 ± 1.5	0.818
Tumor location			
Middle third	29 (48.3)	28 (46.7)	0.855
Lower third	31 (51.7)	32 (53.3)	
T stage			
T1	56 (93.3)	56 (93.3)	1.000
T2	3 (5.0)	3 (5.0)	
T3	1 (1.7)	1 (1.7)	
N stage			
N0	52 (86.7)	52 (86.7)	1.000
N1	8 (13.3)	8 (13.3)	
Stage (UICC 7th)			
I	58 (96.7)	58 (96.7)	1.000
II	2 (3.3)	2 (3.3)	

Data are presented as number (%) or mean ± standard deviation

bleeding, which was resolved conservatively, occurred in one patient in the LADG group. Complications in other organ systems, such as the heart and lungs occurred in one patient in the TLDG group and two patients in the LADG group. The mortality rate in both groups was 0%.

Inflammatory and nutritional parameters

The laboratory parameters are shown in Table 5. Inflammatory parameters, such as WBC count, neutrophil count, and CRP did not differ between groups at 1 and 4 days after surgery.

Discussion

Conventionally, three gastrointestinal reconstructions after gastric resection—B-I, B-II, R-Y anastomosis—are performed in laparoscopic distal gastrectomy as well as in ODG [9, 15]. B-I anastomosis is the ideal reconstruction after gastrectomy in terms of maintaining physiological intestinal continuity and technical simplicity using a circular stapler. Therefore, many surgeons prefer this anastomosis compared to B-II or R-Y anastomosis during ODG and

Table 2 Comparison of surgical outcomes between LADG and TLDG

	LADG (n = 60)	TLDG (n = 60)	P value
Operative time (min)	205.0 ± 22.4	197.3 ± 40.1	0.381
Open conversion	0	0	1.000
Intraoperative complications	0	0	1.000
Estimated blood loss (mL)	117.2 ± 81.6	100.5 ± 36.8	0.056
Retrieved lymph nodes	38.3 ± 11.4	39.4 ± 9.8	0.736
Laparotomy wound length	5.4 ± 1.3	3.5 ± 0.9	0.030
Time to first flatus (POD)	2.4 ± 1.2	2.1 ± 0.8	0.088
Time to starting soft diet (POD)	3.3 ± 1.8	3.1 ± 1.0	0.212
Postoperative hospital stay (days)	12.0 ± 3.5	9.4 ± 5.0	0.038

Data are presented as mean ± standard deviation
POD postoperative day

LADG. However, its application may be limited depending on tumor location and the size of the remnant stomach, because a remnant stomach of sufficient length is required to avoid tension in the anastomosis. In addition, delta-shaped anastomosis for intracorporeal gastroduodenostomy requires more precise laparoscopic manipulations than other types of reconstruction [16]. R-Y anastomosis can prevent reflux gastritis and esophagitis and reduces the likelihood of gastric cancer recurrence [17]. However, it is more complex and time-consuming than other types of anastomosis. Moreover, the extensive use of laparoscopic linear staplers can result in higher cost [18]. By comparison, one or two linear staplers are sufficient for intracoporeal gastrojejunostomy. B-II anastomosis is more easily applied in TLDG than B-I or R-Y anastomosis, irrespective of tumor location or of remnant stomach size [5, 19].

This study evaluated the feasibility, invasiveness, and benefit of B-II TLDG by comparing the short-term surgical outcomes in TLDG and LADG groups. In addition, this retrospective study involved a patient cohort matched 1:1 for age, sex, tumor characteristics, and TNM stage to minimize the effects of predisposing factors. Therefore, there were no differences in the baseline characteristics of patients in the two groups. We believe that this statistical method improved the accuracy of the comparison of short-term outcomes according to operative method.

As the number of reports that LADG is less invasive and provides faster recovery than ODG increases, the

expectation that TLDG will also have these advantages over LADG has also increased. Indeed, several studies have compared TLDG and LADG. Song et al. [20] published a prospective, multicenter study, which showed that TLDG was more expensive but provided earlier bowel recovery than LADG and ODG. Ikeda et al. [21] reported that TLDG had several advantages over LADG including a smaller incision, less invasiveness, and better feasibility of a secure ablation. Kinoshita et al. [22] suggested that TLDG results in faster recovery, better cosmetic results, and improved quality of life in the short-term compared with LADG. Consistent with previous studies, our results showed that TLDG has advantages over LADG in terms of incision size and hospital stay. These findings suggest that B-II TLDG has better short-term outcomes than B-II LADG. In addition, there were no differences in the rates of postoperative and anastomosis-related complications between the TLDG and LADG groups. Large Korean and Japanese cohort studies have reported postoperative complication rates of 12.7% and 13.1%, respectively, for LADG [23, 24]. In this study, the postoperative complication rates were identical in the TLDG and LADG groups (5.8%). One case (1.7%) of anastomosis-related complications was found in the LADG group. Thus, we suggest that TLDG can be a safe and reliable procedure for gastric cancer.

We hypothesized that TLDG would be less invasive and be associated with improved postoperative inflammation and recovery of internal organs including the gastrointestinal tract, because, as well as a minilaparotomy at the epigastrium, pulling out of the stomach for extracorporeal anastomosis was not needed in TLDG, unlike LADG. Postoperative changes in WBC count, neutrophil count and CRP were determined to evaluate the inflammatory response. While several previous

Table 3 Surgical outcomes in obese patients (BMI ≥25)

	LADG (n = 20)	TLDG (n = 20)	P value
Operation time	218.2 ± 12.1	201.7 ± 17.5	0.054
Postoperative complications	0	0	1.000
Postoperative hospital stay (day)	11.2 ± 3.6	10.4 ± 2.1	0.51

Data are presented as mean ± standard deviation

Table 4 Comparison of postoperative complications between LADG and TLDG

	LADG (n = 60)	TLDG (n = 60)	P value
Overall postoperative morbidity	5 (8.3)	5 (8.3)	1.000
Type			
Paralytic ileus	1 (1.7)	2 (3.3)	0.308
Duodenal stump leakage	1 (1.7)	1 (1.7)	0.986
Anastomotic bleeding	1 (1.7)	0 (0)	0.308
Wound infection	0 (0)	1 (1.7)	0.320
Nonsurgical complications	2 (3.3)	1 (1.7)	0.571
Dindo-Clavien grade			
II	3 (5.0)	3 (5.0)	1.000
IIIa	2 (3.3)	2 (3.3)	1.000
Readmission	1 (1.6)	0 (0)	1.000
Reoperation	0 (0)	0 (0)	-
Hospital death	0 (0)	0 (0)	-

Data are presented as number (%)

Table 5 Comparison of inflammatory markers between LADG and TLDG

	LADG (n = 60)	TLDG (n = 60)	P value
WBC count (10^9/L)			
Preoperative	6.4 ± 1.7	6.5 ± 1.6	0.586
Postoperative day 1	10.3 ± 1.4	10.1 ± 1.2	0.250
Postoperative day 4	7.2 ± 1.2	6.9 ± 1.5	0.641
Neutrophil count (%)			
Preoperative	56.6 ± 7.4	55.3 ± 7.4	0.152
Postoperative day 1	82.7 ± 5.7	79.7 ± 3.3	0.224
Postoperative day 4	66.5 ± 5.6	62.6 ± 6.3	0.538
CRP (mg/L)			
Preoperative	0.6 ± 0.7	0.6 = 0.8	0.250
Postoperative day 1	5.2 ± 2.9	4.8 ± 1.2	0.295
Postoperative day 4	7.7 ± 6.5	7.4 = 5.6	0.792

Data are presented as or mean ± standard deviation

studies have reported lower WBC counts and CRP levels in TLDG compared with LADG [20, 21], our results showed no differences between groups. Therefore, additional studies using more sensitive inflammation markers, such as interlukin-6 (IL-6) and tumor necrosis factor (TNF) alpha are required to determine the superiority of TLDG in this respect.

In LADG, extracorporeal anastomosis is conducted in a limited working space with limited visual field, thus making it a difficult procedure, especially on obese patients. Extension of the laparotomy is necessary to obtain a better view for secure anastomosis on obese patients. In BMI > 25 kg/m^2 patients, the operation time was shorter in the TLDG group than in the LADG group although it was not statistically significant. This finding indicates possibility that extracorporeal anastomosis needs more time because of the limited working space with restricted vision on obese patients. In this study, both TLDG and LADG were performed safely with few complications regardless of BMI. However, for obese patients, TLDG can provide more adequate working space with good visual field for the anastomosis.

Our study has several limitations. First, it was a retrospective study. Comparison between two groups was performed with limited data. More information could be collected if more variable biomarkers were used to examine, in particular, the relative invasiveness of the procedures. Second, the study size was small. However, this study was designed with a matched cohort. The enrolled patients were matched for age, sex, BMI, comorbidities, and tumor characteristics, which we would expect to compensate somewhat for its small size. Third, the surgeon's learning curve may influence the data of this study, as enrollee selection depended upon the time period when the surgery was performed. However, as

mentioned above, the surgeons already had significant experience in laparoscopic gastrectomy prior to the cases enrolled in this study. Also, as TLDG involves the same procedures as LADG for radical gastrectomy, with lymph node dissection preceding anastomosis, we believe that the effect of different operative periods should not be significant.

Conclusion

In this study, surgical outcomes of B-II TLDG showed it to be feasible compared with those of B-II LADG. TLDG has several advantages over LADG, such as a smaller incision, a shorter hospital stay, and more convenience during surgery. However, prospective randomized controlled studies are still needed to confirm that B-II TLDG can be used as a standard procedure for LDG.

Abbreviations
B-I: Billroth-I; B-II: Billroth-II; BMI: Body mass index; LADG: Laparoscopic-assisted distal gastrectomy; ODG: Open distal gastrectomy; R-Y: Roux-en-Y; SD: Standard deviation; TLDG: Totally laparoscopic distal gastrectomy

Acknowledgements
No additional investigators were involved in this research.

Funding
No funding.

Authors' contributions
JK, KJ and HC contributed equally to this work. KJ and HC performed the operations. JK and KJ collected and analyzed the data. JK wrote the manuscript and KJ assisted in drafting the manuscript and reviewed the article. All authors read and approved the final manuscript.

Competing interests
The authors declare that they have no competing interests.

References
1. Tanimura S, Higashino M, Fukunaga Y, Takemura M, Tanaka Y, Fujiwara Y, et al. Laparoscopic gastrectomy for gastric cancer: experience with more than 600 cases. Surg Endosc. 2008;22(5):1161–4.
2. Lee JH, Yom CK, Han HS. Comparison of long-term outcomes of laparoscopy-assisted and open distal gastrectomy for early gastric cancer. Surg Endosc. 2009;23(8):1759–63.
3. Huscher CG, Mingoli A, Sgarzini G, Sansonetti A, Di Paola M, Recher A, et al. Laparoscopic versus open subtotal gastrectomy for distal gastric cancer: five-year results of a randomized prospective trial. Ann Surg. 2005;241(2):232–7.
4. Kim YW, Baik YH, Yun YH, Nam BH, Kim DH, Choi IJ, et al. Improved quality of life outcomes after laparoscopy-assisted distal gastrectomy for early gastric cancer: results of a prospective randomized clinical trial. Ann Surg. 2008;248(5):721–7.
5. Zhang C, Xiao W, Chen K, Zhang Z, Du G, Jiang E, et al. A new intracorporeal Billroth II stapled anastomosis technique in totally laparoscopic distal gastrectomy. Surg Endosc. 2015;29(6):1636–42.
6. Goh P, Tekant Y, Kum CK, Isaac J, Shang NS. Totally intra-abdominal laparoscopic Billroth II gastrectomy. Surg Endosc. 1992;6(3):160.
7. Kanaji S, Harada H, Nakayama S, Yasuda T, Oshikiri T, Kawasaki K, et al. Surgical outcomes in the newly introduced phase of intracorporeal anastomosis following laparoscopic distal gastrectomy is safe and feasible compared with established procedures of extracorporeal anastomosis. Surg Endosc. 2014;28(4):1250–5.

8. Han G, Park JY, Kim YJ. Comparison of short-term postoperative outcomes in totally laparoscopic distal gastrectomy versus laparoscopy-assisted distal gastrectomy. J Gastric Cancer. 2014;14(2):105–10.

9. Kim JJ, Song KY, Chin HM, Kim W, Jeon HM, Park CH, et al. Totally laparoscopic gastrectomy with various types of intracorporeal anastomosis using laparoscopic linear staplers: preliminary experience. Surg Endosc. 2008;22(2):436–42.

10. Woo J, Lee JH, Shim KN, Jung HK, Lee HM, Lee HK. Does the Difference of Invasiveness between Totally Laparoscopic Distal Gastrectomy and Laparoscopy-Assisted Distal Gastrectomy Lead to a Difference in Early Surgical Outcomes? A Prospective Randomized Trial. Ann Surg Oncol. 2015;22(6):1836–43.

11. Lee SH, Kim IH, Kim IH, Kwak SG, Chae HD. Comparison of short-term outcomes and acute inflammatory response between laparoscopy-assisted and totally laparoscopic distal gastrectomy for early gastric cancer. Ann Surg Treat Res. 2015;89(4):176–82.

12. Japanese Gastric Cancer A. Japanese gastric cancer treatment guidelines 2010 (ver. 3). Gastric Cancer. 2011;14(2):113–23.

13. Washington K. 7th edition of the AJCC cancer staging manual: stomach. Ann Surg Oncol. 2010;17(12):3077–9.

14. Dindo D, Demartines N, Clavien PA. Classification of surgical complications: a new proposal with evaluation in a cohort of 6336 patients and results of a survey. Ann Surg. 2004;240(2):205–13.

15. Hosogi H, Kanaya S. Intracorporeal anastomosis in laparoscopic gastric cancer surgery. J Gastric Cancer. 2012;12(3):133–9.

16. Jeong O, Jung MR, Park YK, Ryu SY. Safety and feasibility during the initial learning process of intracorporeal Billroth I (delta-shaped) anastomosis for laparoscopic distal gastrectomy. Surg Endosc. 2015;29(6):1522–9.

17. Kojima K, Yamada H, Inokuchi M, Kawano T, Sugihara K. A comparison of Roux-en-Y and Billroth-I reconstruction after laparoscopy-assisted distal gastrectomy. Ann Surg. 2008;247(6):962–7.

18. Inokuchi M, Kojima K, Yamada H, Kato K, Hayashi M, Motoyama K, et al. Long-term outcomes of Roux-en-Y and Billroth-I reconstruction after laparoscopic distal gastrectomy. Gastric Cancer. 2013;16(1):67–73.

19. Chen K, Xu X, Mou Y, Pan Y, Zhang R, Zhou Y, et al. Totally laparoscopic distal gastrectomy with D2 lymphadenectomy and Billroth II gastrojejunostomy for gastric cancer: short- and medium-term results of 139 consecutive cases from a single institution. Int J Med Sci. 2013;10(11):1462–70.

20. Song KY, Park CH, Kang HC, Kim JJ, Park SM, Jun KH, et al. Is totally laparoscopic gastrectomy less invasive than laparoscopy-assisted gastrectomy?: prospective, multicenter study. J Gastrointest Surg. 2008;12(6):1015–21.

21. Ikeda O, Sakaguchi Y, Aoki Y, Harimoto N, Taomoto J, Masuda T, et al. Advantages of totally laparoscopic distal gastrectomy over laparoscopically assisted distal gastrectomy for gastric cancer. Surg Endosc. 2009;23(10):2374–9.

22. Kinoshita T, Shibasaki H, Oshiro T, Ooshiro M, Okazumi S, Katoh R. Comparison of laparoscopy-assisted and total laparoscopic Billroth-I gastrectomy for gastric cancer: a report of short-term outcomes. Surg Endosc. 2011;25(5):1395–401.

23. Kitano S, Shiraishi N, Uyama I, Sugihara K, Tanigawa N. Japanese Laparoscopic Surgery Study G: A multicenter study on oncologic outcome of laparoscopic gastrectomy for early cancer in Japan. Ann Surg. 2007;245(1):68–72.

24. Kim W, Song KY, Lee HJ, Han SU, Hyung WJ, Cho GS. The impact of comorbidity on surgical outcomes in laparoscopy-assisted distal gastrectomy: a retrospective analysis of multicenter results. Ann Surg. 2008;248(5):793–9.

24

Is pneumatic balloon dilation safe and effective primary modality of treatment for post-sleeve gastrectomy strictures? A retrospective study

Aneesh Shrihari Dhorepatil, Daniel Cottam*, Amit Surve, Walter Medlin, Hinali Zaveri, Christina Richards and Austin Cottam

Abstract

Background: The optimal treatment of sleeve strictures has not been agreed upon at the current time. At our institution, we began using pneumatic balloon dilation to help resolve these obstructions in 2010. Herein we report our experience with pneumatic balloon dilation for the treatment of sleeve strictures.

Methods: From Jan 2010 to Dec 2016 we retrospectively reviewed our prospectively kept database for patients who developed a Laparoscopic Sleeve Gastrectomy (LSG) stricture within 90 days of surgery. If the stricture was found, then we dilated all our patients initially at 30 mm at 10 PSI for 10-20 min (14.5 min average) and increased the balloon size (30-40 mm) and duration (10-30 min) in subsequent sessions if the first session was unsuccessful.

Results: The review found that 1756 patients underwent either LSG or the first step of a Laparoscopic Duodenal Switch (LDS) (1409 LSG & 356 LDS). Of the 1756 patient 33 patients (24 underwent LSG, and 9 underwent LDS) developed a stricture as a complication of LSG. The average age of the patients was 46.4 (±9.6) years, and the average BMI was 43.7 (±6.4). The most common location for stricture was mid-body of the sleeve (54.5%). The average time from the primary surgery to diagnosis and first pneumatic dilation was 5.6 months (± 6.8) and 5.9 months (± 6.6) respectively. We successfully used pneumatic dilation in 31 (93.9%) of these patients to relieve the stricture.

Conclusion: We conclude that pneumatic dilation is an effective procedure in patients with post sleeve gastrectomy stricture.

Keywords: Laparoscopic sleeve gastrectomy, Loop-duodenal switch, Strictures, Pneumatic balloon dilation, Endoscopic management, Bariatric

Background

Prevalence of laparoscopic sleeve gastrectomy (LSG) for morbid obesity increased from 0 to 37% of the total world interventions for weight loss surgery between 2003 and 2013 [1]. This increase in popularity is attributed to its lower complication rates and safety as a procedure [2].

Despite the LSG's rapidly rising popularity, strictures have remained an ongoing problem with an occurrence rate of 0.1–3.9% [1]. Strictures are usually divided into

early strictures and late strictures. Patients with early strictures present within the first few weeks following the surgery complaining of dysphagia, vomiting, food intolerance, rapid weight loss, and regurgitation of either food or saliva. These are often pseudo strictures caused either as a result of post-operative edema or hematoma formation.

Late strictures, which occur > 1 month from the time of surgery are usually true strictures [3]. They are usually caused by ischemia, retraction due to scarring, or misalignment during stapling [3].

Treatment of LSG strictures is controversial. When to intervene, when to dilate, with what to dilate, and when

* Correspondence: drdanielcottam@yahoo.com
Bariatric Medicine Institute, 1046 East 100 South, Salt Lake City, UT 84102, USA

to place metallic stents are all active areas of debate [4]. When these non-invasive methods fail, when to perform surgery and which type of surgery to perform, whether it's a simple seromyotomy or strictureplasty or more invasive approaches to some bypass procedure, all lack consensus [5, 6].

In this article, we share one of the largest case series of LSG strictures treated with pneumatic balloon dilation as a primary modality of treatment. We also present a sustainable management plan using pneumatic balloon dilation as the primary modality of treatment for LSG strictures.

Methods

This study has been approved by Quorum Review- Independent review board (QR# 31353), prior to data collection. 1409 cases of LSG and 356 cases of LDS were retrospectively reviewed from a prospectively collected database from Jan 2010 to Dec 2016. Demographic data for all patients was collected. This included pre-operative BMI, age, weight, and co-morbidities.

Thirty-three patients (1.8%) that presented with dysphagia, nausea, vomiting, or food intolerance after LSG or LDS with documented stricture on endoscopy or upper gastrointestinal (UGI) contrast study were considered eligible for pneumatic dilation. An area of narrowing, slow passage, or frank obstruction on an UGI were defined as a stricture. Similarly, a stricture was defined as a small, unsurpassable stretch of the lumen when using a 9.8 mm endoscope with or without symptoms, especially if the lumen is 6 mm or less [3]. We included all patients who demonstrated a stricture of gastric origin and underwent at least 20 mm of dilation into the study. We excluded all patients with strictures of non-gastric origin and patients undergoing a revision surgery of gastric bypass.

We used endoscopic pneumatic balloon dilation as a primary modality of treatment and repeated the procedure if symptoms did not resolve. Patients were informed of a surgical alternative in cases requiring repeated dilations.

Technique of pneumatic dilation

We performed all our endoscopies under general anesthesia. Initially, an endoscope is passed down to the level of the stricture under direct vision. The stricture's position is then confirmed on fluoroscopy and marked with a simple paper clip on the anterior abdominal wall. After confirming the stricture, the scope is then passed distally to the stricture and into the distal small bowel. A MAXXWIRE (MeritMedica Endotek) metallic guide-wire is passed through the scope and using fluoroscopic guidance placed in the distal small bowel, and the EGD scope is removed

keeping the guide-wire in place. Then using the guidewire and fluoroscopic guidance we slide the Rigiflex II Balloon (Boston Scientific, Marlborough, Massachusetts) into position using the previously placed paper clip as a reference.

The balloon is then inflated under fluoroscopic and endoscopic visualization to 30 mm for an average of 14.5 min per patient. Optical view through the balloon and re-inspection endoscopy was used to confirm the resolution of the stricture. Depending on clinical improvement and the patients' decision, repeat dilations were performed up to a maximum of 40 mm, with a minimum interval of 2 weeks between 2 dilations.

Technique for LSG and LDS [7]

All surgeries were done by the three surgeons at the Bariatric Medicine Institute at a single hospital in Salt Lake City with identical technique. Out technique for both the LSG and LDS has been described previously [7].

Briefly, the LSG is created by stapling alongside a 40 French bougie. No patient in the study had his or her staple line oversewn or staple line reinforced. The staple line in all patients is started approximately 5 cm from the pylorus and ended at the angle of His. Each patient has a visual inspection of the hiatus to evaluate for a hiatal hernia with the simultaneous repair if a defect is found.

The loop duodenal switch procedure begins with an identical technique as a LSG. Following this, the gastroepiploic vessels are divided from the end of the sleeve staple line past the pylorus to the point where the perforating vessels from the pancreas enter the duodenum. This is 2 to 4 cm beyond the pylorus. The duodenum is divided with an Endo GIA stapler (Medtronic). Then the ileocecal valve is identified, and 300 cm of small bowel are measured and marked for point of anastomosis. The small bowel is then connected to the proximal duodenum.

Results

Out of 1756 patients who underwent sleeve gastrectomy or LDS, 33 patients were included in this study. Twenty-seven patients were female, and 6 patients were male. The average age of the patients was 46.4 ($\pm$9.6) years, and the average BMI was 43.7 ($\pm$6.4).

Sixty-five percent of the patients followed up at 1 year and the excess body weight loss (EBWL%) at 1 year was 66.1% (62.6–69.7%).

24 patients underwent laparoscopic sleeve gastrectomy, and 9 patients underwent a LDS. Of 33 patients, 15 patients (45.4%), 5 patients (15.1%), and 9 patients (27.2%) had diabetes mellitus (DM), positive smoking history, and hiatal hernia repair, respectively. After endoscopy and/or Upper GI series, in 54.5%(18/33)

patients the stricture was localized to the Mid-Body, 30.2%(10/33) were noted to have it at the incisura, and 15.2%(5/33) had it in the upper 1/3 of the sleeve. The average time from surgery to diagnosis was 5.6 months ±6.8 months. The average duration of primary surgery to the first pneumatic dilation was 5.9 months (+/− 6.6). The average duration from primary surgery to the second dilation was 8.6 months (+/− 7.1). Overall only 2 patients from the study group were dilated 3 times. The average duration of primary surgery to the third dilation was 19 months (+/− 19.7). The average balloon size used for the first dilation was 32.1 mm(+/− 6.8); for the second dilation it was 35 mm (+/− 5.2); and for the third dilation it was 40 mm.

The mean duration of dilation was 14.5 min (+/− 7.5 min). In the 21 patients who required a single dilation for symptom resolution, the mean duration was 15.6 min (+/− 6.6). Of the 8 patients that required a second dilation for symptom resolution, the mean duration of dilation in the first dilation was 14.6 min (+/− 8.3) and in their second dilation was 20 min (+/− 8 min). The 2 patients who required 3 dilations for symptom resolution were dilated for 10 min during the first dilation; 22.5 min (+/− 10.6 min) during their second dilation, and 30 min during their third dilation. 93.9% (31/33) patients had complete resolution of symptoms after pneumatic balloon dilation. 67.7% (21/31) required only 1 dilation, 25.8% (8/31) required 2 dilations, and 6.4% (2/31) required 3 dilations. Of the remaining 6.1% (2/33) patients, 1 patient required surgical intervention for symptom resolution, and 1 patient required a fcSEMS stent.

The location of the stricture, operative details, and the outcomes following pneumatic dilation can be seen in Table 1.

Discussion

Strictures following a LSG is a very rare complication with a reported incidence of 0.1–3.9% [1]. Due to this rarity, there are few studies which thoroughly explore its management. Strictures usually present about 6 weeks after surgery [8], and are characterized by persistent dysphagia, nausea, vomiting, and food regurgitation following surgery. Early identification and management lead to better outcomes [8]. Our study is one of the largest case series detailing the magnitude of the complication and explores the efficacy of pneumatic balloon in its management.

According to many authors, the most common site of stricture is at the incisura [5, 9–11], but we observed that the most common location of the stricture was at the Mid-Body of the narrow sleeve (54.5%) followed by the incisura (30.2%) and then the upper 1/3rd of the sleeve (15.2%). This correlates with similar studies

conducted by Donatelli et al. [12] and Rebibo et al. [13]. The question as to why we have more strictures in the mid-body just like Donatelli and Rebibo we believe relates to technique, specifically, the way the assistant pulls on the stomach while stapling. However, since the rate of stricture formation was only 2%, it will be several years and almost a thousand patients before we can definitively say whether or not our change in technique has made a difference.

Excess body weight loss achieved at 1 year after LSG can range from 50 to 70% [7, 14, 15]. We believe with early recognition and treatment, the presence of a stricture does not alter the pattern and degree of excess body weight loss achieved by LSG. This can be seen in the EBWL% achieved by the patients in this study, which was 66.1%.

Graded Pneumatic Balloon Dilation has been introduced as an effective and safer alternative to surgery for strictures [16, 17]. The primary aim of pneumatic balloon dilation is to pull apart the fibrosed muscular fibers. The pneumatic balloon, due to its rigid structure, achieves the high radial force of expansion [10]. Our study's use of higher initial balloon size and increased duration time ensures the initial few minutes of dilation help tear the muscular fibers while the longer duration overcomes the elasticity of the fibrosis which has invariably occurred at the site of the stricture.

The magnitude of balloon dilation required for most effective management has not yet been defined. Most authors recommend 30 mm as the diameter of the balloon during the initial dilation for effective management of the stricture [3, 11]. Shnell et al. [10] demonstrated a relative lack of clinical success using the 20 mm balloon, and Donatelli et al. [12] and Rebibo et al. [13] showed higher success rates using the 30 mm balloon. In this study, we too used the 30 mm balloon during the first dilation. We believe dilating with up to 40 mm balloon is safe and effective even during the initial dilation. We dilated 8 patients with 40 mm balloons during their initial dilation and reported no adverse events associated with the pneumatic dilation. As far as efficacy is concerned, 50% (4/8) reported resolution of symptoms after a single dilation and 50% (4/8) required repeated dilation. In our experience, the 30 mm balloon is the safer and wiser choice as an initial dilator. We believe there isn't a significant increase in efficacy by using a larger balloon as an initial dilator. The decision to use a larger balloon must be patient specific and should be taken after visualizing the stricture intra-operatively. Further studies comparing the 30 mm balloon and the 40 mm are required to determine the benefit of one over the other.

Compared to other studies, which document up to 1 min as the duration of dilation, this study has

Table 1 Operative Details and Outcomes

Surgery		LSG	LDS	Total
N		24	9	33
MSS		5.1 ± 6.9	6.4 ± 6.3	5.9 ± 6.6
Operative Details of Dilations with avg. dilation (mm) and avg. duration (min)	1st Dilation	15/24 Dilation: 32 ± 7.7 Duration: 15.5 ± 6.3 7/24 Dilation: 31.4 ± 6.9 Duration: 15.2 ± 8.7 1/24 Dilation: 40 Duration: 10	6/9 Dilation: 31.6 ± 4.1 Duration: 15.8 ± 8 1 /9 Dilation: 30 Duration: 10 1/9 Dilation: 40 Duration: 10	
	2nd Dilation	7/24 Dilation: 33.7 ± 5.1 Duration: 20 ± 8.1 1/24 Dilation: 40 Duration: 30	1/9 Dilation: 30 Duration: 30 1/9 Dilation: 40 Duration: 15	
	3rd Dilation	1/24 Dilation: 40 Duration: 30	1/9 Dilation: 40 Duration: 30	
Resolution rate with each dilation	1st Dilation	62.5% (15/24)	66.7% (6/9)	
	2nd Dilation	29.1% (7/24)	11.1% (1/9)	
	3rd Dilation	4.1% (1/24)	11.1% (1/9)	
Overall Outcomes		Resolved: 95.8% (23/24) Unresolved: 4.1% (1/24)	Resolved: 88.9% (8/9) Unresolved: 11.1% (1/9)	Resolved: 93.9% (31/33) Unresolved: 6.1% (2/33)

Abbreviations: N number, MSS months since surgery, LSG Laparoscopic sleeve gastrectomy, LDS Loop duodenal switch

Is pneumatic balloon dilation safe and effective primary modality of treatment for post-sleeve...

161

demonstrated a mean duration of 14.5 min (+/− 7.5 min). The increased duration of dilation leads to increased long-term patency of the previously strictured sleeve. We propose it leads to the lesser need for repeat dilations and lesser need for operative intervention to treat the stricture. We achieved successful resolution of symptoms in 93.9% of our patients only using pneumatic dilation. 67.7% of the patients with reported resolution of symptoms required just a single dilation. This could be the reason for our higher success rate as compared to other studies in the literature [9–12, 18]. Moreover, the patients who achieved symptom resolution after a single dilation were subjected to a longer duration of dilation (15.3 min) as compared to those who required a second dilation (14.6 min) {during their first dilation}. The longer balloon dilation times are not unheard of as Zundel dilated his sleeve strictures for a mean of 20 min [3]. In reality, the basic science and retrospective data are lacking in this regard, and there are no papers comparing dilation time and the incidence of complication. Our paper clearly showed that longer dilation times lead to better outcomes. However, we would never object to the argument that the appropriate dilation time and size are still open for vigorous debate.

Recently, Deslauriers et al. successfully performed dilation in 56% of his patients with sleeve stenosis [19]. Of these, 73% only needed single dilation, while 44% of the patients who were unsuccessful needed conversion to gastric bypass. All the successful cases needed a maximum of 3 interventions. Our success rate was higher and failure rate was lower than the one reported in this study. However, the success rate with single dilation was very similar between the two studies (73% vs 68%). Similarly, Nath A et al. [20] performed hydrostatic balloon dilation in 33 patients with gastric sleeve narrowing. He used 10–18 mm of balloon dilation for 1 min. Resolution was seen in 69% of his patients; 39.4% after first dilation, 15.2% after 2nd dilation and 15.2% after third dilation. Two patients (6%) had no improvement at all. His resolution rate was also lower compared to ours; however, it is important to note that size of his dilation was much smaller compared to the other published studies [10, 12, 13, 21].

Complex strictures sometimes require a different approach. The treatment options include fcSEMS stent and revision surgeries including pyloroplasty, stricturoplasty [22], or revision bariatric surgery [6]. fcSEMS are currently used for short periods to fine-tune narrowed sleeves [4]. Stents are most useful in refractory strictures, which have failed multiple attempts at dilation [4]. Unfortunately, stent migration is a very real complication and is reported in a very high number of cases [4]. This leads to repositioning in a majority of cases and operative stent removal in others.

In this study, we had 1 patient who required a stent. The patient underwent stent placement because of diverticulum formed due to gastric dilation, which required a partial gastrectomy. The patient experienced persistent pain and dysphagia 1 week after stent placement. After endoscopy, it was revealed that the stent had migrated into the esophagus, which had caused an intussusception of the esophagus and had led to an obstruction. We proceeded with endoscopic removal of the stent. The patient reported resolution of symptoms after removal of the stent.

Revision surgeries range from pyloroplasty, stricturoplasty, and seromyotomy to revision bariatric procedures like gastric bypass [6], single anastomosis gastric bypass, revision sleeve gastrectomy and loop duodenal switch. Dapri et al. [5] and Vilallonga et al. [11] have shown promising results of seromyotomies in patients suffering from long stenosis after sleeve gastrectomies. Some surgeons have approached the refractory strictures with more conservative techniques like a circular gastro-gastrostomy [23] or a laparoscopic median gastrostomy [24]. We had 1 patient who required revision surgeries for complete resolution of symptoms. The patient suffered from a refractory stricture at the incisura 1 month after a LDS procedure. After 3 unsuccessful attempts at graded pneumatic dilation over 6 months, a decision was taken to perform a partial gastrectomy to resect the gastric dilation caused by the stricture. This significantly controlled her symptoms. But one year later, the patient experienced a significant resurgence in her symptoms which led to the decision to perform a Heineke-Mickulicz stricturoplasty with a gastrogastrostomy. This procedure too had limited success. Finally, a decision was taken to place a transabdominal jejunostomy tube. Currently, the patient is still symptomatic but does not want a further intervention and is fine with her limited ability to eat as long as she has a functioning J tube.

In retrospect, our study could have been improved in many ways. These include the addition of a questionnaire to document resolution of symptoms like the BAROS (Bariatric Analysis and Reporting Outcome System) score [25] and a larger sample size.

Another major limitation of our study is the lack of long-term follow up for some of our patients. Though almost all patients at the time of writing do report resolution of symptoms, a follow up of at least 12 months is needed to rule out the possibility of recurrence.

Last but not least due to a small sample size, we were not able to thoroughly explore the management of refractory strictures. Larger studies are needed to compare fcSEMS versus revision surgery for the effective management of refractory strictures.

Conclusions

The post-operative stricture is a rare complication following VSG, and earlier detection with effective management significantly reduces patient morbidity. Endoscopic treatment with pneumatic balloon dilation has repeatedly proven to be effective and safe as the first line of management for this complication.

In our series, the duration of dilation is as important as balloon size in achieving early resolution of symptoms and avoiding revision surgeries. However, both the timing and size of the balloon should not be considered settled, and we look for other authors to corroborate our findings or further define what can be done when strictures appear in the sleeve patient. Surgical intervention should be considered only after multiple failed attempts at dilation.

Abbreviations

BAROS: Bariatric Analysis and Reporting Outcome System; DM: Diabetes mellitus; EBWL: Excess body weight loss; LAGB: Laparoscopic gastric band; LDS: Laparoscopic Duodenal Switch; LSG: Laparoscopic Sleeve Gastrectomy; UGI: Upper gastrointestinal series

Statement of human and animal rights

All procedures performed in studies involving human participants were in accordance with the ethical standards of the institutional and/or national research committee and with the 1964 Helsinki declaration and its later amendments or comparable ethical standards."

Authors' contributions

Operating or assistant surgeon and reviewed the manuscript: Drs. DC, CR, and WM. Drafting, data collection, data analysis, and interpretation: AD, AS. Data Analysis and interpretation: HZ, AC Manuscript review: AC. All authors read and approved the final manuscript.

Competing interests

DC, the corresponding author reports personal fees and other from Medtronic, outside the submitted work.
Drs. AD, WM, CR, AS and HZ declare that they have no competing interests.
AC declares that he has no competing interests.

References

1. Angrisani L, Santonicola A, Iovino P, Formisano G, Buchwald H, Scopinaro N. Bariatric surgery worldwide 2013. Obes Surg. 2015;25(10):1822–32.
2. Zellmer J, Mathiason M, Kallies K, Kothari S. Is laparoscopic sleeve gastrectomy a lower risk bariatric procedure compared with laparoscopic roux-en-Y gastric bypass? A meta-analysis. Am J Surg. 2014;208(6):903–10.
3. Zundel N, Hernandez J, Neto M, Campos J. Strictures after laparoscopic sleeve gastrectomy. Surg Laparosc Endosc Percutan Tech. 2010;20(3):154–8.
4. Eubanks S, Edwards C, Fearing N, Ramaswamy A, de la Torre R, Thaler K, Miedema B, Scott J. Use of endoscopic stents to treat anastomotic complications after bariatric surgery. J Am Coll Surg. 2008;206(5):935–8.
5. Dapri G, Cadière G, Himpens J. Laparoscopic Seromyotomy for long stenosis after sleeve gastrectomy with or without duodenal switch. Obes Surg. 2009; 19(4):495–9.
6. Bellorin O, Lieb J, Szomstein S, Rosenthal R. Laparoscopic conversion of sleeve gastrectomy to roux-en-Y gastric bypass for acute gastric outlet obstruction after laparoscopic sleeve gastrectomy for morbid obesity. Surg Obes Relat Dis. 2010;6(5):566–8.
7. Cottam A, Cottam D, Roslin M, Cottam S, Medlin W, Richards C, Surve A, Zaveri H. A matched cohort analysis of sleeve gastrectomy with and without 300 cm loop duodenal switch with 18-month follow-up. Obes Surg. 2016;26(10):2363–9.
8. Rosenthal R. International sleeve gastrectomy expert panel consensus statement: best practice guidelines based on experience of >12,000 cases. Surg Obes Relat Dis. 2012;8(1):8–19.
9. Cottam D, Qureshi F, Mattar S, Sharma S, Holover S, Bonanomi G, Ramanathan R, Schauer P. Laparoscopic sleeve gastrectomy as an initial weight-loss procedure for high-risk patients with morbid obesity. Surg Endosc. 2006;20(6):859–63.
10. Shnell M, Fishman S, Eldar S, Goitein D, Santo E. Balloon dilatation for symptomatic gastric sleeve stricture. Gastrointest Endosc. 2014;79(3):521–4.
11. Vilallonga R, Himpens J, van de Vrande S. Laparoscopic Management of Persistent Strictures after Laparoscopic Sleeve Gastrectomy. Obes Surg. 2013;23(10):1655–61.
12. Donatelli G, Dumont J, Pourcher G, Tranchart H, Tuszynski T, Dagher I, Catheline J, Chiche R, Marmuse J, Dritsas S, Vergeau B, Meduri B. Pneumatic dilation for functional helix stenosis after sleeve gastrectomy: long-term follow-up (with videos). Surg Obes Relat Dis. 2016;13(6):943–50.
13. Rebibo L, Hakim S, Dhahri A, Yzet T, Delcenserie R, Regimbeau J. Gastric stenosis after laparoscopic sleeve gastrectomy: diagnosis and management. Obes Surg. 2015;26(5):995–1001.
14. Carlin AM, Arthur M, et al. The Comparative Effectiveness Of Sleeve Gastrectomy, Gastric Bypass, And Adjustable Gastric Banding Procedures For The Treatment Of Morbid Obesity. Annals of Surgery. 2013;257(5):791–7.
15. Casillas RA, et al. Comparative Effectiveness Of Sleeve Gastrectomy Versus Roux-En-Y Gastric Bypass For Weight Loss And Safety Outcomes In Older Adults. Surgery for Obesity and Related Diseases. 2017;13(9):1476–83.
16. Boeckxstaens G, Annese V, Varannes S, Chaussade S, Costantini M, Cuttitta A, Elizalde J, Fumagalli U, Gaudric M, Rohof W, Smout A, Tack J, Zwinderman A, Zaninotto G, Busch O. Pneumatic dilation versus laparoscopic Heller's Myotomy for idiopathic achalasia. N Engl J Med. 2011;364(19):1807–16.
17. Gambardella C, Allaria A, Siciliano G, et al. Recurrent esophageal stricture from previous caustic ingestion treated with 40-year self-dilation: case report and review of literature. BMC gastroenterol. 2018;18(1):68.
18. Ogra R, Kini G. Evolving endoscopic management options for symptomatic stenosis post-laparoscopic sleeve gastrectomy for morbid obesity: experience at a large bariatric surgery unit in New Zealand. Obes Surg. 2014;25(2):242–8.
19. Deslauriers V, Beauchamp A, Garofalo F, et al. Endoscopic management of post-laparoscopic sleeve gastrectomy stenosis. Surg Endosc. 2018; 32(2):601–9.
20. Nath A, Yewale S, Tran T, Brebbia JS, Shope TR, Koch TR. Dysphagia after vertical sleeve gastrectomy: evaluation of risk factors and assessment of endoscopic intervention. World J Gastroenterol. 2016;22(47):10371–9.
21. Agnihotri A, Barola S, Hill C, et al. Endoscopic management of gastric stenosis following laparoscopic sleeve gastrectomy. GIE. 2017;(85, 5):AB276.
22. Sudan R, Kasotakis G, Betof A, Wright A. Sleeve gastrectomy strictures: technique for robotic-assisted strictureplasty. Surg Obes Relat Dis. 2010;6(4):434–6.
23. Parikh M, Gagner M. Laparoscopic revision of Gastrogastric stricture with a Transoral circular stapler. Surg Innov. 2007;14(3):225–30.
24. Kalaiselvan R, Ammori B. Laparoscopic median gastrectomy for stenosis following sleeve gastrectomy. Surg Obes Relat Dis. 2015;11(2):474–7.
25. Oria H, Moorehead M. Updated bariatric analysis and reporting outcome system (BAROS). Surg Obes Relat Dis. 2009;5(1):60–6.

25

Giant duodenal ulcers after neurosurgery for brainstem tumors that required reoperation for gastric disconnection: a report of two cases

Chihoko Nobori[1], Kenjiro Kimura[1*], Go Ohira[1], Ryosuke Amano[1], Sadaaki Yamazoe[1], Hiroaki Tanaka[1], Kentaro Naito[2], Toshihiro Takami[2], Kosei Hirakawa[1] and Masaichi Ohira[1]

Abstract

Background: Despite the efficacy of pharmacotherapy for gastrointestinal ulcers, severe cases of bleeding or perforation due to gastrointestinal ulcers still occur. Giant duodenal ulcer perforation is an uncommon but difficult-to-manage pathology with a high mortality rate. We report two cases of giant duodenal ulcer perforation after neurosurgery for brainstem tumors that needed reoperation for gastric disconnection because of postoperative leakage and bleeding.

Case presentation: Both cases had undergone neurosurgery for brainstem tumors, and the patients were in a shock state for several days with peritonitis due to giant duodenal perforation. In Case 1, antrectomy with Billroth II reconstruction was performed. However, reoperation for gastric disconnection was needed because of major leakage of gastrojejunostomy and jejunojejunostomy. In Case 2, an omental patch, cholecystectomy, and insertion of a bile drainage tube from the cystic duct were performed for the giant duodenal ulcer, but leakage and bleeding from the ulcer edge required reoperation for gastric disconnection.

Conclusions: Brainstem tumors in these cases might have been related to duodenal ulcer perforation with late diagnosis that progressed to severe sepsis. For giant duodenal ulcer perforation with poor general condition, simple closure including omental patch or antrectomy with reconstruction is hazardous. Antrectomy with gastric disconnection, meaning gastrostomy, duodenostomy, feeding jejunostomy and cholecystectomy, is recommended.

Keywords: Giant duodenal ulcer, Gastric disconnection, Brainstem tumor

Background

Cushing reported gastroduodenal ulcers produced by elevated intracranial pressure caused by an intracranial tumor, head injury, or other space-occupying lesion, which have been called Cushing's ulcer [1]. The use of histamine H2-receptor antagonists or proton pump inhibitors can decrease the incidence of Cushing's ulcer and its complications, such as bleeding and perforation. However, cases of severe bleeding or perforation from gastroduodenal ulcers still occur. Generally, duodenal ulcer perforation is a

surgical emergency. Factors such as advanced age, concomitant disease, preoperative shock, large size of the perforation, and delays in presentation and operation have been identified as risk factors for mortality from duodenal ulcer perforation [2]. Gapta et al. classified duodenal ulcer perforations into three groups based on the size of the perforations: 'small' perforations less than 1 cm in diameter; 'large' perforations more than 1 cm but less than 3 cm in diameter; and 'giant' perforations exceeding 3 cm [2]. Small and large perforations are common and relatively easy to manage, resulting in low mortality rates. On the other hand, giant perforations are uncommon but difficult to manage and associated with higher mortality rates. Simple closure or omental patching alone have been

* Correspondence: kenjiro@med.osaka-cu.ac.jp
[1]Department of Surgical Oncology, Osaka City University Graduate School of Medicine, 1-4-3 Asahi-machi, Abeno-ku, Osaka, Japan
Full list of author information is available at the end of the article

reported as unsafe. Two cases of giant duodenal ulcer perforation after neurosurgery that needed re-operation because of postoperative leakage and bleeding are described. Taking these cases into account, we discuss how to cope with perforation of a giant duodenal ulcer that has progressed to sepsis because of late diagnosis.

Case presentations

Case 1 involved a 25-year-old man who had undergone surgical resection of anaplastic ependymoma extending from the brainstem to the fourth ventricle (Fig. 1). Two days after neurosurgery, laboratory data showed an unexpectedly severe inflammatory response (white cell count, 18,900/μL; C-reactive protein (CRP), 12.8 mg/dl). The patient was observed with administration of meropenem.

Two days later, he developed shock and the abdomen appeared severely distended. Vital signs were: temperature, 39.1 °C; heart rate, 130 beats/min; blood pressure, 73/37 mmHg under medication with dopamine 8 μg/kg/min and noradrenaline 0.25 μg/kg/min; and oxygen saturation, 94 % in room air. Laboratory data showed: white cell count, 23,100/μL; platelet count, 32,000/μL; CRP, 5.48 mg/dL. Computed tomography (CT) showed free air and massive ascites (Fig. 2), and emergency surgery was performed under a presumptive diagnosis of gastrointestinal perforation. On laparotomy, 3 L of muddy ascites was removed, and a perforation 3.5 cm in diameter was found in the second portion of the duodenal bulb (Fig. 3). Antrectomy including the ulcerated portion using Billroth II reconstruction with Braun anastomosis, insertion of a duodenal drainage tube from the duodenal stump, and cholecystectomy with insertion of a bile drainage tube from the cystic duct were performed.

Ten days after the ulcer operation, major leakage of the gastrojejunostomy and jejunojejunostomy required re-operation, involving gastric disconnection, gastrostomy, duodenostomy, and feeding jejunostomy. After reoperation, the patient developed multiple-organ failure,

but he recovered with intensive care. Eight months after the reoperation, digestive tract reconstruction surgery was performed using the Roux-en-Y method. Since that reconstruction surgery, the patient has been making satisfactory progress.

Case 2 involved a 62-year-old woman. She had undergone surgical resection of a brainstem hemangioblastoma that progressed acutely after stereotactic radiosurgery (Fig. 4). Six days after neurosurgery, laboratory data revealed an unexpectedly severe inflammatory response (white cell count, 23,100/μL; CRP, 18.5 mg/dL). However, she was observed with administration of cefepime. After another 3 days, she developed shock and the abdomen appeared distended. Vital signs were: temperature, 38.1 °C; heart rate, 140 beats/min; blood pressure, 60/40 mmHg under medication with dopamine 10 μg/kg/min and noradrenaline 0.15 μg/kg/min; and oxygen saturation, 92 % in room air. Laboratory data showed: white cell count, 18,100/μL; platelet count, 29,000/μL; CRP, 4.1 mg/dL. CT showed massive ascites, but no free air at that time (Fig. 5). Aspirated ascites showed intestinal juice, so emergency surgery was performed under a diagnosis of gastrointestinal perforation.

On laparotomy, 4 L of biliary ascites was removed, and a perforation 4 cm in length was found at the duodenal bulb (Fig. 6). An omental patch over the perforation site, insertion of a drainage tube into the duodenum from the anterior wall of the stomach, and cholecystectomy with insertion of a bile drainage tube from the cystic duct were performed. Fifteen days after the ulcer operation, continuous bleeding at the wall edge of the duodenal ulcer required reoperation. Operative findings revealed ulcer bleeding and dehiscence of the perforation site. Gastric disconnection was performed, comprising antrectomy including resection of the ulcerated portion, tube duodenostomy, and tube gastrostomy. The patient also needed intensive care, and her condition improved after 3 months. However, digestive reconstruction surgery has not yet

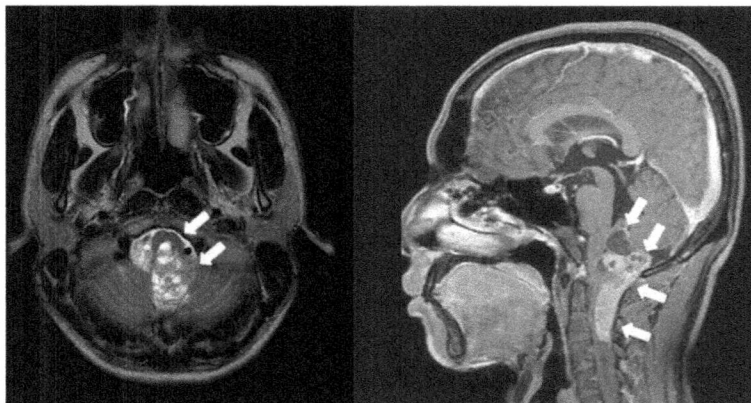

Fig. 1 Head MRI. The MRI scan reveals an anaplastic ependymoma that extended from brainstem to forth ventricle

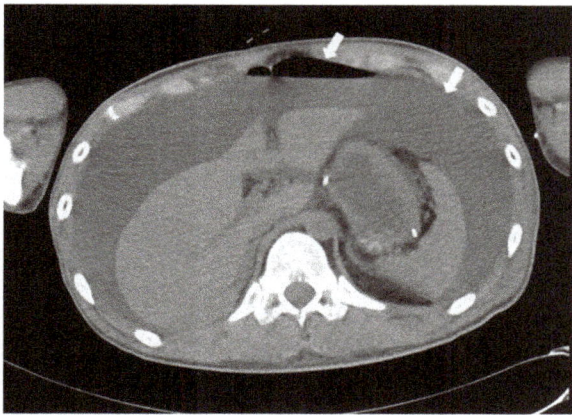

Fig. 2 Abdominal CT. The CT scan reveals a considerable amount of fluid and free air (arrow)

been performed as of the time of writing, as the brain tumor recurred during recovery.

Discussion

In these two cases, the brainstem tumors might have been related to duodenal ulcer perforation that progressed to septicemia. In 1841, Rokitansky suggested for the first time that ulcerative processes of the stomach might involve dysfunction of nervous mechanisms [3]. In 1932, Cushing reported gastroduodenal ulcers produced by elevated intracranial pressure caused by an intracranial tumor, head injury, or other space-occupying lesion. He suggested that such ulcerative processes might be related to diencephalic or brainstem disorders affecting the parasympathetic

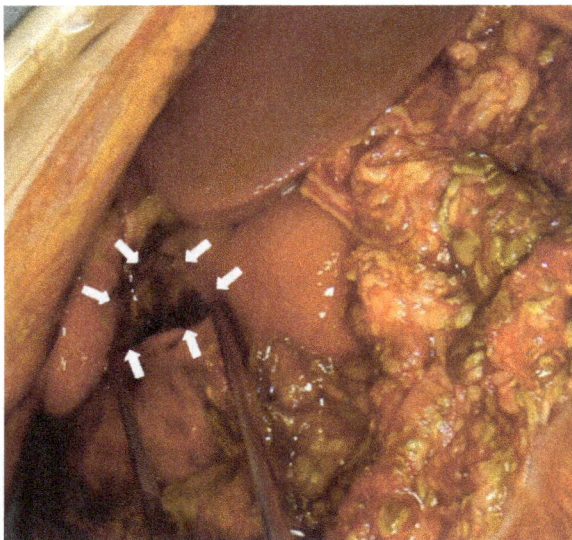

Fig. 3 The intra-operative finding. The perforation 3.5-cm in diameter was found in the second portion of the duodenal bulb

nervous system. Since then, ulcers of this type have been called Cushing's ulcers [1].

The mechanism of ulceration appears to involve three routes from the central nervous system to the stomach: 1) anterior hypothalamus – vagus nerve; 2) posterior hypothalamus – sympathetic nerve; and 3) posterior hypothalamus – anterior pituitary gland – adrenal cortex. Through these three routes, factors that aggravate the stomach are increased or protective factors are decreased. The sympathetic and parasympathetic nervous systems usually maintain a balance of the blood supply, gastric secretion, and gastric motility. Dysfunction of the central nervous system stimulates the hypothalamus, which then stimulates the sympathetic and parasympathetic nervous systems. Stimulation of sympathetic nerves decreases blood supply to the stomach, and stimulation of parasympathetic nerves increases gastric secretion. Moreover, adrenal cortical hormones through the anterior pituitary gland decrease gastric mucus secretion [4–10]. These factors then contribute to the development of gastroduodenal ulcers.

In general, factors such as advanced age, concomitant disease, preoperative shock, large size of the perforation, and delays in presentation and operation have been identified as risk factors for mortality in duodenal ulcer perforation [2]. Based on these factors, several scoring systems have been used to evaluate the condition of the patient with duodenal ulcer perforation, such as the Boey score [11], Mannheim Peritonitis Index [12–14], APACHE II score [15] and Jabalpur score [16]. In particular, the perforation-operation interval seems to represent an important factor for mortality. Mishra et al. reported that the mortality rate is 3 % within 24 h, 57 % from 25 to 72 h, and 80 % over 120 h after duodenal ulcer perforation [16]. Many reports have stated that an interval to operation larger than 24 h increases the mortality rate [17–19], because heavier bacterial contamination occurs in patients with delayed treatment [20]. In the present two cases, decreased level of consciousness was the major cause of delayed diagnosis in both patients. Although gauging the interval since ulcer perforation is difficult, at least 48 h may have elapsed in both cases, given the presence of septic shock. Of the above risk factors, our two cases showed large perforations, delayed diagnosis, concomitant disease, and preoperative shock, as well as advanced age in Case 2. Operations in such cases are generally difficult. Nonetheless, antrectomy with Billroth II reconstruction was performed for Case 1 and omental patching was performed for Case 2. Because gastric disconnection requires a second operation for digestive reconstruction, we hesitated to perform this procedure, but gastric disconnection was unavoidable at the first emergency surgery.

Most duodenal ulcer perforations are less than 1 cm in length, and can be successfully treated with one-layer

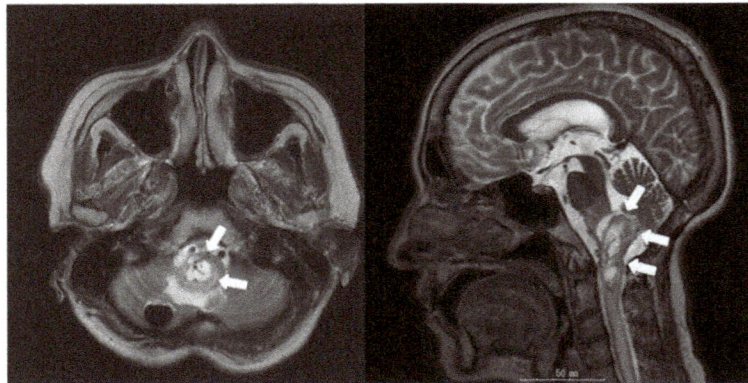

Fig. 4 Head MRI. The MRI scan reveals an a brainstem hemangioblastoma

closure plus a pedicled omental patch (Cellan-Jones technique) or an omental patch repair (Graham technique) [21–23]. On the other hand, giant duodenal ulcers are uncommon, with duodenal ulcer perforation more than 3 cm in length reportedly accounting for about 1.23 % of cases [2]. Giant duodenal ulcers are difficult to manage and are associated with high rates of both morbidity (20–70 %) and mortality (15–40 %) because of the extensive duodenal tissue loss and surrounding tissue inflammation [24]. The Cellan-Jones and Graham techniques often fail to achieve closure of the perforation, resulting in postoperative leakage or gastric outlet obstruction.

Several reports have described surgical procedures for giant ulcers, including partial gastrectomy, jejunal serosal patch [25], free omental plug [26], and jejunal pedicle graft [27]. Lal et al. reported the efficacy of triple-tube-ostomy (tube gastrostomy, retrograde tube duodenostomy, and feeding jejunostomy) with repair of the perforation for large duodenal ulcer perforations [28]. Cranford et al. advocated gastric disconnection with truncal vagotomy,

antrectomy, and triple-tube-ostomy [29]. This surgical approach is considered the most appropriate procedure for giant duodenal ulcer perforation in cases with poor general conditions owing to late diagnosis. Because one of the present cases showed bleeding and leakage from the repaired duodenal ulcer, antrectomy including the ulcerative portion was thought to be necessary for giant duodenal ulcer. In cases with poor general conditions owing to late diagnosis, digestive tract reconstruction is hazardous, and gastric disconnection might be needed. This approach necessitates a second elective operation for digestive reconstruction, but is thought to represent the safest procedure given the high mortality rate of this condition. Moreover, cholecystectomy with insertion of a bile drainage tube from the cystic duct might

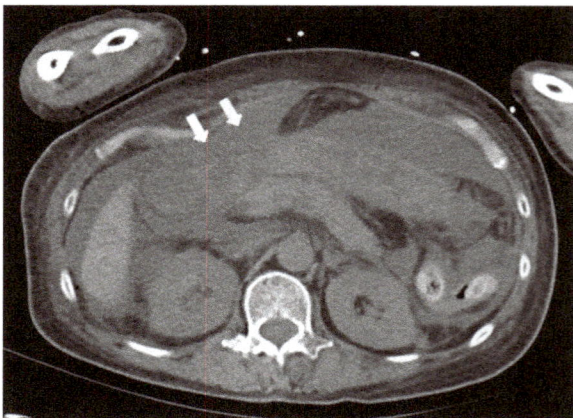

Fig. 5 Abdominal CT. The CT scan reveals massive fluid accumulation and an irregular duodenal wall

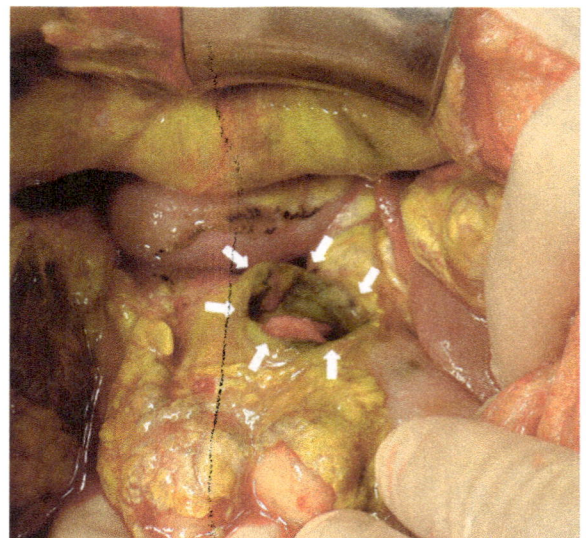

Fig. 6 The intra-operative finding. An 4-cm perforation was noted at the anterior wall of the duodenval bulb

also be necessary in preparation for duodenal stump leakage.

Conclusion

We have reported two cases of giant duodenal ulcer perforation after neurosurgery that needed reoperations because of postoperative leakage and bleeding. For giant duodenal ulcer with poor general condition owing to late diagnosis, simple closure including omental patching or antrectomy with reconstruction is hazardous. Antrectomy with gastric disconnection, which means gastrostomy, duodenostomy, feeding jejunostomy and cholecystectomy, is recommended.

Abbreviations
CRP: C-reactive protein; CT: Computed tomography

Acknowledgements
None.

Funding
No funding was obtained for this study.

Authors' contributions
CN, KK, and GO were involved in data collection, case analysis and writing the manuscript. RA, SY, HT, MO, and KH assisted in drafting the manuscript and reviewed the article. TT and KN performed the first surgeries. All authors read and approved the final manuscript.

Competing interests
The authors declare that they have no competing interests.

Author details
[1]Department of Surgical Oncology, Osaka City University Graduate School of Medicine, 1-4-3 Asahi-machi, Abeno-ku, Osaka, Japan. [2]Department of Neurosurgery, Osaka City University Graduate School of Medicine, 1-4-3 Asahi-machi, Abeno-ku, Osaka, Japan.

References
1. Cushing H. Peptic ulcers and the inter-brain. Surg Gynecol Obste. 1932;55:1–34.
2. Gupta S, Kaushik R, Sharma R, Attri A. The management of large perforations of duodenal ulcers. BMC Surg. 2005;5:15.
3. Rokitansky c. Handbuch der pathologischen Anatomie, vol. 2. Wien: Braumüller & Seidel; 1846.
4. Brooks FP. Stress ulcer: etiology, diagnosis and treatment. Med Clin North Am. 1966;50(5):1447–55.
5. Leonard AS, Long D, French LA, Peter ET, Wangensteen OH. Pendular pattern in gastric secretion and blood flow following hypothalamic stimulation – origin of stress ulcer? Surgery. 1964;56:109–20.
6. Porter RW, Movius HJ, French JD. Hypothalamic influences on hydrochloric acid secretion of the stomach. Surgery. 1953;33(6):875–80.
7. French JD, Porter RW, Von Amerongen FK, Raney RB. Gastrointestinal hemorrhage and ulceration associated with intracranial lesions; a clinical and experimental study. Surgery. 1952;32(2):395–407.
8. Boles RS. Neurogenic factors in production of acute gasatric ulcer. JAMA. 1940;115(21):1771–3.
9. Hernandez DE. The role of brain peptides in the pathogenesis of experimental stress gastric ulcers. Ann N Y Acad Sci. 1990;597:28–35.
10. Spencer JA, Morlock CG, Sayre GP. Lesions in upper portion of the gastrointestinal tract associated with intracranial neoplasms. Gastroenterology. 1959;37(1):20–7.
11. Boey J, Choi SK, Poon A, Alagaratnam TT. Risk stratification in perforated duodenal ulcers. A prospective validation of predictive factors. Ann Surg. 1987;205(1):22–6.
12. Billing A, Frohlich D, Schildberg FW. Prediction of outcome using the Mannheim peritonitis index in 2003 patients. Peritonitis Study Group Br J Surg. 1994;81(2):209–13.
13. Qureshi AM, Zafar A, Saeed K, Quddus A. Predictive power of Mannheim Peritonitis Index. J Coll Physicians Surg Pak. 2005;15(11):693–6.
14. Demmel N, Maag K, Osterholzer G. The value of clinical parameters for determining the prognosis of peritonitis–validation of the Mannheim Peritonitis Index. Langenbecks Arch Chir. 1994;379(3):152–8.
15. Ahuja A, Pal R. Prognostic scoring indicator in evaluation of clinical outcome in intestinal perforations. J Clin Diagn Res. 2013;7(9):1953–5.
16. Mishra A, Sharma D, Raina VK. A simplified prognostic scoring system for peptic ulcer perforation in developing countries. Indian J Gastroenterol. 2003;22(2):49–53.
17. Surapaneni S, Rajkumar S, Reddy AV. The Perforation-Operation time Interval; An Important Mortality Indicator in Peptic Ulcer Perforation. J Clin Diagn Res. 2013;7(5):880–2.
18. Kocer B, Surmeli S, Solak C, Unal B, Bozkurt B, Yildirim O, Dolapci M, Cengiz O. Factors affecting mortality and morbidity in patients with peptic ulcer perforation. J Gastroenterol Hepatol. 2007;22(4):565–70.
19. Tas I, Ulger BV, Onder A, Kapan M, Bozdag Z. Risk factors influencing morbidity and mortality in perforated peptic ulcer disease. Ulus Cerrahi Derg. 2015;31(1):20–5.
20. Boey J, Wong J, Ong GB. Bacteria and septic complications in patients with perforated duodenal ulcers. Am J Surg. 1982;143(5):635–9.
21. Bertleff MJ, Lange JF. Perforated peptic ulcer disease: a review of history and treatment. Dig Surg. 2010;27(3):161–9.
22. Cellan-Jones CJ. A rapid method of treatment in perforated duodenal ulcer. Br Med J. 1929;1(3571):1076–7.
23. Graham RR. The treatment of perforated duodenal ulcers. Surg Gynec Obstet. 1937;64:235–8.
24. Cienfuegos JA, Rotellar F, Valenti V, Arredondo J, Baixauli J, Pedano N, Bellver M, Hernandez-Lizoain JL. Giant duodenal ulcer perforation: a case of innovative repair with an antrum gastric patch. Rev Esp Enferm Dig. 2012; 104(8):436–9.
25. Chaudhary A, Bose SM, Gupta NM, Wig JD, Khanna SK. Giant perforations of duodenal ulcer. Indian J Gastroenterol. 1991;10(1):14–5.
26. Sharma D, Saxena A, Rahman H, Raina VK, Kapoor JP. 'Free omental plug': a nostalgic look at an old and dependable technique for giant peptic perforations. Dig Surg. 2000;17(3):216–8.
27. McIlrath DC, Larson RH. Surgical management of large perforations of the duodenum. Surg Clin North Am. 1971;51(4):857–61.
28. Lal P, Vindal A, Hadke NS. Controlled tube duodenostomy in the management of giant duodenal ulcer perforation: a new technique for a surgically challenging condition. Am J Surg. 2009;198(3):319–23.
29. Cranford Jr CA, Olson R, Bradley 3rd EL. Gastric disconnection in the management of perforated giant duodenal ulcer. Am J Surg. 1988; 155(3):439–42.

26

Laparoscopic-assisted total gastrectomy for early gastric cancer with situs inversus totalis: report of a first case

Mamoru Morimoto[1], Tetsushi Hayakawa[1], Hidehiko Kitagami[1], Moritsugu Tanaka[1], Yoichi Matsuo[2*] and Hiromitsu Takeyama[2]

Abstract

Background: Situs inversus totalis is a relatively rare condition and is an autosomal recessive congenital defect in which an abdominal and/or thoracic organ is positioned as a "mirror image" of the normal position in the sagittal plane. We report our experience of laparoscopic-assisted total gastrectomy with lymph node dissection performed for gastric cancer in a patient with situs inversus totalis.

Case presentation: A 58-year-old male was diagnosed with cT1bN0N0 gastric cancer. There were no vascular anomalies on abdominal angiographic computed tomography with three-dimensional reconstruction. laparoscopic-assisted total gastrectomy was performed with D1+ lymph node dissection, in accordance with the Japanese Gastric Cancer Treatment Guidelines. There were no intraoperative issues, and no postoperative complications.

Conclusions: This was the first report describing laparoscopic-assisted total gastrectomy with the standard typical lymph node dissection in the English literature. We emphasize that the position of trocars and the standing side of the primary surgeon during the lymph node dissection are critical.

Keywords: Situs inversus totalis, Gastric cancer, Laparoscopic-assisted total gastrectomy

Background

Situs inversus totalis (SIT) is a relatively rare condition found in only approximately 1 per 5,000 to 20,000 people [1]. SIT is an autosomal recessive congenital defect in which an abdominal and/or thoracic organ is positioned as a "mirror image" of the normal position in the sagittal plane. Laparoscopic surgery for such patients has been reported upon, with most reports describing laparoscopic cholecystectomy [1]. Reports of advanced laparoscopic surgery in such patients are also increasing in accord with the overall progress of laparoscopic procedures. In 2003, the first case of laparoscopic surgery for a SIT patient with gastric cancer was reported [2]. Only a few cases of laparoscopic assisted distal gastrectomy (LADG) for gastric cancer have been reported [2–8]. However, there are no reports of

laparoscopic assisted total gastrectomy (LATG) for gastric cancer in patients with SIT in the English literature. We herein report a case of LATG with lymph node dissection and esophagojejunostomy using the overlap method in a patient with early gastric cancer and SIT.

Case presentation

A 58-year-old male with SIT was diagnosed with early gastric cancer by an esophagogastroduodenoscopy (EGD) performed at an outside hospital, and was subsequently referred to our hospital for further evaluation and surgical treatment. He was diagnosed with SIT 5 years previously. He had been healthy until this diagnosis with no other underlying disease or any family history of SIT or gastric cancer. History and physical examination revealed right orchidoptosis. Laboratory examination, including tumor markers, showed no abnormal findings. Electrocardiogram (ECG) examination

* Correspondence: matsuo@med.nagoya-cu.ac.jp
[2]Department of Gastroenterological Surgery, Nagoya City University Graduate School of Medical Sciences, Kawasumi 1, Mizuho-cho, Mizuhoku, Nagoya 467-8601, Japan
Full list of author information is available at the end of the article

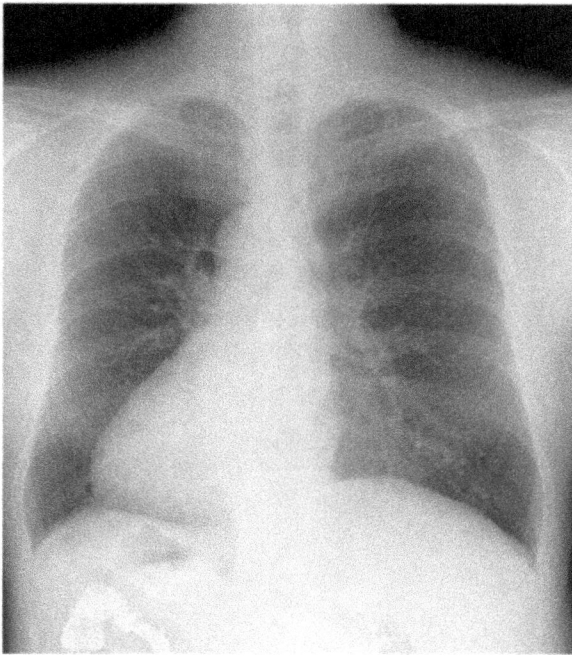

Fig. 1 Dextrocardia was evident on chest radiography from the frontal view

revealed right bundle branch block. Chest x-ray suggested dextrocardia (Fig. 1). Upper gastrointestinal imaging (UGI) and repeat EGD identified a superficial lesion with slight depression (0-IIc) measuring 20 × 25 mm in size on the posterior side of the lesser curvature of the upper gastric body (Fig. 2a, b). The lesion was 3 cm distal to the esophagogastric junction (EGJ). Biopsy revealed poorly differentiated adenocarcinoma. Abdominal computed tomography (CT) showed that all intraabdominal organs were inversely positioned (Fig. 3a). Prior to surgery, abdominal angiographic CT with 3D reconstruction was performed to reveal any other anatomic variations and to verify the locations of the major vasculature. There were no arterial variations (Fig. 3b). Chest and abdominal CT did not reveal any metastases, including none to the liver or lung. Based on findings of the biopsy, UGI, EGD and CT, a 0-IIc lesion of the upper gastric body, clinical stage cT1b, cN0cH0cP0cM0, stage IB according to the Japanese Classification of Gastric Carcinoma was diagnosed [9]. We decided to perform LATG with standard lymph node dissection (D1 + No. 7, 8a, 9) in accordance with the Japanese Gastric Cancer Treatment Guidelines [10].

After general anesthesia was induced, the patient was placed in a supine position. The position of trocars is showed in Fig. 4. First, a 12-mm trocar was placed in the umbilical site, and carbon dioxide was injected into the peritoneal cavity at 10 mmHg. A laparoscope was inserted into the abdomen through the 12-mm trocar. An additional 4 ports were placed in the left and right subcostal positions and lateral abdominal regions. The surgeon was positioned on the right side of the patient for dissection of lymph node basins 5, 6, 7, 8a, and 9 and was positioned on the left side for the dissection of lymph node basins 1, 2, 3, 4sa, 4sb, 4d, and 11p. At the beginning of the operation, the surgeon was positioned on the left side of the patient and the greater omentum was dissected. The location of the spleen was confirmed, and the 4sa node basin (along the short gastric vessels) and 4sb node basin (along the left gastroepiploic vessels) were dissected. The left gastroepiploic vessels were clipped and divided. Next, the surgeon was positioned

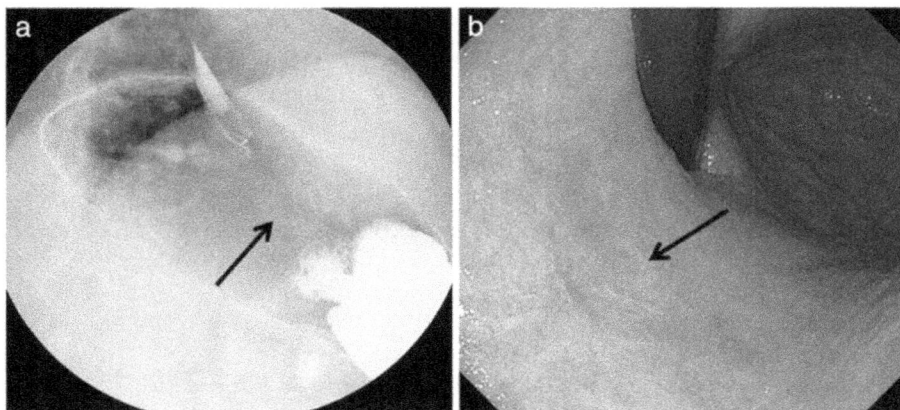

Fig. 2 a, b Upper gastrointestinal endoscopy and gastrointestinal imaging study showed a superficial lesion with a slight depression of the upper gastric body

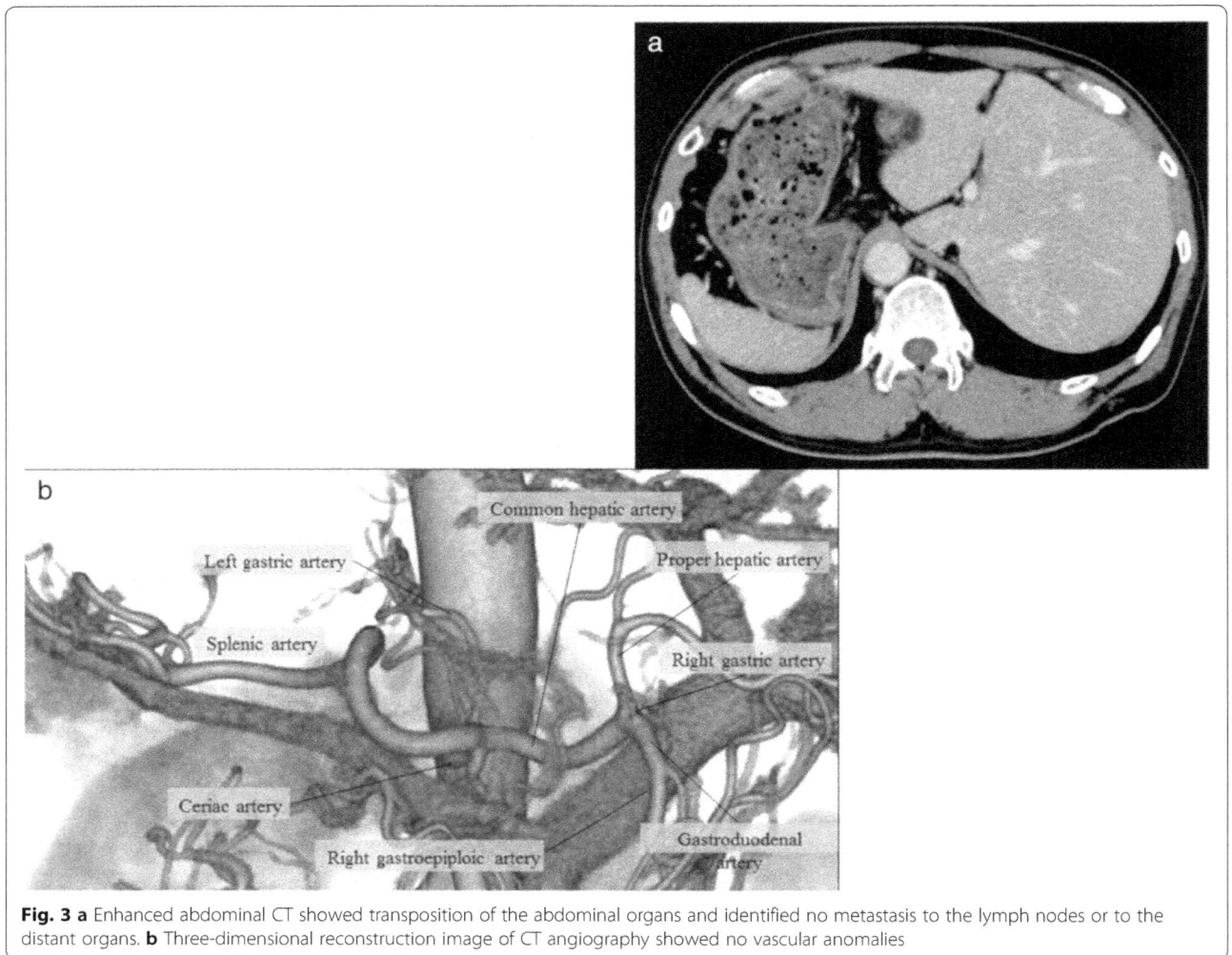

Fig. 3 a Enhanced abdominal CT showed transposition of the abdominal organs and identified no metastasis to the lymph nodes or to the distant organs. **b** Three-dimensional reconstruction image of CT angiography showed no vascular anomalies

on the right side of the patient, and the node basin 6 (infrapyloric lymph nodes) was dissected (Fig. 5a) and the duodenum was transected with a linear stapling device intraperitoneally. Next, the node basins 5 (suprapyloric lymph nodes), 8a [lymph node along the common hepatic artery (CHA)], 9 [lymph node around the celiac artery (CA)], and 7 [lymph node along the left gastric artery (LGA)] were dissected safely (Fig. 5b). Next, the surgeon was positioned on the left side of the patient again, and the node basins 11p [along the proximal splenic artery (SA)], 1 (right pericardial lymph node), 2 (left pericardial lymph node), and 3 (along the lesser curvature) were dissected completely in accord with Gastric Cancer Treatment Guidelines [10] (Fig. 5c). We exposed the abdominal esophagus and transected it at an appropriate resection line using an endoscopic linear stapler. The resected stomach and surrounding fatty tissue including harvested lymph nodes were placed in a plastic specimen bag. The specimen in the bag was retrieved through an extended umbilical port incision. At last, we performed an esophagojejunostomy using the overlap method intraperitoneally (Fig. 5d). Operating time was 359 min, and blood loss was 90 mL. The final pathology showed a poorly differentiated 0-IIc lesion with invasion limited to the mucosa. There was no metastasis in any of the retrieved lymph nodes. The final stage was pT1aN0M0, Stage 1A according to the Japanese Classification of Gastric Carcinoma [9]. There were no immediate postoperative complications, and the patient was discharged 7 days after the operation. The patient is still alive without recurrence or symptoms 4 years after surgery.

Discussion

In this case, we made two important clinical observations. First, 3D reconstruction of an abdominal CT angiography image should be done to examine a blood stream in detail in SIT patients preoperatively. Second,

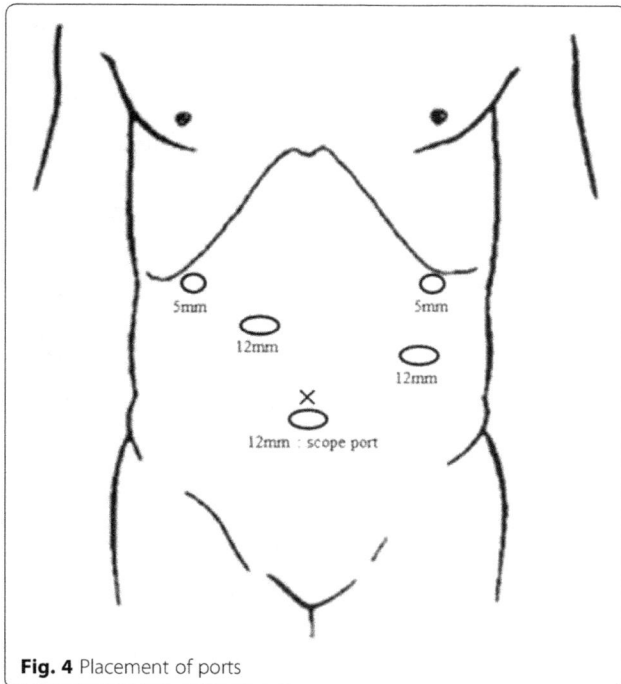

Fig. 4 Placement of ports

the position of trocars and the standing side of the primary surgeon during the dissection of basins 5, 7, 8a, and 9 are critical.

SIT is a rare congenital anomaly. SIT can be accompanied by cardiopulmonary malformations, familial long QT syndrome, total esophageal duplication, agnathia, and a variety of urologic anomalies. Typically, the frequency of cardiovascular anomalies is 10 times greater than in a patient with normal anatomy [6]. In other report, SIT is associated with cardiovascular malformations in 8 % of cases [11]. Therefore, preoperative identification of any abnormal vasculature is important, because abnormal vasculature carries with it the risk of misidentifying anatomy and causing unanticipated injury of important vessels. In our case, major vascular abnormalities were not found. However, it is required to examine a blood stream in 3D reconstruction of an abdominal CT angiography image preoperatively.

Second, the position of trocars and the standing side of the primary surgeon during the dissection of basins 5, 7, 8a, and 9 are critical. Laparoscopic surgery has been performed for SIT patients in numerous case reports, including laparoscopic cholecystectomy [12], laparoscopic colectomy [13], laparoscopic fundoplication [14], and laparoscopic gastric band surgery [15]. In 2003, LADG for gastric cancer in a patient with SIT was successfully performed in Japan, and was the first reported case of its kind [2]. Furthermore, in 2010, LADG with D1 + β lymph-node dissection for early gastric cancer

was successfully performed in Japan [3]. It was the first case of laparoscopic gastrectomy with extended lymph node dissection. The reported cases of laparoscopic gastrectomy for gastric cancer with SIT are listed in Table 1 [2–8]. LATG is not performed as frequently as LADG even in patients without SIT due to the technical difficulty of the laparoscopic approach, particularly the esophagojejunostomy and complete lymph node dissection. The present patient was the first report describing LATG with the standard typical lymph node dissection (D1+) [10] in the English literature. It is a very important element where the surgeon inserts the trocar, and which direction the surgeon operates on from. However, there is no consensus about it until now, because LATG has never been reported for the patients with SIT. Thus, based on our experience, we describe the position of trocars and the standing side of the primary surgeon when the surgeon performs LATG for the patients with SIT.

The surgeon should perform the dissection of basins 5, 7, 8a, 9 from right side of patient same as normal operation. We did not perform the dissection of basins 5, 7, 8a, and 9 from the left side of patient as the surgeon's right hand (dominant hand) using the ultrasonic cut and coagulation instrument can contact the proper hepatic artery (PHA).

This risk is not completely avoided with the surgeon on the right side, however. The ultrasonic cut and coagulation instrument may hit the PHA perpendicularly, and damage the vessels during dissection of basin 5. However, lymph node dissection from the right side of the patient is safer than that from the left side of the patient if we pay attention to the cavitation of the ultrasonic cut and coagulation instrument so as not to damage the vessels.

Furthermore, in normal operation, if the surgeon is right-handed, he inserts the lower right trocar more vertically up and towards the center. That is because he can dissect node basins 7, 8a and 9 precisely and more deeply, and he can reach the spleen using right hand for dissecting lymph node around the splenic artery. In SIT, there is no need to insert the lower right trocar toward the center because there is no spleen in the left side of abdomen. However, the trocar should be inserted in the higher position, because it is difficult to perform the lymph node dissection around the CHA as the pancreas interferes with movement of the right hand. We describe the procedure after the surgeon moves to the left side of the patient. The surgeon should insert the upper left trocar (which is used with the right hand) more toward the center. As a result, the surgeon's hand can reach the spleen and he can avoid the injury of PHA during the dissection of node basins 11p. The diagram of the optimum positions of the trocars in LATG with SIT is shown in Fig. 6.

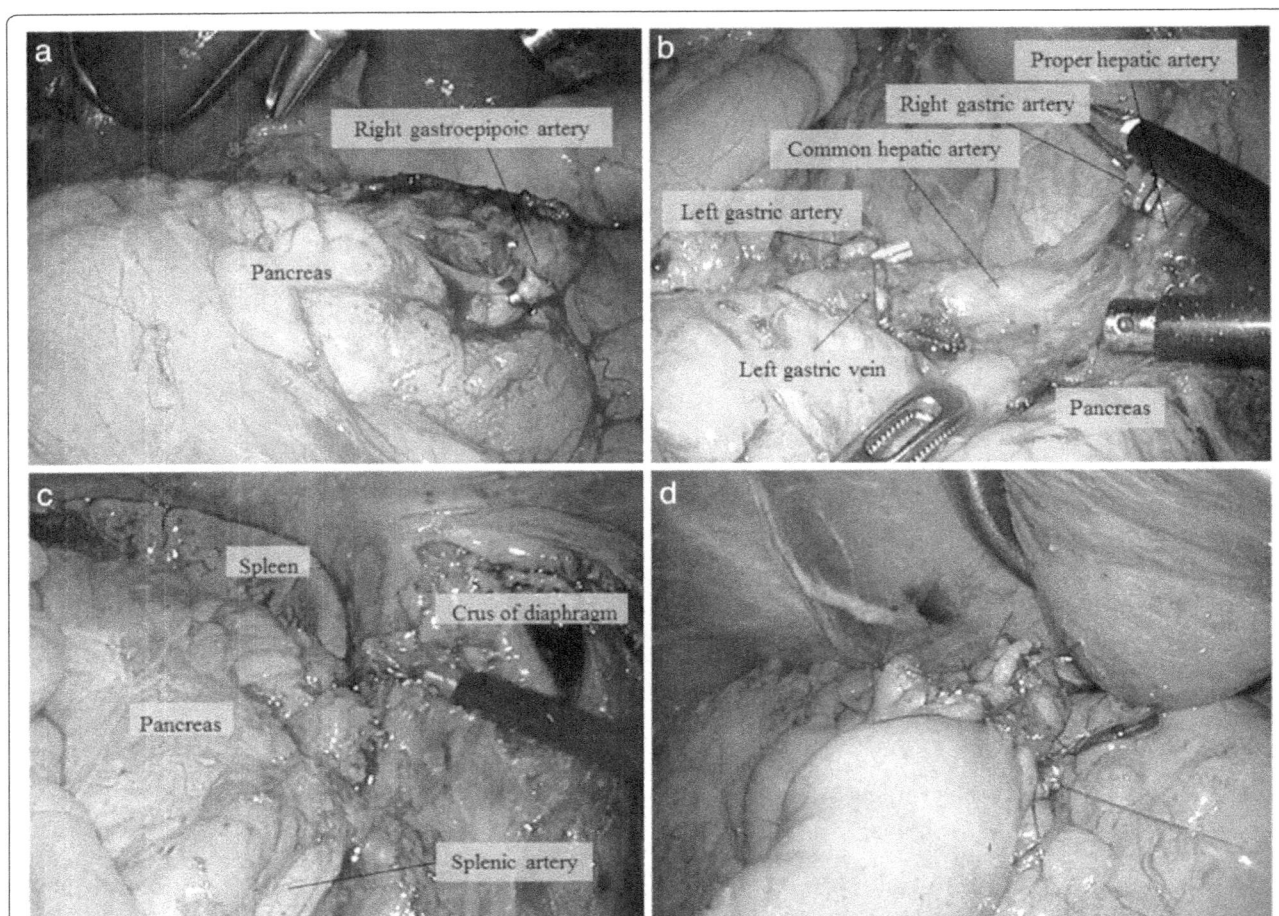

Fig. 5 a Dissection of lymph nodes in lymph node basin 6 (infrapyloric lymph nodes). **b** Dissection of lymph nodes in lymph node basins 8a, 9, and 7 (along the common hepatic artery, the celiac artery, and the left gastric artery). **c** Dissection of lymph node basin 11p (along the splenic artery). **d** Reconstruction via esophagojejunostomy using the overlap method

There are 4 cases in the literature describing the operation done with the surgeon standing in the standard position [4, 5, 7]. One of these authors reported that the mirror image led to confusion during the operation [4]. Furthermore, another of these authors reported that even slight confusion of the anatomy can jeopardize the patient's life, and that only a surgeon experienced with laparoscopic gastrectomy should perform the operation [7]. There is a report of the use of surgical instruments in the non-dominant hand from the opposite side of patient when operating on patients with SIT [6]. We advise against this technique to prevent the damage of major vessels and to ensure adequate node dissection. However, robot-assisted distal gastrectomy (RADG) is an exception to this as the surgeon does not need to change his positon during surgery because of the centered robotic view of the field with easy changing of the instruments between hands [5].

Our procedure of LATG with D1+ dissection and esophagojejunostomy using the overlap method was completed in 359 min with 90 mL blood loss. In other reports of LADG, the median operating time and blood loss were 267 min and 90 mL, respectively. It is logical that total gastrectomy has a longer operative time given the more extensive dissection necessary compared to distal gastrectomy. Also, the esophagojejunostomy using overlap method was carried out from the left side of the patient, we could perform it safely. As in our procedure, lymph node dissection and esophagojejunostomy can be performed safely and efficiently by coordinating the position of trocars, and alternating the standing side of the primary surgeon over the course of the case.

Conclusions

In conclusion, there has been marked improvement of the surgical technique and instruments used in

Table 1 Previous reports of laparoscopic surgery for gastric cancer with SIT

No.	Author	Age	Sex	Anomalies of blood vessels	Operation	Lymoh node dissection*	Position of surgeon	Operating time (min)	Blood loss (ml)	Stage**	Post operation
1	Yamaguchi (2003)	76	M	ND	LADG	ND	ND	ND	ND	ND	ND
2	Futawatari (2010)	53	M	no anomalies	LADG	D1 + β	left side (opposite the usual side)	300	350	IA	no complications
3	Seo (2011)	60	M	no anomalies	LADG	D1 + β	right side (same the usual side)	200	70	IB	no complications
4	Kim (2012)	47	M	no anomalies	RADG	D1 + β	same the usual side	300	ND	IIIB	no complications
5	Fujikawa (2013)	60	F	no anomalies	LADG	ND	opposite the usual side	234	5	IB	mechanical obstruction (re-operation)
6	Min (2013)	52	M	the CHA from SMA 2 branches from the LGA	LADG	D1+	same the usual side	220	100	IB	no complications
7		68	M	no anomalies	LADG	D1+	same the usual side	117	50	IA	no complications
8	Sumi (2014)	42	M	the LHA from the SMA	LADG	D1 + No.7, 8a, 9	opposite the usual side	313	90	IB	no complications
9	Our case	58	M	no anomalies	LATG	D1+	opposite the usual side (except for no.5, 7,8a, 9)	359	90	IA	no complications
										IA	no complications

*According to Japanese gastric cancer treatment guidelines 2010 (ver. 3)
**According to Japanese classification of gastric carcinoma: 3rd English edition

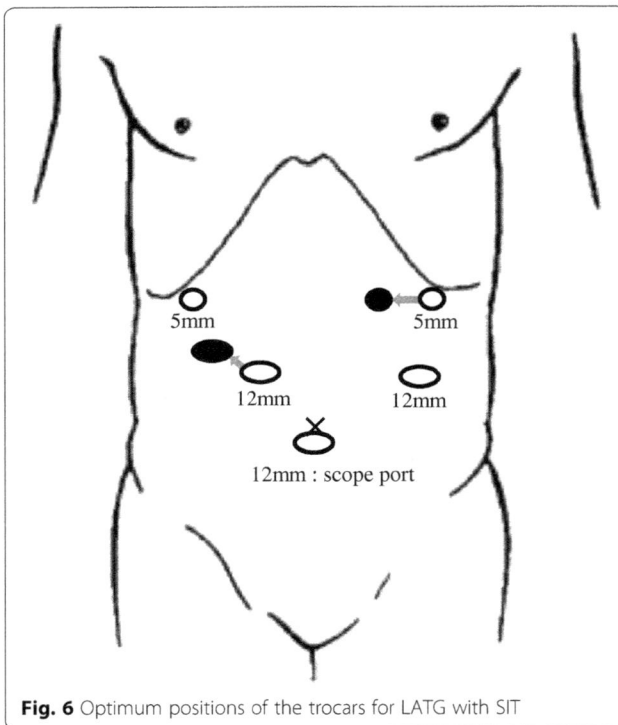

Fig. 6 Optimum positions of the trocars for LATG with SIT

laparoscopic surgery recently. Since the LATG was performed at our hospital more than 200 times, the operating team has become very comfortable with performing it. While performing LATG with SIT, we have encountered some problems present. Thus, we have described the important technical aspects of LATG with lymph node dissection for patients with gastric cancer and SIT, namely recognition of the anatomy, with particular attention to the vasculature as determined by preoperative 3D reconstruction of an abdominal CT angiography image. Furthermore, it was important to simulate the position of the trocar insertion, and the change of the position of the primary surgeon preoperatively.

Abbreviations

SIT: Situs inversus totalis; LATG: Laparoscopic-assisted total gastrectomy; 3D: Three-dimensional; LADG: Laparoscopic-assisted distal gastrectomy; EGD: Esophagogastroduodenoscopy; ECG: Electrocardiogram; UGI: Upper gastrointestinal imaging; EGJ: Esophagogastric junction; CT: Computed tomography; CHA: Common hepatic artery; CA: Celiac artery; LGA: Left gastric artery; SA: Splenic artery; PHA: Proper hepatic artery; RADG: Robot-assisted distal gastrectomy; SMA: Superior mesenteric artery; LHA: Left hepatic artery; DG: Distal gastrectomy; TG: Total gastrectomy; PG: Proximal gastrectomy; ND: Not described.

Competing interest

The authors declare that they have no competing interests.

Authors' contributions

All six authors were involved in planning, data collection, analysis of case and writing the manuscript. MM, TH, and HK performed surgical procedures. MM and MT managed the patients. MM collected data and wrote the paper. YM and HT reviewed it. All authors approved the final manuscript.

Acknowledgement

The authors acknowledge all the ward staff who took care of the patient.

Author details

[1]Department of Surgery, Kariya Toyota General Hospital, Kariya, Japan.
[2]Department of Gastroenterological Surgery, Nagoya City University Graduate School of Medical Sciences, Kawasumi 1, Mizuho-cho, Mizuhoku, Nagoya 467-8601, Japan.

References

1. Nursal TZ et al. Laparoscopic cholecystectomy in a patient with situs inversus totalis. J Laparoendosc Adv Surg Tech A. 2001;11(4):239–41.
2. Yamaguchi S et al. Laparoscope-assisted distal gastrectomy for early gastric cancer in a 76-year-old man with situs inversus totalis. Surg Endosc. 2003;17(2):352–3.
3. Futawatari N et al. Laparoscopy-assisted distal gastrectomy for early gastric cancer with complete situs inversus: report of a case. Surg Today. 2010;40(1):64–7.
4. Seo KW, Yoon KY. Laparoscopy-assisted distal gastrectomy for early gastric cancer and laparoscopic cholecystectomy for gallstone with situs inversus totalis: a case report. J Korean Surg Soc. 2011;81 Suppl 1:S34–8.
5. Kim HB et al. Robot-assisted distal gastrectomy for gastric cancer in a situs inversus totalis patient. J Korean Surg Soc. 2012;82(5):321–4.
6. Fujikawa H et al. Laparoscopy-assisted distal gastrectomy for an early gastric cancer patient with situs inversus totalis. Int Surg. 2013;98(3):266–70.
7. Min SH et al. Laparoscopic distal gastrectomy in a patient with situs inversus totalis: a case report. J Gastric Cancer. 2013;13(4):266–72.
8. Sumi Y et al. Laparoscopy-assisted distal gastrectomy in a patient with situs inversus totalis. JSLS. 2014;18(2):314–8.
9. Japanese Gastric Cancer Association. Japanese classification of gastric carcinoma: 3rd English edition. Gastric Cancer. 2011;14(2):101–12.
10. Japanese Gastric Cancer Association. Japanese gastric cancer treatment guidelines 2010 (ver. 3). Gastric Cancer. 2011;14(2):113–23.
11. Fonkalsrud EW, Tompkins R, Clatworthy Jr HW. Abdominal manifestations of situs inversus in infants and children. Arch Surg. 1966;92(5):791–5.
12. Machado NO, Chopra P. Laparoscopic cholecystectomy in a patient with situs inversus totalis: feasibility and technical difficulties. JSLS. 2006;10(3):386–91.
13. Fujiwara Y et al. Laparoscopic hemicolectomy in a patient with situs inversus totalis. World J Gastroenterol. 2007;13(37):5035–7.
14. Koo KP. Laparoscopic Nissen fundoplication in a patient with situs inversus totalis: an ergonomic consideration. J Laparoendosc Adv Surg Tech A. 2006;16(3):271–3.
15. Samaan M et al. Laparoscopic adjustable gastric banding for morbid obesity in a patient with situs inversus totalis. Obes Surg. 2008;18(7):898–901.

27

Severe abdominopelvic actinomycosis with colon perforation and hepatic involvement mimicking advanced sigmoid colon cancer with hepatic metastasis: a case study

Song Soo Yang and Yeong Cheol Im[*]

Abstract

Background: Actinomycosis is a rare chronic invasive disease caused by *Actinomyces* spp. Although abdominopelvic actinomycosis, which involves the colon and the pelvic organs extensively, has been frequently reported, abdominopelvic actinomycosis presenting with colon perforation and hepatic involvement concurrently has yet to be reported.

Case presentation: A 55-year-old woman presented at the emergency room with squeezing epigastric pain. Palpation of the abdomen revealed a hard mass with no acute peritoneal signs. Vital signs were normal range except for tachycardia. Initial laboratory testing revealed leukocytosis, anemia, elevated C-reactive protein (CRP), hypoalbuminemia; and normal AST/ALT and BUN/creatinine. CT scan of the abdomen-pelvis revealed a microperforations of the sigmoid colon, abscess in the left lower quadrant and hepatic lesion. Furthermore, there was a large infiltrating conglomerated mass invading the urinary bladder, left adnexa, sigmoid, left inguinal canal and left pelvic wall area. Ultrasound revealed an intra-uterine device (IUD). All these findings initially raised a suspicion of malignancy such as advanced cancer of the colon with liver metastasis. Despite the rarity of the disease, actinomycosis were not excluded because of the IUD found on ultrasound. Parenteral antibiotics and percutaneous drainage of abdomen abscess as well as fasting with total parental nutrition were prescribed for sigmoid perforation and abscess. After 10 days of conservative treatment, no remarkable change was detected in conglomerated mass invading pelvis. Furthermore, the finding of newly developed mechanical small bowel obstruction warranted surgery. Exploratory laparotomy was performed for the removal of perforated colon, obstructive small bowel and organs involved and postoperative histology confirmed a diagnosis of colonic actinomycosis. The patient made an uneventful recovery and was started on a 6-month course of penicillin.

Conclusions: Abdominopelvic actinomycosis presenting with colon perforation and hepatic involvement is extremely rare; however, it is clinically similar to advanced colon cancer with liver metastasis, therefore, complicating the preoperative diagnosis. A diagnosis of abdominopelvic actinomycosis should be considered in patients with a history of IUD and chronic abdominal pain, along with an abdominal mass or cutaneous abscess. If surgery is indicated, preoperative empirical antibiotic therapy for actinomycosis and frozen biopsy during surgery may be considered.

Keywords: Abdominopelvic actinomycosis, Colon perforation, Liver involvement

* Correspondence: driyc@hotmail.com
Department of Surgery, Ulsan University Hospital, University of Ulsan College of Medicine, 877, Bangeojinsunhwando-ro, Dong-gu, Ulsan 44033, Republic of Korea

Background

Actinomycosis is a rare chronic invasive disease and *Actinomyces israelii* is the most prevalent species, anaerobic gram-positive bacteria that normally colonize oral, digestive and urogenital tracts in humans [1]. Breach of tissue integrity in mucosal lesions facilitates invasion of local structures and organs, leading to pathogenic co-infection with other organisms. All the tissues and organs may be infected, but four main clinical types of infection can be distinguished, depending on the primary site of infection: cervicofacial, thoracic, abdominopelvic, and disseminated disease [2]. Abdominopelvic actinomycosis is a rare disease encompassing abdominal infection, intrauterine devices (IUD)-related pelvic abscesses, infections of appendix, rectum and liver [3]. When it is associated with gastrointestinal organs, it is similar to chronic inflammatory bowel disease or malignancy, especially colon cancer [4]. Although abdominopelvic actinomycosis, which involves the colon and the surrounding pelvic organs extensively, has been frequently reported, abdominopelvic actinomycosis presenting with colon perforation and hepatic involvement concurrently has yet to be reported.

Here, we report a severe case of abdominopelvic actinomycosis with sigmoid colon perforation and hepatic lesion mimicking advanced colon cancer with liver metastasis.

Case presentation

A 55-year-old woman with no specific medico-surgical history presented at the emergency room with a 1-day history of squeezing epigastric abdominal pain. Patient also complained of a thick turbid yellowish discharge in the left inguinal area that was intermittently drained for some years.

Vital signs were normal range except for tachycardia (pulse rate, 110/min). Palpation of the abdomen revealed a wood-like hard mass in the left lower quadrant with minimal tenderness and no acute peritoneal signs warranting emergent surgery. A visible scar was noted in the left inguinal area without any discharge.

Initial laboratory testing revealed marked leukocytosis (white blood cells, 24,730 cells/mm^3), anemia (hemoglobin concentration of 6.9 g/dL), elevated C-reactive protein (CRP) 32.05 mg/dL (reference range, 0–0.5 mg/dL), hypoalbuminemia (albumin, 2.5 g/dL); and normal AST/ALT and BUN/creatinine. CT scan of the abdomen-pelvis revealed a microperforation of the sigmoid colon, abscess in the left lower quadrant, a hepatic lesion and bilateral hydronephrosis. Furthermore, there was a large infiltrating heterogenous hyperattenuating conglomerated mass invading the urinary bladder, left adnexa, sigmoid, left inguinal canal and left pelvic wall area (Fig. 1). Ultrasound revealed an intra-uterine device (IUD) (Fig. 2). All these findings initially raised a suspicion of malignancy such as advanced cancer of the colon or ovary with liver metastasis. Despite the rarity of the disease, infectious diseases such as actinomycosis were not excluded because of the IUD found on ultrasound. Colonoscopy or percutaneous needle biopsy was not performed for accurate diagnosis due to suspected colon perforation and the small bowel enclosed mass.

Since the patient showed minimal peritoneal irritation and stable vital signs, and extensive organ resection was expected due to invasion of bladder and ureters, treatment was initially conservative rather than primary debulking surgery. The antibiotic regimen was always

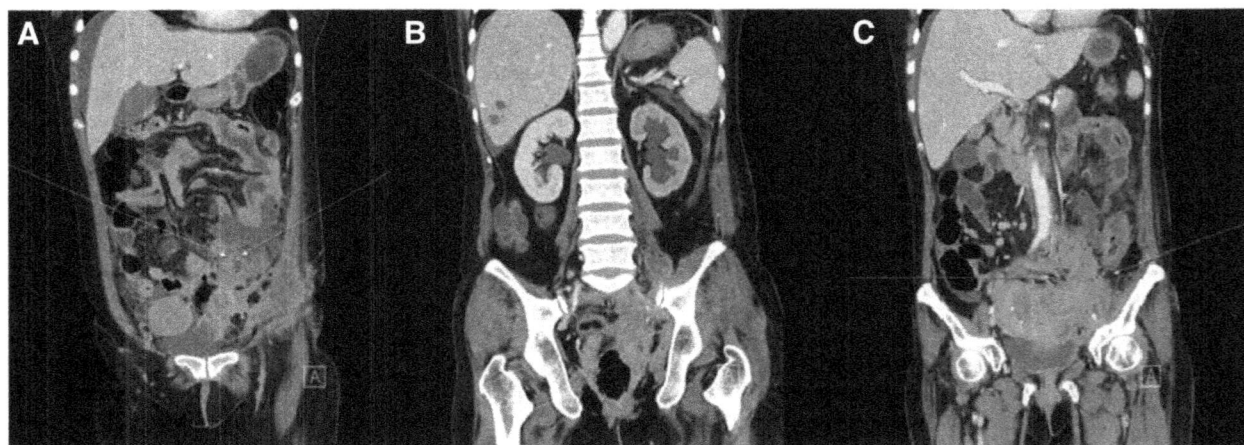

Fig. 1 CT finding at the emergency room. **a** CT scan of the abdomen-pelvis revealed a microperforation (*arrow*) of the sigmoid colon and abscess in the left lower quadrant. **b** CT scan showed a hepatic lesion (*arrow*) and bilateral hydronephrosis. **c** There was a large infiltrating heterogenous hyperattenuating conglomerated mass invading the urinary bladder, left adnexa, sigmoid, left inguinal canal and left pelvic wall area (*arrow*)

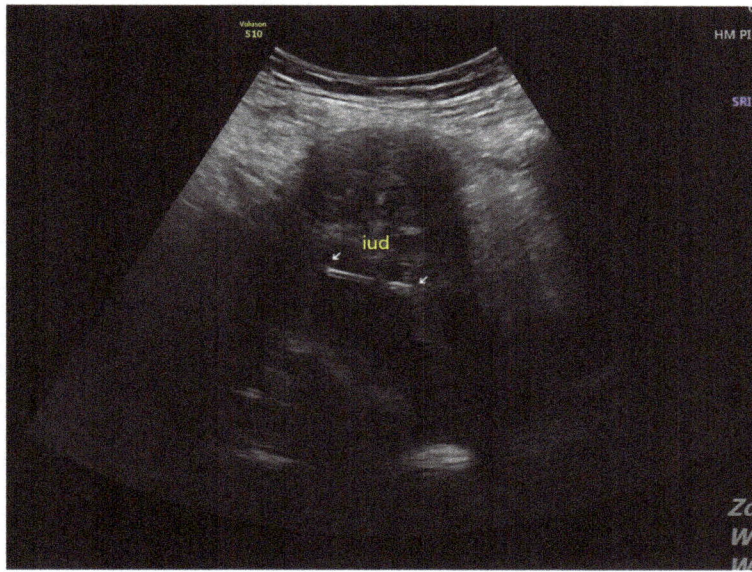

Fig. 2 Ultrasound revealed an intra-uterine device (IUD)

determined based on the infectious disease diagnosis after hospitalization. Parenteral antibiotics (ceftriaxone +metronidazole+azithromycin) and fasting with total parental nutrition were prescribed for sigmoid perforation. Because there was a huge left abdominal abscess (11X8X3cm) that could spread to other spaces and cause generalized peritonitis, the imaging-guided percutaneous abscess drainage was performed.

After 10 days of conservative treatment, a repeat CT scan of the abdomen-pelvis showed improvement in abdominal abscess and liver lesion. However, no remarkable change was detected in conglomerated mass invading pelvis. Furthermore, the finding of newly developed mechanical small bowel obstruction warranted surgery.

Exploratory laparotomy was performed for the removal of perforated colon, obstructive small bowel and organs involved. Abscess of the sigmoid colon involved the uterus, adnexa, loop of small bowel and distal colon with severe adhesion between the mass and pelvic organs including the uterus, small and large bowels, and bladder. The abscess compressed the left ureter and caused ureteral dilatation. En-bloc excision of the mass was performed using Hartmann's procedure, bilateral salpingo-oophorectomy, small bowel resection and appendectomy. The gynecologist decided not to resect uterus because of severe fibrotic adhesion in the pelvis and transvaginal IUD removal failed repeatedly due to severe adhesion.

Since the frozen section excluded malignancy, a double J catheter was inserted into both the ureters without resection. Although *Actinomyces* spp. failed to grow in preoperative cultures, postoperative permanent histology confirmed a definitive diagnosis of colonic actinomycosis, which showed the granular colonies of bacteria, commonly termed sulfur granule, with aggregates of filamentous bacteria and neutrophils (Fig. 3) and abscess with invasion into the uterus and ovaries.

After surgery, the parenteral antibiotic regimen was changed to tigecycline, amikacin, metronidazole and Penicillin G. Three days after surgery, bowel movement was restored and vital signs were stabilized, which decreased the abdominal pain. The patient made an uneventful recovery and was started on a 6-month course

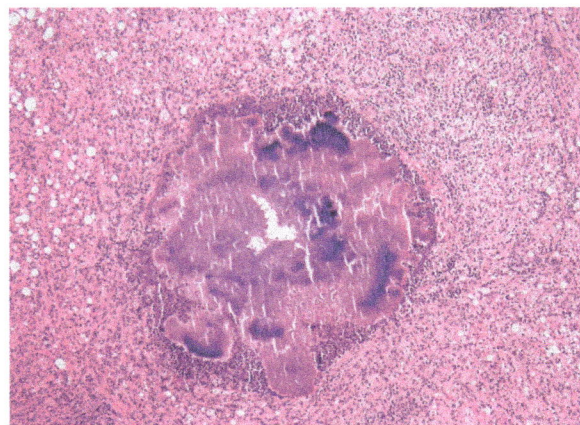

Fig. 3 This histologic section showed the granular colonies of bacteria, commonly termed sulfur granule, with aggregates of filamentous bacteria and neutrophils. H&E × 100

of penicillin. At 1-year follow-up, the patient was well and free from disease.

Discussion and conclusions

Abdominopelvic actinomycosis is one of the main clinical types according to the site of infection. It is a rare disease, but it leads to tissue granulation, dense fibrosis and abscess, resulting in a hard pelvic mass compressing the urinary bladder, ureter and rectum [5]. Previous studies of actinomycosis showed bowel strictures or hydronephrosis [6, 7]. However, whatever the origin of infection, colon perforation is a rare event. There is a case that a single perforation of the transverse colon at the hepatic flexure caused by obstructing sigmoid colon mass was managed by emergency surgery and subsequent histologic examination revealed actinomycosis [8]. In our case, the precise factors underlying spontaneous colon perforation are unclear. However, it is assumed that the high pressure of the proximal colon due to the colorectal stricture as well as persistent inflammation of the sigmoid colon wall due to actinomycosis triggered colon perforation.

Hepatic actinomycosis (HA) is also a very rare form of abdominal actinomycosis and often, it is a secondary infection following abdominal infection. HA constitutes 15% of abdominal actinomycosis, and 5% of all actinomycosis [9–11]. The clinical features, diagnosis and treatment of colonic and hepatic actinomycosis in previous cases were shown in Table 1.

In the present unusual case, the patient presented with signs and symptoms mimicking advanced colon cancer with liver metastasis. Few studies have demonstrated other clinical features such as mimicking colon cancer, large mass with perforation, hydronephrosis and involvement of adjacent tissues. However, there are no reports showing all the features including colon perforation, rectal stricture, hydronephrosis, ascites and hepatic involvement.

Abdominopelvic actinomycosis does not produce the characteristic disease signs or symptoms and usually manifests as a slowly growing mass, which may be associated with altered bowel habits, nausea, vomiting and cramping pain [12]. Patients with hepatic involvement present mostly with chronic or subacute and non-specific symptoms including anorexia, weight loss, fever and night sweats [11, 13]. The nonspecific findings complicate the differential diagnosis of abdominopelvic actinomycosis from other chronic diseases such as chronic granulomatous infection, inflammatory bowel disease, and pelvic inflammatory diseases. Furthermore, it often presents as a mass either clinically or radiologically, which is not easily distinguishable from malignancies [12, 14, 15].

Several reports show abdominopelvic actinomycosis mimicking malignancies [16, 17]. Due to the

misdiagnosis, several previous cases were treated with neoadjuvant chemotherapy [17–19]. Hepatic actinomycosis is also difficult to distinguish from primary hepatocellular carcinoma and metastatic liver cancer [20].

In addition, because the preoperative diagnosis is rarely considered and is established only in less than 10% of cases, the diagnosis is based on clinical manifestations and imaging findings [12, 21]. Since the cultures of *Actinomyces* species show very low yield, histopathological examination is the most utilized diagnostic method worldwide, which is generally conducted after surgical intervention due to an initial diagnostic error [4, 12, 22]. Sulfur granules were observed in the purulent material in 50% of cases. Although these might not be pathognomonic of actinomycosis, the presence of sulfur granules is highly suggestive of the diagnosis [23, 24].

In our case, colon perforation with liver lesion resembled advanced colon cancer with liver metastasis. Radiologically, actinomycosis was considered, but colon cancer with liver metastasis was not excluded.

Treatment of abdominopelvic actinomycosis depends on the extent of the disease and the patient's condition. Long-term treatment with penicillin is the standard medical therapy for uncomplicated cases [25]. Indeed, *Actinomyces* spp. are usually extremely susceptible to beta-lactams, and especially Penicillin G or amoxicillin. Clindamycin, tetracycline, and erythromycin are alternatives in cases of allergy to penicillin [12]. Piperacillin-tazobactam or a carbapenem (imipenem or meropenem) may be an appropriate alternative [26]. The need for surgery must be assessed on an individual basis and surgery may be a valid option for patients who do not respond to medical treatment [26].

Treatment of HA mainly involves surgical or puncture drainage, hepatic resection, and postoperative treatment with anti-infectives [9, 20].

This particular case is interesting in several aspects.

First, although preoperative antibiotic therapy was administered only for 2 weeks, a significant reduction in inflammation due to actinomycosis was detected during surgery. The bladder and ureter, which were expected to be sacrificed, were preserved. Ureteral dilatation and hydronephrosis were resolved following insertion of a temporary double-J stent, and antibiotic therapy as reported previously [27–29].

Second, the exclusion of malignant tumors in frozen biopsy during surgery also facilitated the demarcation of the extent of surgery. In most of the previous cases, abdominopelvic mass was considered as a malignant tumor before surgery, and the diagnosis of actinomcycosis was made after surgery [2, 4, 8, 18, 19, 28–31]. However, in our case, by excluding the malignant tumor through the frozen biopsy during surgery, we could avoid unnecessary extensive surgery.

Table 1 Overview of previous reported case of colonic and hepatic actinomycosis

Reference	Year	Total cases	Involved sites	Mean age	Gender	Symptoms	IUD	Leukocytosis	Anemia	Presumptive diagnosis	Confirmatory test	Treatment
Colonic actinomycosis												
4	1995	1	Left colon	41	Female	Abdominal pain, nausea, constipation	+	–	+	Tumor of colon or retroperitoneum	Histologic diagnosis of surgical specimen	Complete excision of mass with colectomy + actinomycosis medication
30	2000	1	Transverse colon	37	Female	Abdominal pain with a sensation of fullness	–	–	+	Colon cancer	Histologic diagnosis of surgical specimen	Colectomy + actinomycosis medication
2	2000	4	Sigmoid, rectum	48.8 (38–55)	Male: 2 case Female: 2 case	Abdominal pain, constipation, weight loss, indigestion	+(1 female)	All case: +	n.av	colorectal cancer	Histologic diagnosis of surgical specimen: 3 case Biopsy: 1 case	3 case: colectomy + actinomycosis medication 1 case: actinomycosis medication
19	2000	1	Rectosigmoid, right colon, uterus, adnexa,	49	Female	Abdominal pain, constipation, vomiting	+	n.av	n.av	Colon cancer	Histologic diagnosis of surgical specimen	Colectomy + ovary excision + actinomycosis medication
28	2000	1	Rectosigmoid, right ureter	63	Male	Abdominal pain, constipation, malaise, weight loss	n.ap	+	–	colon cancer	Biopsy	Diverting sigmoidostomy + ureteral stent + actinomycosis medication
29	2002	1	Sigmoid, uterus, adnexa, right ureter	63	Female	Abdominal pain, fever	+	+	–	Pelvic actinomycosis or malignancy	Histologic diagnosis of surgical specimen	Total hysterectomy, bilateral salphigo-oophorectomy, adhesiolysis around urter + actinomycosis medication
8	2004	1	Sigmoid	39	Male	Abdominal pain	n.ap	+	n.av	Colon perforation due to obstructing colon cancer	Histologic diagnosis of surgical specimen	Colectomy, ileostomy + actinomycosis medication
31	2006	1	Sigmoid, both adnexa	38	Female	Abdominal pain, constipation, fever	+	+	n.av	Crohns disease or sigmoid tumor	Histologic diagnosis of surgical specimen	Colectomy + bilateral salphingo-oophorectomy + actinomycosis medication
18	2008	1	Rectosigmoid, uterus, adnexa, left ureter	42	Female	Pelvic discomfort, constipation	+	–	+	Advanced Ovarian cancer	Histologic diagnosis of surgical specimen	Neoadjuvant chemotherapy +total hysterectomy, bilateral salphingo-oophorectomy, rectosigmoid resection + ureteral stent + actinomycosis medication
Hepatic actinomycosis												
20	1997	11	Right lobe: 1 case Left lobe: 2 case Central area: 1 case	55 (20–86)	Male: 7 case Female: 4 case	Fever: 9/11 (81.9%) Abdominal pain: 6/11 (54.5%) Palpable mass:	n.av	+: 7/9 (77.8%)	+: 2/9 (22.2%)	Liver tumor: 6/11 (54.5%) Liver abscess: 5/11	Histologic diagnosis of surgical specimen: 6/11 (54.5%)	Liver resection + actinomycosis medication: 5/11 (45.5%) Surgical or percutaneous

Table 1 Overview of previous reported case of colonic and hepatic actinomycosis (*Continued*)

Reference	Year	Total cases	Involved sites	Mean age	Gender	Symptoms	IUD	Leukocytosis	Anemia	Presumptive diagnosis	Confirmatory test	Treatment
			No data: 7 case			4/11 (36.4%) Back pain: 2/11 (18.2%) Nausea, vomiting: 2/11 (18.2%) Anorexia: 1/11 (9%) Diarrhea: 1/11 (9%) No clinical sign: 1/11 (9%)				(45.5%)	Biopsy: 1/11 (9%) Sulfur granule in pus: 2/11 (18.2%) Actinomyces culture: 2/11 (18.2%)	drainage + actinomycosis medication: 5/11 (45.9%) Liver resection only: 1/11 (9%)
11	2010	1	Liver (both lobe)	70	Male	Fever, abdominal pain, anorexia, weight loss	n.ap	+	+	Hepatic metastasis	Biopsy	Actinomycosis medication
10	2011	1	Right lobe, single lesion	65	Male	Incidental finding of regular surveillance after pancreatic adenocarcinoma	n.ap	–	n.av	Metastatic liver tumor	Histologic diagnosis of surgical specimen	Liver resection + actinomycosis medication
9	2011	1	Liver (right lobe), ovary	41	Female	Abdominal pain	+	+	+	Ovarian cancer with hepatic metastasis	Histologic diagnosis of surgical specimen	Rt. Salpingo-oophorectomy + IUD removal + actinomycosis medication
3	2012	1	Liver(multiple nodules on surface), spleen	37	Male	Fever, abdominal pain	n.ap	+	–	Spleen abscess	Histologic diagnosis of surgical specimen	Splenectomy + liver biopsy + actinomycosis medication
13	2014	1	Left lobe	55	Male	Abdominal pain, weight loss	n.ap	–	–	Liver tumor	Histologic diagnosis of surgical specimen	Liver resection + actinomycosis medication
		32 (data of analysis in literature)	Right lobe: 19/29 (65.5%) Both lobe: 8/29 (27.6%) Left lobe: 2/29 (6.9%)	45.5 (5–86)	Male: 19 (59%) Female: 13 (41%)	Fever: 25/27 (92.6%) Weight loss: 15/25 (60%)	2 (6.3%)	+: 27/29 (93.1%)	+: 17/24 (70.8%)	Liver tumor: 20/28 (71.4%) Hepatophyta: 8/28 (28.6%) Liver hydatidosis: 2/28 (7.1%) Inflammatory pseudotumor: 1/28 (3.65%) Tuberculosis: 1/2 (3.65%)	Gram staining: 22/27 (81.5%) Histologic diagnosis of sulfur granule: 22/31 (71%) Actinomyces culture: 10/20 (50%)	Only actinomycosis medication: 14/32 (43.8%) Surgical or percutaneous drainage + actinomycosis medication: 12/32 (37.5%) Liver resection + actinomycosis medication: 6/32 (18.7%)

n.av. not available, *n.ap* not applicable

Therefore, we recommend the use of preoperative empirical antibiotics and exclusion of malignant tumors during surgery via frozen biopsy. Such a strategy reduces the extent of surgery and postoperative complications in patients, with actinomycosis indistinguishable from malignant tumor before surgery.

In conclusion, abdominopelvic actinomycosis presenting with colon perforation and hepatic involvement is extremely rare; however, it is clinically similar to advanced colon cancer with liver metastasis, therefore, complicating the preoperative diagnosis. A diagnosis of abdominopelvic actinomycosis should be considered in patients with a history of IUD and chronic abdominal pain, along with an abdominal mass or cutaneous abscess. If surgery is indicated, preoperative empirical antibiotic therapy for actinomycosis and frozen biopsy during surgery may be considered.

Author's ex-post considerations

- A diagnosis of abdominopelvic actinomycosis should be considered in patients with a history of IUD, even though concurrent hepatic mass was detected.
- If the patient's condition allows, the use of preoperative empirical antibiotics should be considered for at least 2 weeks to decrease the extent of surgery and postoperative complications.
- If surgery is indicated, exclusion of malignant tumors via intraoperative frozen biopsy facilitated the determination of the extent of surgery.

Abbreviations
ALT: Alanine transaminase; AST: Aspartate transaminase; BUN: Blood urea nitrogen; CRP: C-reactive protein; CT: Computer tomography; HA: Hepatic actinomycosis; IUD: Intra-uterine device

Authors' contributions
SSY and YCI drafted the manuscript. Both authors have read and approved the manuscript, and ensure that this is the case.

Competing interests
The authors declare that they have no competing interests.

References
1. Berardi R. Abdominal actinomycosis. Surg Gynecol Obstet. 1979;149:257–66.
2. Son SH, Kim BS, Huh KC, Park SK. Abdominal actinomycosis initially diagnosed as a colorectal cancer or periappendiceal abscess. Korean J Gastrointest Endosc. 2000;21(3):717–22.
3. Wang H-K, Sheng W-H, Hung C-C, Chen Y-C, Liew P-L, Hsiao C-H, Chang S-C. Hepatosplenic actinomycosis in an immunocompetent patient. J Formos Med Assoc. 2012;111(4):228–31.
4. Kaya E, Yilmazlar T, Emiroğlu Z, Zorluoğlu A, Bayer A. Colonic actinomycosis: report of a case and review of the literature. Surg Today. 1995;25(10):923–6.
5. Fiorino AS. Intrauterine contraceptive device-associated actinomycotic abscess and Actinomyces detection on cervical smear. Obstet Gynecol. 1996;87(1):142–9.
6. Bae JJ, Kim JH, Park YK, Lee DJ, Koh MW, Lee TH, Lee SH. A clinical analysis of pelvic actinomycosis. Korean J Obstet Gynecol. 2007;50(8):1132–40.
7. Hyung WJ, Kim MW, Kim MK, Chang DY, Jeon MK, Lee ES. 4 cases of pelvic actinomycosis associated with intrauterine contraceptive device. Korean J Obstet Gynecol. 2005;48(2):509–18.
8. Norwood MG, Bown MJ, Furness PN, Berry DP. Actinomycosis of the sigmoid colon: an unusual cause of large bowel perforation. ANZ J Surg. 2004;74(9):816–8.
9. Kim YS, Lee BY, Jung MH. Metastatic hepatic actinomycosis masquerading as distant metastases of ovarian cancer. J Obstet Gynaecol Res. 2012;38(3):601–4.
10. Wayne MG, Narang R, Chauhdry A, Steele J. Hepatic actinomycosis mimicking an isolated tumor recurrence. World J Surg Oncol. 2011;9(1):70.
11. Kanellopoulou T, Alexopoulou A, Tiniakos D, Koskinas J, Archimandritis AJ. Primary hepatic actinomycosis mimicking metastatic liver tumor. J Clin Gastroenterol. 2010;44(6):458–9.
12. Garcia-Garcia A, Ramirez-Duran N, Sandoval-Trujillo H, Romero-Figueroa MDS. Pelvic Actinomycosis. Can J Infect Dis Med Microbiol. 2017;2017:9428650.
13. Yang XX, Lin JM, Xu KJ, Wang SQ, Luo TT, Geng XX, Huang RG, Jiang N. Hepatic actinomycosis: report of one case and analysis of 32 previously reported cases. World J Gastroenterol. 2014;20(43):16372–6.
14. Lim DR, Hur H, Min BS, Baik SH, Kim NK. Intrauterine contraceptive device-related actinomycosis infection presenting as ovarian cancer with carcinomatosis. Surg Infect. 2014;15(6):826–8.
15. Weese WC, Smith IM. A study of 57 cases of actinomycosis over a 36-year period: a diagnostic 'failure' with good prognosis after treatment. Arch Intern Med. 1975;135(12):1562–8.
16. Hoffman M, Roberts W, Solomon P, Gunasekarin S, Cavanagh D. Advanced actinomycotic pelvic inflammatory disease simulating gynecologic malignancy. A report of two cases. J Reprod Med. 1991;36(7):543–5.
17. Koshiyama M, Yoshida M, Fujii H, Nanno H, Hayashi M, Tauchi K, Kaji Y. Ovarian actinomycosis complicated by diabetes mellitus simulating an advanced ovarian carcinoma. Eur J Obstet Gynecol Reprod Biol. 1999;87(1):95–9.
18. Lee YK, Bae JM, Park YJ, Park SY, Jung SY. Pelvic actinomycosis with hydronephrosis and colon stricture simulating an advanced ovarian cancer. J Gynecol Oncol. 2008;19(2):154–6.
19. Yeguez JF, Martinez SA, Sands LR, Hellinger MD. Pelvic actinomycosis presenting as malignant large bowel obstruction: a case report and a review of the literature. Am Surg. 2000;66(1):85.
20. Sugano S, Matuda T, Suzuki T, Makino H, Iinuma M, Ishii K, Ohe K, Mogami K. Hepatic actinomycosis: case report and review of the literature in Japan. J Gastroenterol. 1997;32(5):672–6.
21. Chan P, Chong S, Ng B, Chan S. Splenic actinomycosis. J R Coll Surg Edinb. 1999;44(5):344.
22. Smith TR. Actinomycosis of the distal colon and rectum. Gastrointest Radiol. 1992;17(1):274–6.
23. Cintron JR, Del Pino A, Duarte B, Wood D. Abdominal actinomycosis. Dis Colon Rectum. 1996;39(1):105–8.
24. Chitturi S, Hui J, Salisbury E, Mitchell D, George J. Abdominal pain in an intrauterine contraceptive device user. Postgrad Med J. 2001;77(911):602.
25. Valour F, Senechal A, Dupieux C, Karsenty J, Lustig S, Breton P, Gleizal A, Boussel L, Laurent F, Braun E, et al. Actinomycosis: etiology, clinical features, diagnosis, treatment, and management. Infect Drug Resist. 2014;7:183–97.
26. Wong V, Turmezei T, Weston V. Actinomycosis. BMJ. 2011;343:d6099.
27. Fulton I, Paterson W, Crucioli V. Pelvic actinomycosis causing ureteric obstruction. BJOG Int J Obstet Gynaecol. 1981;88(10):1044–50.
28. Haj M, Nasser G, Loberant N, Cohen I, Nesser E, Eitan A. Pelvic actinomycosis presenting as ureteric and rectal stricture. Dig Surg. 2000;17(4):414–7.
29. Nasu K, Matsumoto H, Yoshimatsu J, Miyakawa I. Ureteral and sigmoid obstruction caused by pelvic actinomycosis in an intrauterine contraceptive device user. Gynecol Obstet Investig. 2002;54(4):228–31.
30. Kim H, Lee WK, Kim SH, Pak SM, Kim YN, Choi SJ, Kim EH, Choi YW, Lee YU. A case of abdominal actinomycosis. Korean J Gastroenterol Endo. 2000;20(4):307–11.
31. Valko P, Busolini E, Donati N, Chimchila Chevili S, Rusca T, Bernasconi E. Severe large bowel obstruction secondary to infection with Actinomyces israelii. Scand J Infect Dis. 2006;38(3):231–4.

28

Ascending Cholangitis secondary to migrated embolization coil of gastroduodenal artery pseudo-aneurysm a case report

Haithem Zaafouri[1*], Anis Hasnaoui[1], Sonia Essghaeir[2], Dhafer Haddad[1], Meriam Sabbah[3], Ahmed Bouhafa[1], Jamel Kharrat[3] and Anis Ben Maamer[1]

Abstract

Background: Gastroduodenalartery (GDA) pseudo-aneurysms are very rare. Their clinical importance lies in the eventuality of rupture, causing bleeding and ultimately exsanguination.

Case presentation: We report the case of a man, with prior history of biliary surgery, presenting with haemobilia secondary to a rupture of GDA pseudo-aneurysm eroding the main bile duct. The patient was treated with coil embolization. This technique is considered to be safe. However, on the long term, some complications may occur. In our case, the patient presented with cholangitis subsequent to coil migration in the lower bile duct. This situation was managed using endoscopic retrograde cholangiopancreatography (ERCP) allowing coil extraction with favorable evolution.

Conclusions: GDA pseudo-aneurysms are very rare. Bleeding, secondary to the rupture of these lesions, is a serious complication that could lead to death. Diagnosis and treatment of ruptured GDA pseudo-aneurysms rely on angiography. This method is considered to be safe. Cholangitis secondary to coil migration in the main bile duct is exceedingly rare,but remains an eventuality that physicians should be cognizant of.

Keywords: Gastroduodenal artery, Pseudo-aneurysm, Haemobilia, Embolization coil, Cholangitis

Background

Splanchnic artery aneurysms are rare entities. They are mainly cited in literature as case reports rendering their prevalence hard to determine [1]. Aneurysms of the gastroduodenal artery (GDA) are the least common [2]. Their clinical importance resides in the fact that they can be rapidly fatal if ruptured. The management of these conditions relies on endovascular embolization. This technique is considered to be safe. However, on the long term, seldom complications may occur. We report a case of upper gastrointestinal bleeding secondary to a ruptured pseudo-aneurysm of the gastroduodenal artery after choledochotomy, treated with endovascular

embolization, and subsequent migration of a coil in the main bile duct, causing severe cholangitis.

Case presentation

A 55-year-old man, with previous history of alcohol consumption, presented to our institution with a 6-day history of right upper quadrant pain, fever and progressive jaundice. Physical examination showed a temperature of 38 °C, a pulse rate of 98/min, a blood pressure of 10/7 cm Hg, scleral icterus and right upper quadrant pain with no rebound. Laboratory blood tests showed a leukocyte count of 12,300/ml, C-reactive protein of 215 mg/l, a conserved renal function. His liver function tests revealed a total bilirubin of 130 umol/l, an alanine transaminase (ALT) of 213 U/l, a gamma-glutamyltranspeptidase (γ-GT) of 686 U/l and an alkaline phosphatase (ALP) of 284 U/l. Amylase level and

---
* Correspondence: zaafouri.haithem@hotmail.fr
[1]Department of General Surgery Habib Thameur Hospital, Ali Ben Ayed Street's 2037 Montfleury, Tunis, Tunisia
Full list of author information is available at the end of the article

prothrombin time were normal. Abdominal ultrasonography foundcholelithiasis and a mild dilatation of both the extrahepatic and intrahepatic biliary tract. The obstacle was not identified. CT scan confirmed the presence of several stones impacted in the common bile duct, upstream biliary tree dilatation, and an enlarged pancreatic head with adjacent peripancreatic inflammation. We retained the diagnosis of acute pancreatitis with ascending cholangitis. The patient was admitted and antibiotics were then intravenously administered. Twenty-four hours later, he had an endoscopic retrograde cholangiopancreatography (ERCP) with sphincterotomy and stones extraction with favorable evolution (Fig. 1). The patient was discharged 3 days later.

A laparoscopic cholecystectomy was scheduled, after regression of peripancreatic inflammation, 3 months later. Due to dissection difficulties, we converted to a Kocher's incision to complete the cholecystectomy. Transcystic cholangiography showed residual stones. We performed choledocotomy with two stones retrieval and T-tube choledochostomy. Immediate post-operative course was uneventful and T-tube cholangiography was normal. The patient was discharged in the 5th post-operative day.

Two weeks later, the patient presented with hematemesis and melena. On examination, he had icterus, blood pressure of 12/8 cm Hg and a pulse of 85 beats per minute. On digital rectal examination, he had melena. There was no blood exteriorization from the T-tube. Blood tests showed a hemoglobin level at 96 g/l, a total bilirubin of 46 umol/l, an ALT of 225 U/l, a γ-GT of 516 U/l. He underwent upper gastrointestinal endoscopy showing mycotic esophagitis and erosive bulbitis with no active bleeding. Lateral duodenoscopy revealed no bleeding from the papilla. CT scan showed infiltration of subhepatic fat and magnetic resonance cholangiopancreatography was normal. During hospitalization, the patient was hemodynamically stable, without further drop in hemoglobin level. He was discharged with an appointment to our outpatient department.

After 1 month of being discharged, the patient presented with recurrence of upper gastrointestinal bleeding and haemobilia with blood exteriorization from the T-tube. On examination, he was hemodynamically stable, he had scleral icterus and right upper quadrant pain. On digital rectal examination, he had melena. Hemoglobin level was at 85 g/l and his liver function tests revealed icteric cholestasis. A CT-angiography was performed showing a pseudoaneurysm of the gastroduodenal arterywith probable erosion of the main bile duct (Fig. 2).

In the third day post admission,a massivebleeding and hemorrhagic shock occurred. Hemoglobin level was at 40 g/l. The patient was admitted to the intensive care department. After resuscitation and transfusion his condition was relatively stabilized, and he was addressed for urgent embolization. Coeliac arteriography confirmed the bleeding from the pseudo-aneurysm of the gastroduodenal artery. Embolization using three coils achieved successful hemostasis with preserved permeability of the gastroduodenal artery. The immediate post-embolization period passed without any complications. The patient was discharged 6 days later after T-tube removal. Then he was lost to follow-up.

Twenty months later, the patient presented with Charcot's triad. Physical examination showed a temperature of 40 °C, heart rate of 120/min, blood pressure of 14/9 cmHg, icterus and right upper quadrant tenderness. On blood tests, leukocyte count was 22,770/ml, C-reactive protein level260 mg/l, and conserved renal function. His liver function tests revealed a total bilirubin of 355 umol/l, conjugated bilirubin of 195 umol/l, an ALT of 215 U/l, a γ-GT of 729 U/l and an alkaline phosphatase of 126 U/l. Prothrombin time was 50%. On ultrasonography, we noted dilatation of both the extrahepatic and intrahepatic biliary tract. CT scan revealed a hyper-dense obstacle of the lower bile duct (Fig. 3).

ERCP showed the presence, in the lower bile duct, of an intraluminal coil and stones, with upstream biliary tree dilatation (Fig. 4). An extraction of the coil and fragmented stones was carried out and vacuity of bile ducts was attained. Following this, the patient recovered uneventfully and was discharged 8 days later.

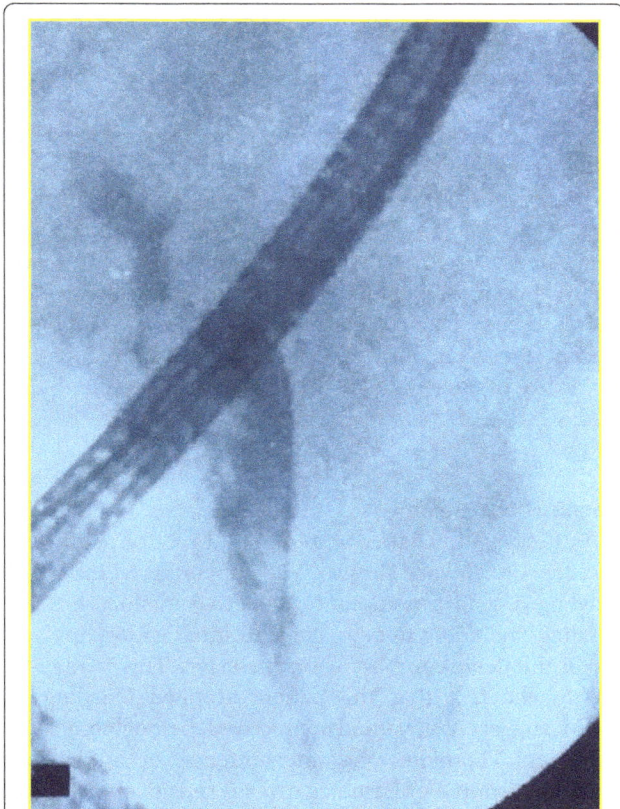

Fig. 1 ERCP showing stones in the main bile duct

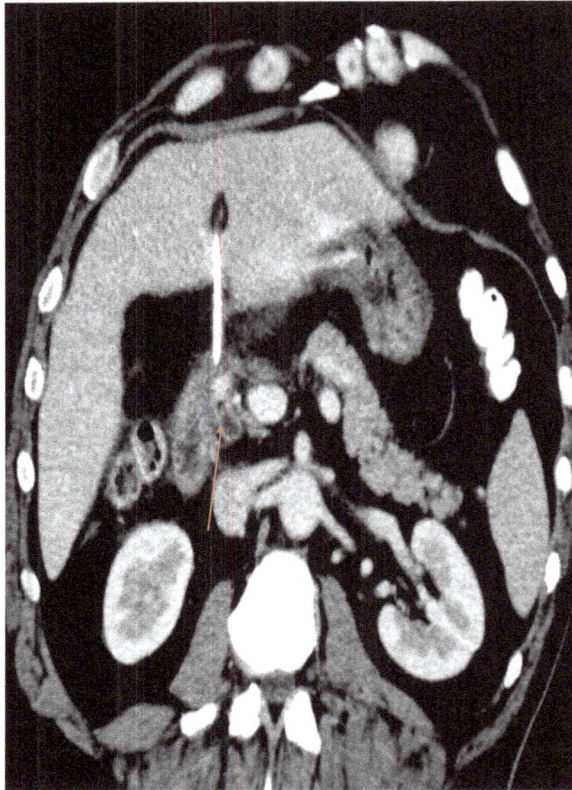

Fig. 2 CT-angiography showing a pseudo-aneurysm of the gastro-duodenal artery with probable erosion of the main bile duct

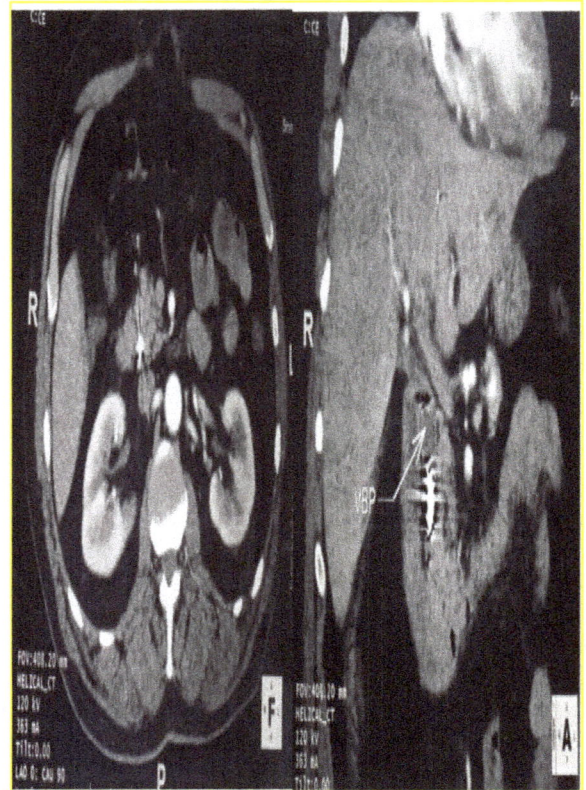

Fig. 3 Axial (*Left picture*) and Frontal (*right picture*) CT-scan images, showing a hyper-dense obstacle in the bile duct

Discussion

Etiology of GDA pseudo-aneurysms

Aneurysms of GDA are very rare. They are estimated to be less than 1.5% of all splanchnic artery aneurysms [2]. They are divided into two types: True aneurysms and pseudo-aneurysms like our case. GDA pseudo-aneurysms are generally secondary to acute or chronic pancreatitis, cholangitis, traumatic or iatrogenic causes [3–6]. All these factors were present in our case. It is most likely that the iatrogenic factor in an inflammatory environment precipitated the formation of the pseudo-aneurysm. This is the second case of GDA pseudo-aneurysm after choledochotomy in the English literature. The first case was reported byEkeland and al in 1974 [7].

Symptomatology

GDA pseudo-aneurysms could remain silent for a long time and be revealed accidentally in an imaging study. On the contrary, theycould be symptomatic. Revelation modes are mainly compression, and bleeding. Bleeding is considered to be the most serious complication, as it can rapidly lead to a hemorrhagic shock, and ultimately death. It can occur after the rupture of the pseudo-aneurysm in the peritoneum, the retroperitoneum or in the gastrointestinal tract by way of the duodenum or the bile duct causing haemobilia like in our case [8].

Rupture of a GDA pseudo-aneurysm in the main bile duct is exceedingly rare. Only few cases in the literature have been reported [4]. Symptoms of haemobilia are, classically, abdominal pain, upper gastrointestinal hemorrhage and jaundice. The complete triad known as Quincke's triad occurred only in 22% of 222 cases of haemobilia, in the review of Green and al. [9]. Our patient presented this triad, which adds to the particularities of this case.

Diagnosis and treatment

In our case, the patient presented to our institution, 2 weeks after biliary surgery, with upper gastrointestinal bleeding. Usedexplorations to detect an etiology for this bleeding, including upper gastrointestinal endoscopy and lateral duodenoscopy, were inconclusive. This is may be due to the fact that the patient stopped bleeding as would suggest the hemodynamic and hemoglobin level stabilities. Therefore, the intermittence of a bleeding could be a source of false negatives if sensitive diagnostic tools are not used. In the recent literature, only 12% of haemobilia cases were diagnosed endoscopically [10].

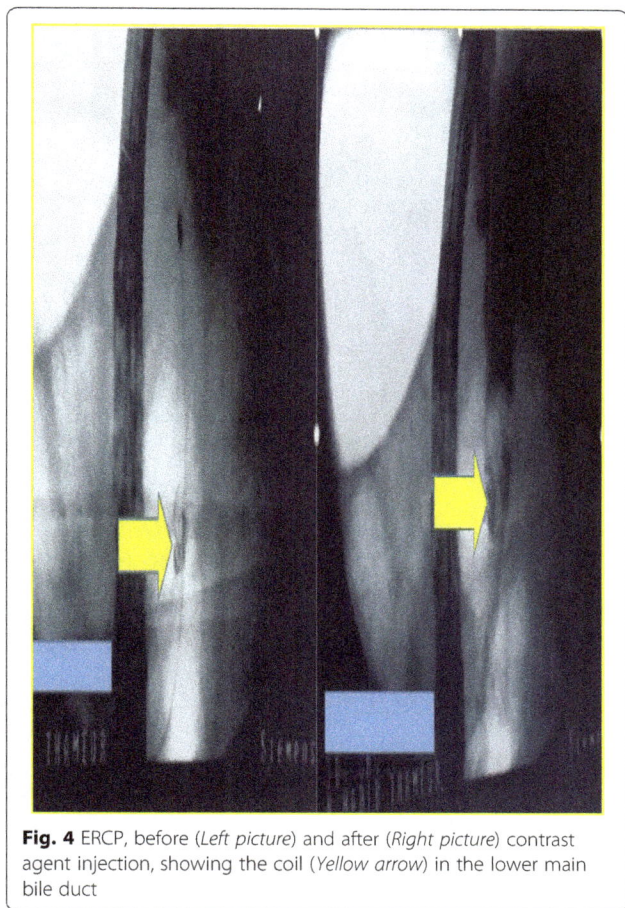

Fig. 4 ERCP, before (*Left picture*) and after (*Right picture*) contrast agent injection, showing the coil (*Yellow arrow*) in the lower main bile duct

Arteriography is the most valuable diagnostic test to detect Splanchnic artery aneurysms and the exact location of bleeding [11, 12]. However, this technique requires a trained interventional radiologist. CT angiography and magnetic resonance angiography could be also used in the diagnostic arsenal, when arteriography is not available, with high threshold of detection of Splanchnic artery aneurysms [13].

Management of GDA pseudo-aneurysms relies either on surgery or angiographic embolization. The latter, if available, is considered the safer and more effective option, especially in the active bleeding patient [13, 14]. Success rate is estimated to be around 80 to 100% [9]. A variety of embolic agents have been used. In our case, we used three metallic coils with preserved permeability of the gastroduodenal artery. Nevertheless,surgery remains the only option for proximal GDA pseudo-aneurysms [4] and should be considered if angiographic embolization fails or is unavailable or contraindicated [15, 16].

Rare complication after GDA embolization
After embolization of Splanchnic artery aneurysms, some complications could occur. In the short term, accidentalembolization of the wrong vessel with ensuing infarction is may be the most serious complication. In the long term, complications are rare. In our case, 20 months after embolization, the patient presentedwith cholangitis secondary to coil migration from the embolized GDA pseudo-aneurysm. To our knowledge, this is the first case to be published in the English literature. Some cases of cholangitis after coil embolization of hepatic arteries were reported [17–19]. The best management of these conditions is through ERCP, especially in severe cholangitis like in our case. AS for surgery, it could be indicated after ERCP failure.

Conclusion
GDA pseudo-aneurysms are very rare. Bleeding, secondary to the rupture of these lesions, is a serious complication that could lead to death. Thus, surgeons must keep a high index of suspicion, in the set of patients with history of biliary surgery, presenting with upper gastrointestinal bleeding. Diagnosis and treatment of ruptured GDA pseudo-aneurysms, rely on angiography. This method is considered to be safe. Cholangitis secondary to coil migration in the main bile duct is exceedingly rare,but remains an eventuality that physicians should be cognizant of.

Abbreviations
ALP: Alkaline phosphatase; ALT: Alanine transaminase; ERCP: Endoscopic retrograde cholangiopancreatography; GDA: Gastroduodenal artery; γ-GT: Gamma-glutamyltranspeptidase

Acknowledgements
All the authors contributed to this work. The idea of the publication of this paper came after discussion between Haithem ZAAFOURI and Sonia ESSGAHEIR.
Anis HASNAOUI, Meriam SABBAH and Dhafer HADDAD participated in acquisition and interpretation of data.
Haithem ZAAFOURI and Anis HASNAOUI participated in the writing of paper. Finally, all Professors Ahmed BOUHAFA, Jamel KHARRAT and Anis BEN MAAMER approved the final version of manuscript.

Funding
We have no conflict of interest to declare.

Authors' contributions
Conception and design of study: HZ, SE. Acquisition of data: AH, DH. Data analysis and interpretation: MS. Drafting of manuscript: HZ and AH. Approval of final version of manuscript: AB, JK and ABM.

Competing interests
The authors declare that they have no competing interests.

Author details
[1]Department of General Surgery Habib Thameur Hospital, Ali Ben Ayed Street's 2037 Montfleury, Tunis, Tunisia. [2]Department of Radiology Habib Thameur Hospital, Tunis, Tunisia. [3]Department of Gastroenterology Habib Thameur Hospital, Tunis, Tunisia.

References

1. Saltzberg SS, Maldonado TS, Lamparello PJ, et al. Is endovascular therapy the preferred treatment for all visceral artery aneurysms? Ann Vasc Surg. 2005;19(4):507–15.
2. Messina LM, Shanley CJ. Visceral artery aneurysms. Surg Clin North Am. 1997;77(2):425–42.
3. Welling TH, Williams DM, Stanley JC. Excessive oral amphetamine use as a possible cause of renal and splanchnic arterial aneurysms: a report of two cases. J Vasc Surg. 1998;28(4):727–31.
4. Fodor M, Fodor L, Ciuce C. Gastroduodenal artery pseudoaneurysm ruptured in the common bile duct. Acta Chir Belg. 2010;110(1):103–5.
5. Lo Bue S, Denoel A. Gastroduodenal artery pseudoaneurysm after cholecystectomy. Acta Chir Belg. 2003;103(4):416–41.
6. Mawaddah A, Abrar N, Reda J, Yousef Q, Murad A. Delayed hemobilia due to hepatic artery pseudo-aneurysm: a pitfall of laparoscopic cholecystectomy. BMC Surg. 2016;16:59.
7. Ekeland A, Ofstad E, Stiris G. Hemobiliapseudoaneurysm in the gastroduodenal artery following choledochotomia. A Case report. Acta Chir Scand. 1974;140(5):422–7.
8. Sessa C, Tinelli G, Porcu P, et al. Treatment of visceral artery aneurysms: a description of a retrospective series of 42 aneurysms in 34 patients. Ann Vasc Surg. 2004;18:695–703.
9. Green MH, Duell RM, Johnson CD, Jamieson NV. Haemobilia. Br J Surg. 2001; 88:773–86.
10. Napolitano V, et al. A severe case of hemobilia and biliary fistula following an open urgent cholecystectomy. World J Emerg Surg. 2009;4:37.
11. Mandel R, Jaques P, Sanofsky S, Matthew A. Non-operative management of peripancreatic arterial aneurysms. Ann Surg. 1987;205:126–8.
12. Bohl JL, Dossett LA, Grau AM. Gastroduodenal artery pseudoaneurysm associated with haemosuccuspancreaticus and obstructive jaundice. J Gastrointest Surg. 2007;11:1752–4.
13. Horton KM, Smith C, Fishman EK. MDCT and 3D CT angiography of splanchnic artery aneurysms. AJR Am J Roentgenol. 2007;189(3):641–7.
14. Madanur MA, et al. Pseudoaneurysm following laparoscopic cholecystectomy. Hepatobiliary Pancreat Dis Int. 2007;6(3):294–8.
15. Tsu-Te L, Ming-Chih H, Han-Chieh L, Full-Young C, Shou-Dong L. Life-threatening hemobilia caused by hepatic artery pseudoaneurysm: a rare complication of chronic cholangitis. World J Gastroenterol. 2003;9(12):2883–4.
16. Cattan P, et al. Hemobilia caused by a pseudoaneurysm of the hepaticartery diagnosed by EUS. Gastrointest Endosc. 1999;49(2):252–5.
17. Turaga KK, Amirlak B, Davis RE, Yousef K, Richards A, Fitzgibbons RJ. Cholangitis after coil embolization of an iatrogenic hepatic artery pseudoaneurysm: an unusual case report. Surg Laparosc Endosc Percutan Tech. 2006;16(1):36–8.
18. Zervos X, Molina E, Larsen MF. Cholangitis secondary to migrated metallic coils in the common bile duct. Acta Gastroenterol Latinoam. 2013;43(2):146–8.
19. Soondoos R, Manju DC, Khaled A, Glen S, Neil DM. Vascular coil erosion into hepaticojejunostomy following hepatic arterial embolisation. BMC Surg. 2015;15:51.

29

Comparing the short-term outcomes of intracorporeal esophagojejunostomy with extracorporeal esophagojejunostomy after laparoscopic total gastrectomy for gastric cancer

Ke Chen, Yang He, Jia-Qin Cai, Yu Pan, Di Wu, Ding-Wei Chen, Jia-Fei Yan, Hendi Maher and Yi-Ping Mou[*]

Abstract

Background: Totally laparoscopic distal gastrectomy (TLDG) using intracorporeal anastomosis has gradually developed due to advancements in laparoscopic surgical instruments. However, totally laparoscopic total gastrectomy (TLTG) with intracorporeal esophagojejunostomy (IE) is still uncommon because of technical difficulties. Herein, we evaluated various types of IE after TLTG in terms of the technical aspects. We compared the short-term operative outcomes between TLTG with IE and laparoscopy-assisted total gastrectomy (LATG) with extracorporeal esophagojejunostomy (EE).

Methods: Between March 2006 and December 2014, a total of 213 patients with gastric cancer underwent TLTG and LATG. Overall, 92 patients underwent TLTG with IE, and 121 patients underwent LATG with EE. Generally, there are two methods of IE: mechanical staplers (circular or linear staplers) and hand-sewn sutures. Surgical efficiencies and outcomes were compared between two groups. We also described various types of IE using a subgroup analysis.

Results: The mean operation times were similar in the two groups, as was the number of retrieved lymph nodes. However, the mean estimated blood loss of TLTG was statistically lower than LATG. There were no significant differences in time to first flatus, the time to restart oral intake, the length of the hospital stay after operation, and postoperative complications. Four types of IE have been applied after TLTG, including 42 cases of hand-sewn IE. The overall mean operation time and the mean anastomotic time in TLTG were 279.5 ± 38.4 min and 52.6 ± 18.9 min respectively. There was no case of conversion to open procedure. Postoperative complication occurred in 16 patients (17.4 %) and no postoperative mortality occurred.

Conclusions: IE is a feasible procedure and can be safely performed for TLTG with the proper laparoscopic expertise. It is technically feasible to perform hand-sewn IE after TLTG, which can reduce the cost of the laparoscopic procedure.

Keywords: Laparoscopic gastrectomy, Intracorporeal anastomosis, Hand-sewn, Stomach neoplasms

* Correspondence: mouyiping@126.com
Department of General Surgery, Sir Run Run Shaw Hospital, School of Medicine, Zhejiang University, 3 East Qingchun Road, Hangzhou 310016 Zhejiang Province, China

Background

Gastric cancer is the second leading cause of cancer related deaths and the fourth most common form of cancer worldwide. Nearly 70 % of all new cases and deaths occur in developing countries, and about 40 % of those occur in Eastern Asia [1, 2]. Since the introduction of laparoscopy-assisted distal gastrectomy (LADG) for gastric cancer in 1994 [3], LADG has become widely used for tumors located in the lower stomach with satisfactory surgical outcomes. However, the inclusion of the auxiliary incision in LADG makes it divergent from the minimally invasive treatment concept pursued in minimally invasive surgery. During the past decade, some studies have demonstrated the safety and feasibility of totally laparoscopic gastrectomy with intracorporeal reconstruction [4–6]. We have also reported that totally laparoscopic distal gastrectomy (TLDG) with intracorporeal reconstruction is better than laparoscopy-assisted distal gastrectomy (LADG) with extracorporeal reconstruction as it has improved outcomes such as better cosmesis, earlier bowel movements, less pain, and shorter hospital stays [7, 8]. These advantages are attributed to the less invasiveness of totally laparoscopic surgery. However, regarding to the laparoscopic total gastrectomy (LTG), many surgeons have preferred the "laparoscopy-assisted" type because of the high technical demand of intracorporeal esophagojejunostomy (IE). In addition to the relatively low incidence of upper gastric carcinoma in East Asia [2], TLTG for upper and middle gastric cancer has not been generalized. As the development of laparoscopic instruments, various types of IE using linear or circular staplers have recently been reported [4]. A growing number of surgeons are beginning to pay attention to TLTG and accept it. Nevertheless, to the best of our knowledge, there have been no studies that clarify the best approach. On the basis of our laparoscopic experience gained from laparoscopy gastric and pancreatic surgery, and other laparoscopic operations [7–14], we were encouraged to develop TLTG with various types of IE for the treatment of upper and middle gastric cancer. In this article, we present our experiences and short-term clinical outcomes of TLTG with various types of IE using laparoscopic staplers or hand-sewn purse-string suture technique. We also compare those outcomes of patients with laparoscopy-assisted total gastrectomy (LATG) from our center to further clarify the safety and feasibility of IE.

Methods

Patients

The patients in this research come from the gastric cancer database from March 2006 to December 2014 in the Department of General Surgery. A total of 213 patients underwent LTG with Roux-en-Y reconstruction for gastric cancer. During this period, patients were divided into two groups according to reconstructive methods, such as intra-corporeal or extra-corporeal reconstruction. All of these patients were diagnosed with gastric adenocarcinoma in the upper and middle stomach before surgery and they underwent LTG with modified D2 lymph node dissection. American Joint Committee on Cancer (seventh edition) and TNM classification serve as the criterion for clinical and pathologic staging. This research has been approved by the Zhejiang University's Ethics Committee. Informed consent was obtained from each patient preoperatively after they were given a detailed explanation of the two procedures-TLTG and LATG. All of the patients agreed to participate in the study.

Surgical procedure

Our previous essays issued before have elaborated on the lymphadenectomy in detail. With the patient in the supine position, mobilization of the stomach and en bloc systematic lymph node dissection were performed via five trocars under a pneumoperitoneum. Based on the Gastric Cancer Treatment Guidelines 2010 by the Japanese Gastric Cancer Association, which contained not only number D_1 dissection but also number 7, 8, 9, 10, 11p, 11d, and 12a dissection, lymphadenectomy was conducted.

Methods of IE

1. Conventional circular stapler-anvil approach (Type A group) :The stomach was pulled up and a purse-string suture was located at 1 cm above the incision line, which was decided in advance (Figs. 1a and 2a). The harmonic scalpel made a hole at the esophagogastric junction. The anvil was placed in the esophageal stump through the hole. It was then sewn up with the purse-string suture (Figs. 1b and 2b). Then, esophagogastric junction was separated and the stomach was removed. The circular stapler was placed in the jejunum via the jejunal stump and adhered to the anvil (Figs. 1c and 2c). The esophagojejunostomy was finished after the circular stapler was heated (Fig. 1d). Finally, the jejunal stump was closed with endoscopic linear staplers (Fig. 2d).

2. Linear stapler side-to-side approach (Type B group): On the end of the jejunum, a small opening was made 10 cm away from the stump and the stump was subsequently extended to the esophagus, where there was a small opening on one side. A side-to-side antiperistaltic esophagojejunostomy was carried out subsequently with linear staplers (Figs. 3a and 4a, b). Finally, the entry hole and esophagus were closed with staplers (Figs. 3b and 4c, d).

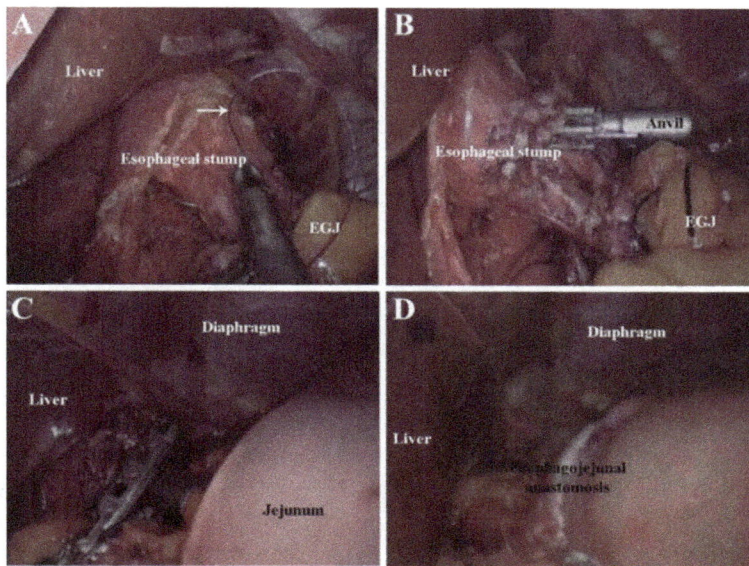

Fig. 1 Conventional circular stapler-anvil method. **a** The purse-string suture (white arrow) was placed in the esophagus. **b** The anvil was introduced into the esophageal stump through the hole. **c** The circular stapler was introduced into the jejunum through the jejunal stump and attached with the anvil. **d** The circular stapler was fired and the esophagojejunostomy was completed

3. Linear stapler delta-shaped approach (Type C group): An endoscopic linear stapler divided the esophagogastric junction and made several small holes on the margin of the esophageal stump and the jejunum. The rear walls of the esophageal stump

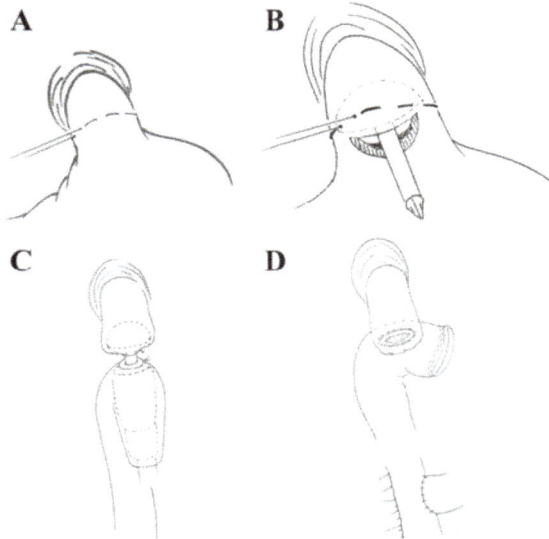

Fig. 2 Conventional circular stapler-anvil method (schematic diagram). **a** The purse-string suture (white arrow) was placed in the esophagus. **b** The anvil was introduced into the esophageal stump through the hole. **c** The circular stapler was introduced into the jejunum through the jejunal stump and attached with the anvil. **d** The circular stapler was fired and the esophagojejunostomy was completed

and the jejunum approached each other and were then connected by the endoscopic linear stapler (Figs. 5a and 6a). Subsequently, the staple line was examined for any potential faults and hemostasis was confirmed. The ordinary opening was pulled up with stay sutures (Figs. 5b and 6b), and was closed with two applications of the linear stapler (Figs. 5c and 6c), leading to the reconstruction of the intracorporeal alimentary tract (Figs. 5d and 6d).

4. Hand-sewn end-to-side approach (Type D group): The jejunal loop was introduced to approach the esophageal stump. The jejunum was attached to the esophageal stump with several serosal muscularis interrupted sutures, which are located at the rear part of the esophageal stump (Figs. 7a and 8a). During this process, one hole was made on the anti-mesenteric side of the jejunum and the other hole was made on the esophageal stump (Fig. 8b). Several full-thickness continuous sutures were used to sew up the posterior wall (Figs. 7b and 8c). Then, a full-thickness continuous suture closed the anterior wall (Figs. 7c and 8d). Interrupted sutures reinforced the seromuscular layer in order to reduce pressure. (Fig. 7d).

Postoperative management

All of the patients stayed in the general ward after surgery. The nasogastric tube was removed at the end of the case in the operating room. Before patients could tolerate a liquid diet, they relied on total parenteral

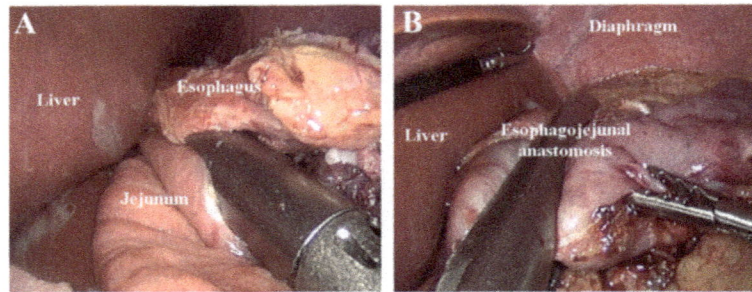

Fig. 3 Linear stapler side-to-side method. **a** Each jaw of the linear stapler was inserted into the holes on the esophageal stump and the jejunum and then the linear stapler was fired. **b** The entry hole and esophagus were closed using the stapler

nutrition (TPN). When patients were able to tolerate a liquid diet, they were gradually given a semiliquid diet. In order to be discharged from the hospital patients had to adapt to a semiliquid diet, have a normal blood work panel and temperature, and could not suffer from obvious discomfort. Follow-ups were conducted every 3 months for 2 years, every 6 months for the following 3 years. Most patient's regular follow-ups included a physical examination, laboratory tests (including CA19-9, CA72-4, and CEA levels), chest radiography, ultrasonography or CT, and endoscopy. All patients were checked on for the rest of their lives or until June 30, 2015, when the follow-up ends.

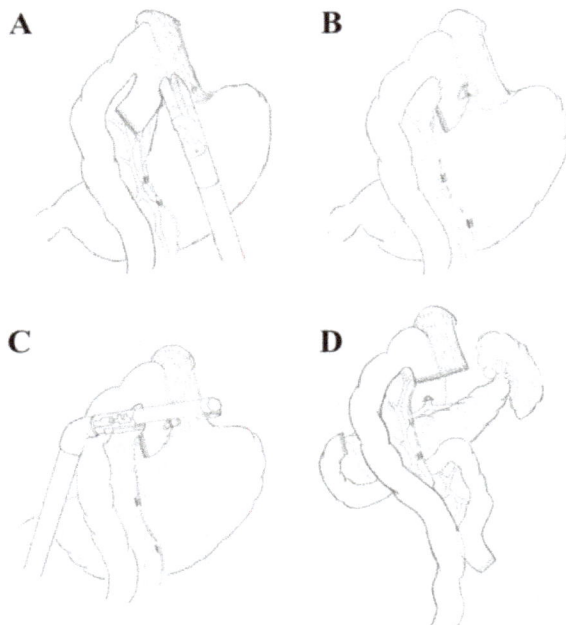

Fig. 4 Linear stapler side-to-side method (schematic diagram). **a** and **b** Each jaw of the linear stapler was inserted into the holes on the esophageal stump and the jejunum and then the linear stapler was fired. **c** and **d** The entry hole and esophagus were closed using the stapler

Statistical analysis
All statistical analyses were performed using the Statistical Package for the Social Sciences (SPSS®) version 18.0 (SPSS, Inc. Chicago, IL, United States). The differences in the measurement data were compared using the Student's t test, and comparisons between groups were tested using the $\chi 2$ test or the Fisher exact probability test. $P < 0.05$ was considered statistically significant.

Results
Comparison of the clinicopathologic characteristics
There was no conversion to an open procedure, and all procedures were completed under the given conditions. Demographics and clinicopathological characteristics are listed in Table 1. Of the 213 patients, 92 underwent TLTG, and 121 patients underwent LATG. There were no significant differences in age, gender, body mass index, the American Society of Anesthesiologists (ASA) physical status classification, presence of comorbid disease, or tumor stage.

Comparison of surgical and postoperative outcomes
The outcomes of the operative procedures and postoperative recovery are listed in Table 2. The mean operation time was similar (225.2 ± 41.5 min vs. 220.3 ± 43.5 min, $P = 0.40$) in both groups, but the estimated blood loss of TLTG was statistically lower than LATG (153.1 ± 57.3 mL vs. 132.3 ± 60.4 mL, $P = 0.01$). The proximal margin distance and number of retrieved lymph nodes were not significantly different between the two groups. The time to first flatus was similar between the groups (3.3 ± 1.1 d vs. 3.5 ± 1.1 d, $P = 0.19$), as was the time to restart oral intake after surgery (4.6 ± 1.2 d vs. 4.7 ± 1.3, $P = 0.56$). There was also no difference in the length of the hospital stay after surgery (9.7 ± 2.36 d vs. 9.5 ± 3.3, $P = 0.60$).

The postoperative complications are listed in Table 3. There was no in-hospital mortality and 30-d mortality. Complications developed in 23 (19.0 %) of patients in the LATG group and 16 (17.4 %) of patients in the

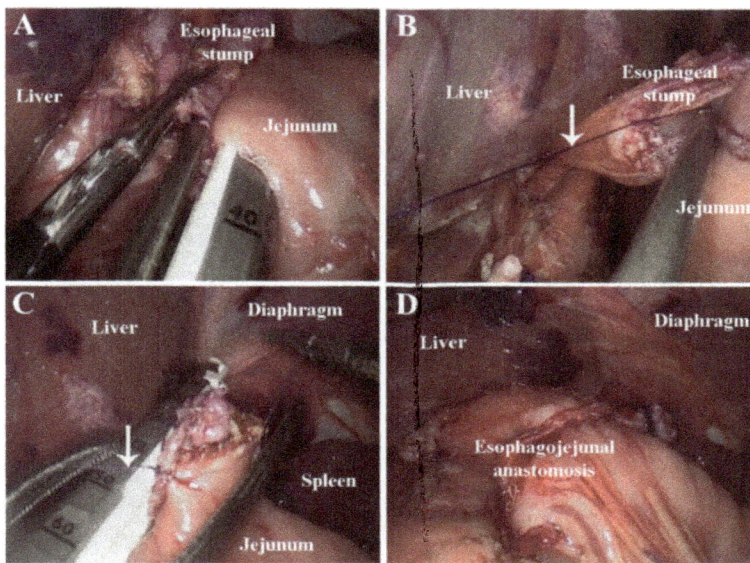

Fig. 5 Linear stapler delta-shaped method. **a** Small holes were created along the edge of the esophageal stump and the jejunum which were approximated and joined with the endoscopic linear stapler. **b** Stay sutures (white arrow) were placed to lift the common opening. **c** The common opening was then closed with two applications of the linear stapler. **d** Reconstruction of the intracorporeal alimentary tract was completed

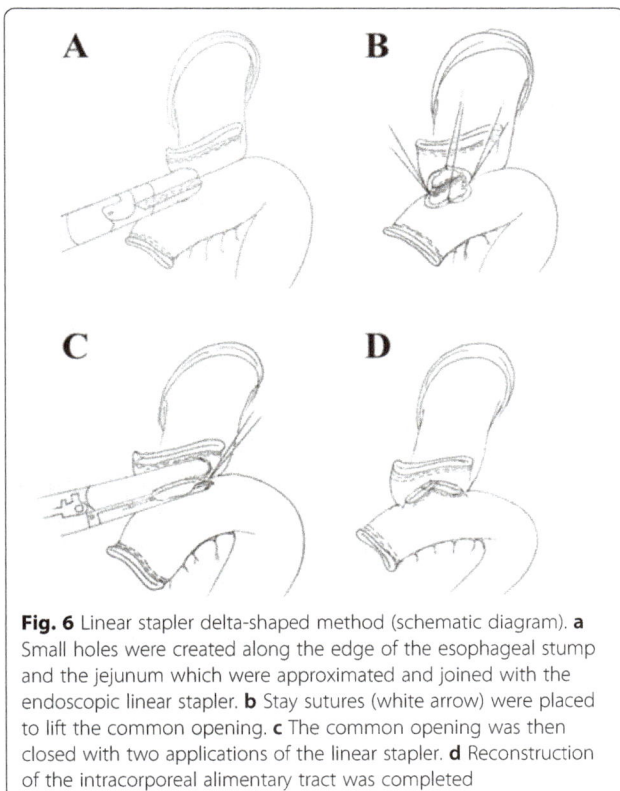

Fig. 6 Linear stapler delta-shaped method (schematic diagram). **a** Small holes were created along the edge of the esophageal stump and the jejunum which were approximated and joined with the endoscopic linear stapler. **b** Stay sutures (white arrow) were placed to lift the common opening. **c** The common opening was then closed with two applications of the linear stapler. **d** Reconstruction of the intracorporeal alimentary tract was completed

TLTG group. There was no significant difference between the two groups regarding the postoperative morbidity. One patient in the LATG group underwent reoperation due to anastomotic leakage. Three patients in the TLTG group underwent reoperation, one for anastomotic leakage, one for anastomotic stricture, and one for intracorporeal hemorrhage.

Subgroup analysis for patients who underwent TLTG
The types of anastomotic methods were type A in 18 patients, type B in 22 patients, type C in 10 patients and type D in 42 patients. The mean anastomotic time was 57.5 ± 18.5, 40.0 ± 11.2, 39.0 ± 3.9 and 60.7 ± 17.5 min for these four groups respectively. Intraoperative blood loss, number of retrieved lymph nodes, and postoperative recovery were similar among the four groups. Five patients in type A group, five in type B group, two in type C group, and four in type D group had postoperative morbidity. The operative findings and subsequent postoperative clinical course data are shown in Tables 4 and 5.

Discussion
Laparoscopic-assisted total gastrectomy (LATG) is the most common type of laparoscopic total gastrectomy (LTG), in which lymph nodes are removed with the aid of a laparoscope. Then in order to promote the resection of the specimen and the reconstruction of the digestive tract, an epigastrium assistant incision is created. Totally laparoscopic total gastrectomy (TLTG) is another type of LTG, without extra incisions or touching of the tumor. It reduces the traumatic stress of

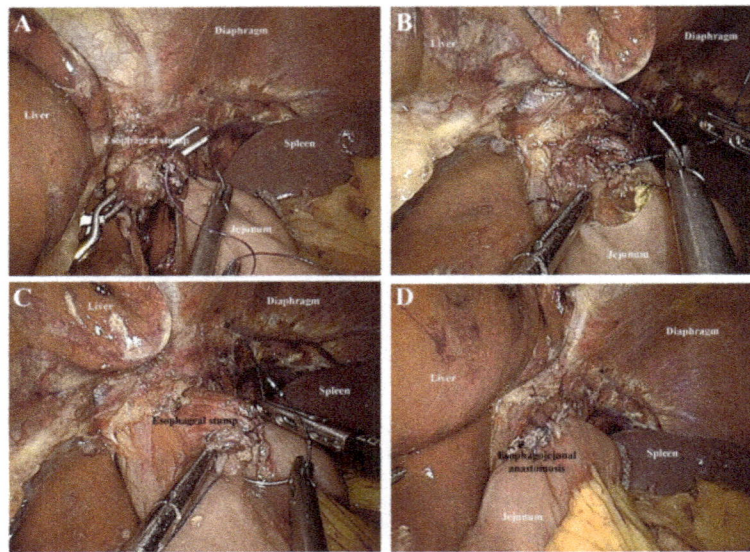

Fig. 7 Hand-sewn end-to-side method. **a**: The jejunum was anchored to the esophageal stump by several serosal muscularis interrupted sutures placed in the posterior layer of the esophageal stump. **b**: Several full-thickness interrupted sutures closed the posterior wall. **c**: A full-thickness continuous suture carried out the closure of the anterior wall. **d**: The seromuscular layer was strengthened with interrupted sutures to reduce tension

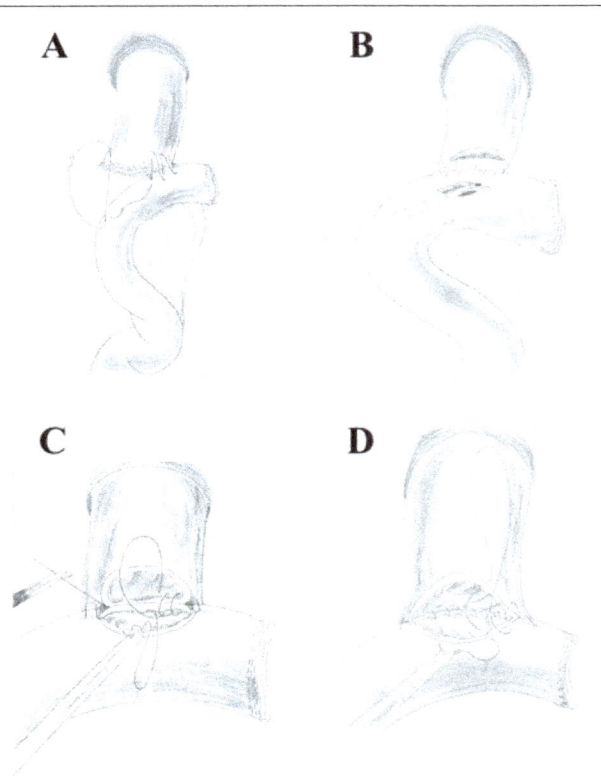

Fig. 8 Hand-sewn end-to-side method (schematic diagram). **a** The jejunum was anchored to the esophageal stump by several serosal muscularis interrupted sutures placed in the posterior layer of the esophageal stump. **b** Make an incision in the esophagus and jejunum stump respectively. **c** Several full-thickness interrupted sutures closed the posterior wall. **d** A full-thickness continuous suture carried out the closure of the anterior wall

surgical patients, as it only involves trocar wounds. In the beginning we wished to overcome the drawbacks of cumbersome reconstruction by adopting extracorporeal anastomosis. In 2007, we thought we could improve the surgery procedure, so we started to perform intracorporeal anastomosis followed by LTG. The security and feasibility of both TLTG and LATG in the treatment of gastric cancer located in upper and middle stomach are verified by the research.

LATG is the most commonly used version of LTG. Compared to traditional open gastrectomy, most studies have reported that LATG can achieve better cosmesis, shorter hospital stays and faster postoperative recovery [15–18]. Because the reconstruction step of TLTG is tricky, operating safety is a continuing worry for surgeons. In our study, the operation time of TLTG was slightly shorter than that of LATG and the intraoperative blood loss of the TLTG group was less than that in the LATG group. Those differences might have been due to the time required for mini-laparotomy, which is time-consuming. Also, anastomosis through small skin incisions created by hand manipulation may increase blood loss. However, considering that LATG was performed during the early period of the surgeon's experience and TLTG was performed during the late period, this time difference appears to be acceptable. Our results also revealed that the overall complications were similar between the two groups. Thus, we believe laparoscopic surgeons with ample experience could be able to achieve a safe and effective digestive tract reconstruction using the TLTG method with a complication rate comparable to that observed with LATG.

Table 1 Comparison of the clinicopathological characteristics

		LATG (n = 121)	TLTG (n = 92)	P value
Age (years)		59.8 ± 11.3	58.7 ± 10.7	0.47
Gender	Male	88	62	0.40
	Female	33	30	
BMI index (kg/m²)		22.8 ± 3.1	23.0 ± 3.2	0.65
Comorbidity	Absence	80	65	0.48
	Presence	41	27	
ASA classification	I	63	54	0.49
	II	53	33	
	III	5	5	
Tumor size (cm)		3.4 ± 1.7	3.7 ± 1.9	0.23
Histology	Differentiated	70	59	0.35
	Undifferentiated	51	33	
TNM stage	IA/IB	51/23	25/21	0.25
	IIA/IIB	15/7	12/11	
	IIIA/IIIB/IIIC	7/8/10	12/5/6	

According to our experience, TLTG is different from LATG in many ways. First of all, intracorporeal reconstruction adopting endoscopic staplers or hand-sewing techniques can achieve a tension-free anastomosis and reduce unnecessary damage to the surrounding tissue. Secondly, TLTG can be described as a "no touch tumor" operation. It avoids the direct contact and extrusion of tumors. The advantages of this method are that it decreases or avoids stimulation of the lesion and conforms to the principles of tumor-free technique and non-touch radical excision of gastric cancer. Thirdly, TLTG requires a small incision instead of the minilaparotomy. In the case of LATG, there is always an auxiliary 6–7 cm incision under the xiphoid. For obese patients, the incision may be as long as 8–10 cm. By contrast, in the case of TLTG, with the soft hypogastrium wall, the physician can simply broaden the incision for the 10 mm trocar under the umbilicus to a 3–4 cm semicircle incision near the navel so that the sample can be extracted in an appropriate way. On the one hand, the smaller incisions would be less traumatic and less invasive, on the other hand, it avoids the difficulty in reconstruction of anastomosis due to limited operation field especially for obese patients [19].

In our study, we have adopted two methods of IE, including mechanical staples and the hand-sewn suture technique. However, the mechanical anastomosis presented many technical problems including exposure difficulties, impossible reinforced suturing variation in the diameter of the esophagus, and a weak point in double stapling [20, 21]. Due to the technical difficulties of laparoscopic anastomosis and concern regarding

Table 2 Comparison of surgical outcomes and postoperative recovery

	LATG (n = 121)	TLTG (n = 92)	P value
Operation time (min)	225.2 ± 41.5	220.3 ± 43.5	0.40
Blood loss (mL)	153.1 ± 57.3	132.3 ± 60.4	0.01
Number of retrieved lymph nodes	28.7 ± 7.5	29.9 ± 7.6	0.25
Proximal resection margin (cm)	4.6 ± 1.4	4.9 ± 1.5	0.13
Time to first flatus (days)	3.3 ± 1.1	3.5 ± 1.1	0.19
Time to starting oral intake (days)	4.6 ± 1.2	4.7 ± 1.3	0.56
Postoperative hospital stay (days)	9.7 ± 2.3	9.5 ± 3.3	0.60

Table 3 Comparison of postoperative complications

Variable	LATG (n = 121)	TLTG (n = 92)	P value
Total complication	23	16	0.76
Anastomotic leakage	1	1	1.00
Anastomotic stricture	2	3	0.65
Intracorporeal hemorrhage	1	2	0.58
Abdominal abscess	4	1	0.39
Pulmonary infection	3	1	0.64
Stasis	3	2	1.00
Pancreatic leakage	2	1	1.00
Ileus	3	1	0.64
Lymphorrhea	1	1	1.00
Wound infection	3	1	0.64
Pulmonary embolism	0	1	0.43
Reoperation	1	3	0.32
Mortality	0	0	

Table 4 Surgical outcomes of 92 patients who underwent TLTG

	Type A (n = 18)	Type B (n = 22)	Type C (n = 10)	Type D (n =42)	Total (n = 92)
Operation time (min)	305.6 ± 45.9 (250–380)	266.8 ± 38.7 (230–360)	278.0 ± 16.2 (250–300)	285.4 ± 36.1 (240–420)	279.5 ± 38.4 (230–420)
Anastomotic time (min)	57.5 ± 18.5 (35–90)	40.0 ± 11.2 (25–60)	39.0 ± 3.9 (35–45)	60.7 ± 17.5 (45–105)	52.6 ± 18.9 (25–105)
Blood loss (mL)	80.6 ± 29.4 (50–160)	86.4 ± 39.7 (50–200)	87.0 ± 24.5 (50–120)	82.6 ± 33.7 (50–180)	83.1 ± 33.2 (50–200)
Retrieved lymph nodes	30.9 ± 5.8 (25–45)	34.6 ± 4.1 (25–42)	34.8 ± 6.1 (28–47)	36.1 ± 13.7 (24–69)	35.6 ± 8.9 (24–69)
First flatus (day)	4.2 ± 0.8 (3–5)	3.6 ± 1.3 (2–7)	3.4 ± 0.8 (2–5)	3.5 ± 0.7 (2–5)	3.7 ± 0.9 (2–7)
Liquid diet (days)	5.2 ± 0.8 (4–6)	4.9 ± 1.1 (3–7)	4.6 ± 0.7 (4–6)	4.5 ± 0.9 (3–7)	4.8 ± 0.9 (3–7)
Soft diet (days)	6.7 ± 1.3 (5–11)	6.3 ± 1.1 (5–8)	6.6 ± 0.8 (5–8)	6.5 ± 2.0 (5–15)	6.6 ± 1.5 (5–15)
Postoperative hospital stay (days)	10.9 ± 2.9 (9–20)	10.2 ± 2.4 (8–17)	10.1 ± 2.9 (8–18)	9.2 ± 1.5 (7–17)	10.0 ± 2.3 (7–20)

Data are means ± standard deviations (range)

anastomotic complications using the stapling method, we were encouraged to use the intracorporeal hand-sewn end-to-side esophagojejunostomy. In our study, 42 patients underwent the intracorporeal hand-sewn esophagojejunostomy. For this subgroup the mean operation time is 285.4 min with a mean blood loss of 82.6 ml. The time to the first flatus and oral intake were 3.5 days and 4.8 days, and the mean postoperative hospital stay was 10.0 days. A recent literature review provided the surgical results of TLTG [22]. The mean surgical time and mean blood loss were 254.2 min and 114.0 ml. The time to the first flatus and time to restart oral intake were 3.3 days and 5.0 days, and the mean postoperative hospital stay was 12.0 days. From the comparison and our acceptable results of mortality and complication rate, the fact that the intracorporeal hand-sewn esophagojejunostomy after TLTG is safe and feasible has been verified. However, when using hand-sewn method, the surgeon has to be skilled at laparoscopic suture technique and the operation tends to take a long time. Our experience indicates that progressive practice can effectively shorten the learning time. For example, surgeons can first practice on the simulator, then practice on animal models and simple suture under laparoscopy and turn to laparoscopic gastrointestinal anastomosis in the end. In the meantime, intracorporeal hand-sewn suture can be simplified with certain novel laparoscopic tools. Knotless barbed sutures (V-Loc™; Covidien Mansfield, MA, USA) can reduce the time of anastomosis and guarantee the security of anastomosis, without involving permanent traction during the entire anastomosis procedure.

Conclusion

In conclusion, TLTG with intracorporeal anastomosis is a secure and feasible method for the treatment of gastric cancer. With improved cosmesis, less blood loss and rapid recovery, TLTG generates favorable effects. Surgeons choose certain intracorporeal methods according to their preference and experience. Hand-sewn end-to-side esophagojejunostomy is an optimal intracorporeal anastomosis approach.

Table 5 Postoperative complication of 92 patients who underwent TLTG

	Type A (n = 18)	Type B (n = 22)	Type C (n = 10)	Type D (n =42)	Total (n = 92)
Postoperative complication	5	5	2	4	16
anastomotic leakage	1				
anastomosis stricture	1	2			
intracorporeal hemorrhage		1	1	1	
stasis	1		1		
lymphorrhea	1				
pulmonary embolism	1				
abdominal abscess		1			
pulmonary infection		1			
ileus				1	
pancreatic leakage					1
wound infection					1

Abbreviations

ASA: American Society of Anesthesiologists.; BMI: body mass index; EE: extracorporeal esophagojejunostomy; IE: intracorporeal esophagojejunostomy; LATG: laparoscopy-assisted total gastrectomy; LTG: laparoscopic total gastrectomy; TLTG: totally laparoscopic total gastrectomy; TNM: tumor-node-metastasis; TPN: total parenteral nutrition.

Competing interests

The authors declare that they have no competing interests.

Authors' contributions

Y-PM, KC, and J-FY performed the operation. YP, DW, and J-QC wrote the manuscript. J-QC, YH and D-WC collected data. HM polished the English language. Y-PM proofread and revised the manuscript. All authors read and approved the final manuscript.

Acknowledgements

This work was supported by grants of Natural Science Foundation of Zhejiang Province (No. LY12H16026); Department of education of Zhejiang Province (No. Y201326835); and Chinese Medical Technology Foundation of Zhejiang Province (No. 2012ZA087), China.

References

1. Jemal A, Bray F, Center MM, Ferlay J, Ward E, Forman D. Global cancer statistics. CA Cancer J Clin. 2011;61:69–90.
2. Bertuccio P, Chatenoud L, Levi F, Praud D, Ferlay J, Negri E, Malvezzi M, La Vecchia C. Recent patterns in gastric cancer: a global overview. Int J Cancer. 2009;125:666–73.
3. Kitano S, Iso Y, Moriyama M, Sugimachi K. Laparoscopy-assisted Billroth I gastrectomy. Surg Laparosc Endosc. 1994;4:146–8.
4. Kim JJ, Song KY, Chin HM, Kim W, Jeon HM, Park CH, Park SM. Totally laparoscopic gastrectomy with various types of intracorporeal anastomosis using laparoscopic linear staplers: preliminary experience. Surg Endosc. 2008;22:436–42.
5. Bouras G, Lee SW, Nomura E, Tokuhara T, Nitta T, Yoshinaka R, Tsunemi S, Tanigawa N. Surgical outcomes from laparoscopic distal gastrectomy and Roux-en-Y reconstruction: evolution in a totally intracorporeal technique. Surg Laparosc Endosc Percutan Tech. 2011;21:37–41.
6. Bracale U, Rovani M, Bracale M, Pignata G, Corcione F, Pecchia L. Totally laparoscopic gastrectomy for gastric cancer: meta-analysis of short-term outcomes. Minim Invasive Ther Allied Technol. 2012;21:150–60.
7. Chen K, Xu X, Mou Y, Pan Y, Zhang R, Zhou Y, Wu D, Huang C. Totally laparoscopic distal gastrectomy with D_2 lymphadenectomy and Billroth II gastrojejunostomy for gastric cancer: short- and medium-term results of 139 consecutive cases from a single institution. Int J Med Sci. 2013;10:1462–70.
8. Chen K, Mou YP, Xu XW, Pan Y, Zhou YC, Cai JQ, Huang CJ. Comparison of short-term surgical outcomes between totally laparoscopic and laparoscopic-assisted distal gastrectomy for gastric cancer: a 10-y single-center experience with meta-analysis. J Surg Res. 2015;194:367–74.
9. Chen K, Mou YP, Xu XW, Cai JQ, Wu D, Pan Y, Zhang RC. Short-term surgical and long-term survival outcomes after laparoscopic distal gastrectomy with D_2 lymphadenectomy for gastric cancer. BMC Gastroenterol. 2014;14:41.
10. Xu X, Chen K, Zhou W, Zhang R, Wang J, Wu D, Mou Y. Laparoscopic transgastric resection of gastric submucosal tumors located near the esophagogastric junction. J Gastrointest Surg. 2013;17:1570–9.
11. Pan Y, Mou YP, Chen K, Xu XW, Cai JQ, Wu D, Zhou YC. Three cases of laparoscopic total gastrectomy with intracorporeal esophagojejunostomy for gastric cancer in remnant stomach. World J Surg Oncol. 2014;12:342.
12. Cai J, Mou YP, Pan Y, Chen K, Xu XW, Zhou Y. Immunoglobulin G4-associated cholangitis mimicking cholangiocarcinoma treated by laparoscopic choledochectomy with intracorporeal Roux-en-Y hepaticojejunostomy. World J Surg Oncol. 2014;12:363.
13. Cai JQ, Chen K, Mou YP, Pan Y, Xu XW, Zhou YC, Huang CJ. Laparoscopic versus open wedge resection for gastrointestinal stromal tumors of the stomach: a single-center 8-year retrospective cohort study of 156 patients with long-term follow-up. BMC Surg. 2015;15:58.
14. Yan JF, Xu XW, Jin WW, Huang CJ, Chen K, Zhang RC, Harsha A, Mou YP. Laparoscopic spleen-preserving distal pancreatectomy for pancreatic neoplasms: a retrospective study. World J Gastroenterol. 2014;20:13966–72.
15. Kim KH, Kim YM, Kim MC, Jung GJ. Is laparoscopy-assisted total gastrectomy feasible for the treatment of gastric cancer? A case-matched study. Dig Surg. 2013;30:348–54.
16. Lee SR, Kim HO, Son BH, Shin JH, Yoo CH. Laparoscopic-assisted total gastrectomy versus open total gastrectomy for upper and middle gastric cancer in short-term and long-term outcomes. Surg Laparosc Endosc Percutan Tech. 2014;24:277–82.
17. Lu J, Huang CM, Zheng CH, Li P, Xie JW, Wang JB, Lin JX, Chen QY, Cao LL, Lin M. Short- and long-term outcomes after laparoscopic versus open total gastrectomy for elderly gastric cancer patients: a propensity score-matched analysis. J Gastrointest Surg. 2015;19:1949–57.
18. Chen K, Xu XW, Zhang RC, Pan Y, Wu D, Mou YP. Systematic review and meta-analysis of laparoscopy-assisted and open total gastrectomy for gastric cancer. World J Gastroenterol. 2013;19:5365–76.
19. Kim MG, Kawada H, Kim BS, Kim TH, Kim KC, Yook JH, Kim BS. A totally laparoscopic distal gastrectomy with gastroduodenostomy (TLDG) for improvement of the early surgical outcomes in high BMI patients. Surg Endosc. 2011;25:1076–82.
20. Offodile 2nd AC, Feingold DL, Nasar A, Whelan RL, Arnell TD. High incidence of technical errors involving the EEA circular stapler: a single institution experience. J Am Coll Surg. 2010;210:331–5.
21. Marangoni G, Villa F, Shamil E, Botha AJ. OrVil™-assisted anastomosis in laparoscopic upper gastrointestinal surgery: friend of the laparoscopic surgeon. Surg Endosc. 2012;26:811–7.
22. Umemura A, Koeda K, Sasaki A, Fujiwara H, Kimura Y, Iwaya T, Akiyama Y, Wakabayashi G. Totally laparoscopic total gastrectomy for gastric cancer: literature review and comparison of the procedure of esophagojejunostomy. Asian J Surg. 2015;38:102–12.

30

Metachronous solitary splenic metastasis arising from early gastric cancer: a case report and literature review

Tsutomu Namikawa[1*], Yasuhiro Kawanishi[1], Kazune Fujisawa[2], Eri Munekage[1], Masaya Munekage[1], Takahito Sugase[1], Hiromichi Maeda[3], Hiroyuki Kitagawa[1], Tatsuya Kumon[4], Makoto Hiroi[2], Michiya Kobayashi[3,5] and Kazuhiro Hanazaki[1]

Abstract

Background: The metastasis of malignant tumors to the spleen is rare, and only a small percentage of cases can be treated surgically, as splenic metastases generally occur in the context of multivisceral metastatic cancer at a terminal stage. We report a rare case of metachronous solitary splenic metastasis arising from early gastric cancer.

Case presentation: A 75-year-old man was initially referred to our hospital for examination of gastric cancer, diagnosed at a medical check-up. Esophagogastroduodenoscopy showed a slightly elevated lesion with a central irregular depression in the upper-third of the stomach. Biopsy specimens of the lesion showed a moderately-differentiated adenocarcinoma, and abdominal computed tomography showed no evidence of distant metastases. Endoscopic submucosal dissection was performed, with histological confirmation of a moderately-differentiated adenocarcinoma invading the submucosal layer. The patient subsequently underwent laparoscopic total gastrectomy with regional lymph node dissection, resulting in no residual carcinoma and no lymph node metastasis. Computed tomography, 28 months later, showed a well-defined mass measuring 4.2 cm in diameter in the spleen, and the patient underwent a splenectomy, since there was no evidence of further metastatic lesions in any other organs. Histological examination confirmed the diagnosis of a poorly-differentiated adenocarcinoma originating from the previous gastric cancer. The patient was alive 2 months after surgical resection of the splenic metastasis without any recurrence.

Conclusion: To the best of our knowledge, this is only the second case of a solitary splenic metastasis from early gastric cancer to be reported in the English literature. The present case suggests surgical resection may be the preferred treatment of choice for patients with a solitary splenic metastasis from gastric cancer.

Keywords: Gastric cancer, Splenic metastasis, Gastrectomy, Solitary metastasis, Splenectomy

Background

The splenic metastasis arising from other malignancies is rare disease, which surgical treatment is often difficult due to presentation as multivisceral metastatic status in an advance progressed stage [1]. Previous literature demonstrated that the incidence of splenic metastasis from other solid malignancies including sarcoma or carcinoma was only 1.3% in a series of 1280 splenectomies

[2]. Although splenic metastasis may originate from various organs, it has been reported that the most common primary organs of splenic metastases are breast, lung, colorectal, and ovarian carcinomas [3]. On the other hand, early gastric cancer (EGC) defined as a lesion confined to the mucosa or submucosa, independent of the lymph node metastasis, has favorable outcomes without hematogenous recurrence by the optimal surgical treatment [4].

In this report, we describe the case of a 77-year-old man who presented 28 months after gastrectomy for EGC, with a solitary splenic metastasis which was

* Correspondence: tsutomun@kochi-u.ac.jp
[1]Department of Surgery, Kochi Medical School, Kohasu, Oko-cho, Nankoku, Kochi 783-8505, Japan
Full list of author information is available at the end of the article

successfully treated by a splenectomy. The clinical characteristics of previously reported cases are also discussed.

Case presentation

A 75-year-old Japanese man was referred to our hospital for further examination of gastric cancer diagnosed at a medical check-up. His past medical history revealed that he had undergone endoscopic submucosal dissection (ESD) 2 years earlier for EGC confined to the mucosa. On admission, his laboratory results, as well as serum carcinoembryonic antigen and cancer antigen 19–9 were almost within normal limits. Esophagogastroduodenoscopy revealed an elevated lesion with a central irregular depression in the upper-third of the stomach, measuring 2.2 cm, which proved to be a well-differentiated adenocarcinoma on biopsy (Fig. 1).

Abdominal computed tomography (CT) showed no evidence of distant metastases and we performed ESD under a clinical diagnosis of EGC. The histological findings showed a well-differentiated adenocarcinoma coexisting with a solid-type poorly-differentiated adenocarcinoma, invading the submucosal layer more than 2 mm (Fig. 2). Therefore, in accordance with Japanese gastric cancer treatment guidelines [5], the patient subsequently underwent laparoscopic total gastrectomy with regional lymph node dissection, resulting in no residual carcinoma, lymph node metastasis, or lymphovenous invasion. The postoperative course was uneventful, and he was discharged on postoperative day 14.

The patient underwent periodic follow-up physical examinations, which were blood tests and CT performed every 6 months. At 28 months after the operation, abdominal CT revealed a well-defined mass measuring

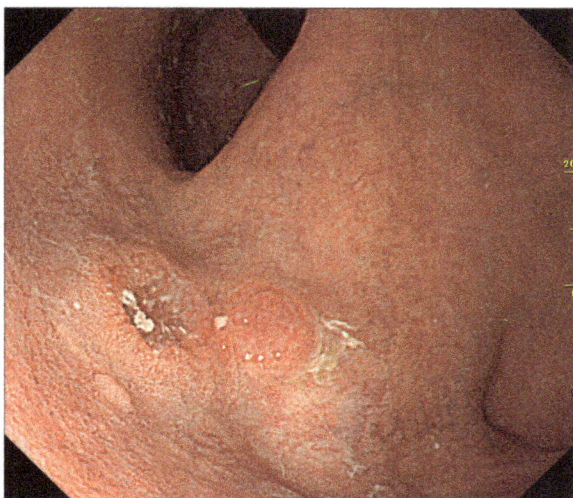

Fig. 2 Histological examination of the resected specimen by endoscopic submucosal dissection showing a well-differentiated adenocarcinoma coexisting with a solid-type poorly-differentiated adenocarcinoma. Stained with hematoxylin and eosin

4.2 cm in diameter in the spleen (Fig. 3, *arrow*). ^{18}F-2-deoxy-2-fluoro-glucose (FDG) positron emission tomography combined with CT imaging showed intense FDG uptake in the splenic mass, with a maximum standardized uptake value of 6.1 (Fig. 4, *arrow*). As there was no evidence of further metastatic lesions in any other organs, a splenectomy was performed. The gross appearance of the surgically-resected specimen showed a discolored surface to the spleen with a slightly irregular surface caused by the tumor (Fig. 5a, *arrow*). On cross-section, the specimen showed a well-circumscribed, solid tumor measuring 5.5 × 4.5 cm in diameter (Fig. 5b).

Histological examination confirmed the diagnosis of a solid-type poorly-differentiated adenocarcinoma, consistent with the features of the primary gastric cancer. The tumor was in the splenic parenchyma and was totally covered with splenic peritoneum (Fig. 6). The results of

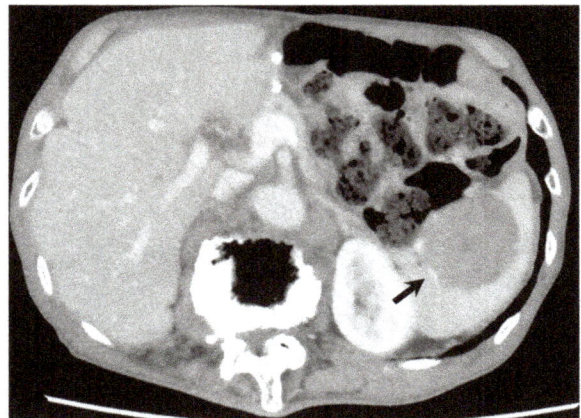

Fig. 1 Esophagogastroduodenoscopy showing a slightly elevated lesion with central depressed area in the upper-third of the stomach

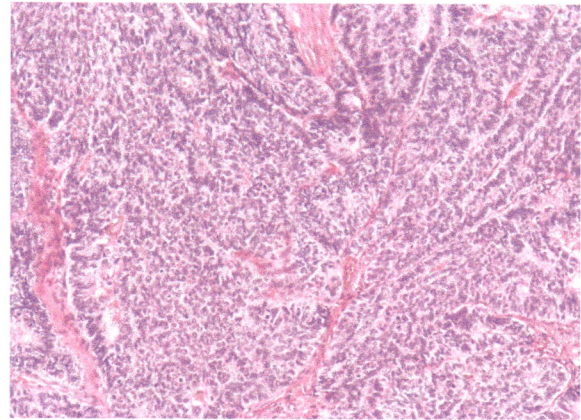

Fig. 3 Abdominal computed tomography showing a well-defined mass in the spleen measuring 4 cm in diameter (*arrow*)

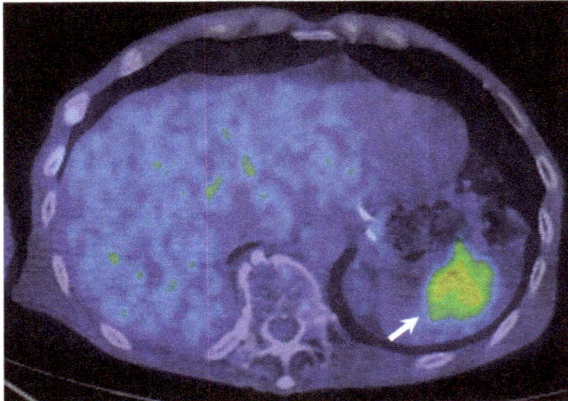

Fig. 4 ^{18}F-2-deoxy-2-fluoro-glucose (FDG) positron emission tomography combined with computed tomography imaging showing the splenic mass with intense FDG uptake *(arrow)*

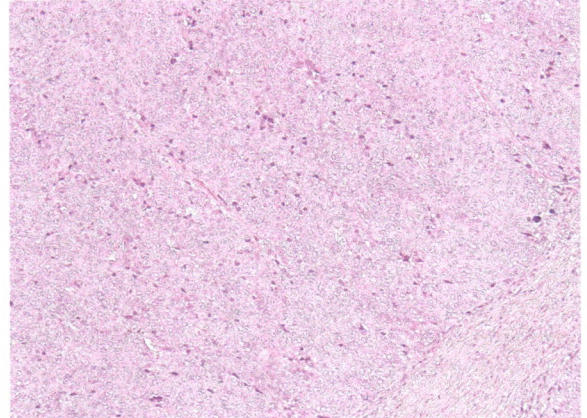

Fig. 6 Histological examination of the resected specimen demonstrating a solid-type poorly-differentiated adenocarcinoma originating from the previous gastric cancer. Stained with hematoxylin and eosin

immunohistochemical investigations of both the primary early gastric cancer and the splenic tumor showed negative immunostaining for chromogranin A, synaptophysin, MUC1, MUC2, MUC5AC, and MUC6. No tumor cells were detected in the lymph nodes of the splenic hilum, and there was no reactivity for human epidermal growth factor receptor 2 in either the primary gastric cancer or splenic metastasis. The postoperative course was uneventful, and the patient has been well without evidence of recurrence for 2 months following the splenectomy.

Discussion and conclusions

This report describes the rare case of a patient with a solitary splenic metastasis arising from EGC, treated by splenectomy. A search of English language publications between 2000 and 2016 was conducted using the

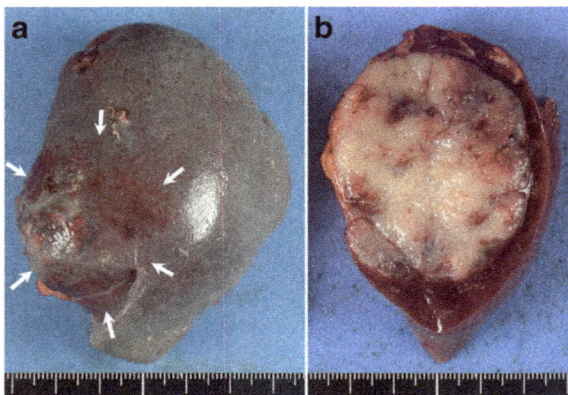

Fig. 5 Gross examination of the surgically resected specimen showing a discolored surface to the spleen caused by the tumor (**a**, *arrows*), which is a well-circumscribed solid tumor measuring 4.2 cm (**b**)

Medline and PubMed databases for articles on splenic metastases from gastric cancer, with the keywords "gastric cancer" and "splenic metastasis". Data on age, gender, tumor location, tumor size, depth of invasion, histological type, treatment, and outcome for each reported case were obtained. To the best of our knowledge, this is only the fourth case of a solitary splenic metastasis arising from gastric cancer, and the second case arising from EGC to be reported in the English literature.

The clinicopathological features of the three previously reported cases [6–8] and the present case are listed in Table 1. The median age of these four patients was 70 years (range, 49–75 years), and all patients were male. Gastric cancer was reported in the upper-third of the stomach in two patients (both EGC), while one patient had a lesion in the middle-third of the stomach, and one had a lesion in the lower-third of the stomach (both advanced gastric cancer).

Treatment consisted of total gastrectomy in one patient, distal gastrectomy in two patients, and proximal gastrectomy in one patient. The two patients with EGC were initially treated endoscopically, such as by endoscopic mucosal resection or ESD. The median tumor size of the primary gastric cancer was 2.2 cm (range, 2.0–6.0 cm), and histological analysis of the gastric tumors revealed intestinal-type carcinomas in all four cases. Regional lymph node metastasis was detected in both cases of advanced gastric cancer and in one case of EGC. The median duration between the initial gastrectomy and the appearance of the splenic metastasis was 39 months (range, 14–60 months). All the patients were treated by surgical resection for the splenic metastasis, and the median tumor size of the splenic metastasis was 6.0 cm (range, 4.5–14 cm). One patient who was initially

Table 1 Clinicopathological data from reported cases of solitary splenic metastasis arising from gastric cancer

| Author | Age | Gender | Primary gastric cancer | | | | | | | Splenic metastasis | | | | Outcome |
			Tumor location	Tumor size (cm)	Gross appearance type	Tumor depth	Lymph node involvement	Histological type	Treatment	Tumor size (cm)	Treatment	Histological type	Duration (months)	
Yamanouchi [6]	65	Male	L	ND	Ulcerated	ss	Positive	Intestinal	DG	4.5	Splenectomy	Intestinal	50	DOD at 40 months
Kawasaki [7]	75	Male	U	2.0	Elevated	sm	Positive	Intestinal	EMR, PG	6.5	Chemotherapy, Splenectomy	Intestinal	14	2 years survival
Deng [8]	49	Male	M	6.0	ND	se	Positive	Intestinal	DG	14	Splenectomy	Diffuse	60	9 months survival
Present case	77	Male	U	2.2	Elevated	sm	Negative	Intestinal	ESD, TG	5.5	Splenectomy	Diffuse	28	2 months survival

Abbreviations: DG distal gastrectomy, *DOD* dead of disease, *EMR* endoscopic mucosal resection, *ESD* endoscopic submucosal dissection, *L* lower-third of the stomach, *M* middle-third of the stomach, *ND* not described, *PG* proximal gastrectomy, *se* serosa, *sm* submucosa, *ss* subserosa, *TG* total gastrectomy, *U* upper-third of the stomach

diagnosed with advanced gastric cancer died from multiple metastases to the liver and peritoneal dissemination 40 months later.

Both the patients with a solitary splenic metastasis arising from EGC were initially treated by endoscopic resection, but subsequently underwent radical gastrectomy with regional lymphadenectomy due to submucosal invasion of the tumor. Lymph node metastasis may contribute to the occurrence of splenic metastases, because it is reported to be the most important risk factor to occur the recurrence of EGC [4, 9, 10]. However, there was no lymph node metastasis or lymphovascular infiltration in our present case, while the previously reported case of EGC showed only one lymph node metastasis. It remains uncertain whether there is any association between initial endoscopic treatment for EGC and splenic metastases. Although a solitary splenic metastasis from gastric cancer is extremely rare, either synchronous or metachronous to the primary tumor, surgical resection might be the effective strategy to treat patients with a solitary splenic metastasis from EGC.

It is a quite difficult issue to diagnose whether the splenic mass lesion is a primary tumor or a metastatic tumor. The differential diagnosis of a splenic mass without the context of active cancerous disease would include a primary splenic lesion, such as lymphoma, hemangioma or lymphangioma. The clinical diagnosis of splenic metastases seems to be largely dependent on the previous history of malignant disease in the patients [8]. Therefore, a splenectomy in the case of a splenic metastasis makes sense, if the metastasis is isolated [1]. Although the reason for the rarity of splenic metastases arising from solid malignant tumors remains uncertain, even though the spleen is a hypervascular organ, the growth of an early blood-borne micrometastasis may contribute its occurrence [3].

A solitary splenic metastasis arising from EGC is extremely rare, as metastases to the spleen are usually found in conjunction with metastases to other organs. However, even in cases of EGC, a solitary metastasis to the spleen should not be discounted during the periodic follow-up examinations of patients with gastric cancer. When treating metastatic or recurrent gastric cancer, clinicians should always consider the adverse clinical effects and stress of surgical resection, however, a splenectomy might be a potentially effective treatment in the case of a solitary metastasis. Further studies and the assessment of additional cases are needed to establish standardized recommendations for the management of this rare entity.

Abbreviations
CT: Computed tomography; EGC: Early gastric cancer; ESD: Endoscopic submucosal dissection

Acknowledgements
We would like to acknowledge with gratitude the contribution of the colleagues of the department of Surgery, Kochi Medical School.

Funding
None.

Authors' contributions
TN and MK designed the study; TN, YK, KF, EM, MM, TS, HM, HK, TK, MH, MK and KH have been involved in drafting the manuscript and revising it critically for important intellectual content; TN and KH finalized the manuscript and submitted the paper for publication. All authors read and approved the final manuscript.

Competing interests
All of the authors have no potential conflicts of interest to disclose with respect to the research, authorship, and publication of this article. All authors received no financial support for the research, authorship, and publication of this article.

Author details
[1]Department of Surgery, Kochi Medical School, Kohasu, Oko-cho, Nankoku, Kochi 783-8505, Japan. [2]Department of Pathology, Kochi Medical School, Kochi, Japan. [3]Cancer Treatment Center, Kochi Medical School Hospital, Kochi, Japan. [4]Department of Surgery, Noichi Central Hospital, Kochi, Japan. [5]Department of Human Health and Sciences, Kochi Medical School, Kochi, Japan.

References
1. Sauer J, Sobolewski K, Dommisch K. Splenic metastases–not a frequent problem, but an underestimate location of metastases: epidemiology and course. J Cancer Res Clin Oncol. 2009;135(5):667–71.
2. Kraus MD, Fleming MD, Vonderheide RH. The spleen as a diagnostic specimen: a review of 10 years' experience at two tertiary care institutions. Cancer. 2001;91(11):2001–9.
3. Compérat E, Bardier-Dupas A, Camparo P, Capron F, Charlotte F. Splenic metastases: clinicopathologic presentation, differential diagnosis, and pathogenesis. Arch Pathol Lab Med. 2007;131(6):965–9.
4. Katai H, Sano T. Early gastric cancer: concepts, diagnosis, and management. Int J Clin Oncol. 2005;10(6):375–83.
5. Japanese Gastric Cancer Association. Japanese gastric cancer treatment guidelines 2014 (ver. 4). Gastric Cancer. 2017;20(1):1–19.
6. Yamanouchi K, Ikematsu Y, Waki S, Kida H, Nishiwaki Y, Gotoh K, Ozawa T, Uchimura M. Solitary splenic metastasis from gastric cancer: report of a case. Surg Today. 2002;32(12):1081–4.
7. Kawasaki H, Kitayama J, Ishigami H, Hidemura A, Kaisaki S, Nagawa H. Solitary splenic metastasis from early gastric cancer: report of a case. Surg Today. 2010;40(1):60–3.
8. Deng Z, Yin Z, Chen S, Peng Y, Wang F, Wang X. Metastatic splenic α-fetoprotein-producing adenocarcinoma: report of a case. Surg Today. 2011;41(6):854–8.
9. Okabayashi T, Kobayashi M, Nishimori I, Sugimoto T, Namikawa T, Onishi S, Hanazaki K. Clinicopathological features and medical management of early gastric cancer. Am J Surg. 2008;195(2):229–32.
10. Namikawa T, Kitagawa H, Iwabu J, Okabayashi T, Sugimoto T, Kobayashi M, Hanazaki K. Clinicopathological properties of the superficial spreading type early gastric cancer. J Gastrointest Surg. 2010;14(1):52–7.

31

Major postoperative complications are associated with impaired long-term survival after gastro-esophageal and pancreatic cancer surgery: a complete national cohort study

Eirik Kjus Aahlin[1,2*], Frank Olsen[3], Bård Uleberg[3], Bjarne K. Jacobsen[3,4] and Kristoffer Lassen[1,2]

Abstract

Background: Some studies have reported an association between complications and impaired long-term survival after cancer surgery. We aimed to investigate how major complications are associated with overall survival after gastro-esophageal and pancreatic cancer surgery in a complete national cohort.

Methods: All esophageal-, gastric- and pancreatic resections performed for cancer in Norway between January 1, 2008, and December 1, 2013 were identified in the Norwegian Patient Registry together with data concerning major postoperative complications and survival.

Results: When emergency cases were excluded, there were 1965 esophageal-, gastric- or pancreatic resections performed for cancer in Norway between 1 January 2008, and 1 December 2013. A total of 248 patients (12.6 %) suffered major postoperative complications. Complications were associated both with increased early (90 days) mortality (OR = 4.25, 95 % CI = 2.78–6.50), and reduced overall survival when patients suffering early mortality were excluded (HR = 1.23, 95 % CI = 1.01–1.50).

Conclusions: Major postoperative complications are associated with impaired long-term survival after gastro-esophageal and pancreatic cancer surgery.

Keywords: Postoperative complications, Surgery, Neoplasms

Background

Major complications after surgery have negative effects on health-related quality of life [1], length-of-stay [2] and resource utilization [2]. Major complications may preclude or delay adjuvant cancer treatment [3]. In addition, long-term survival may be negatively affected [4–7].

Khuri and co-workers [5] found that patients experiencing complications from surgery had a markedly reduced long-term survival even when those who died within 30 days after surgery were excluded from analysis. As summarized in a recent meta-analysis, these findings have been corroborated by several reports, but others again have failed to show this connection [6]. It has been suggested that major complications could have long-standing suppressive effects on a patient's immune system and thereby rendering them more susceptible to cancer recurrence [4, 5, 7–9].

Investigating a possible long-standing detrimental effect of postoperative complications on survival after cancer surgery is challenging: Major complications after modern surgery are relatively uncommon and therefore large cohorts are needed for analysis. There is no consensus on the correct cut-off for early mortality and there may be several factors that affect both susceptibility to complications and decreased overall survival - factors that have to

* Correspondence: eirik.kjus.aahlin@unn.no
[1]Department of GI and HPB surgery, University Hospital of Northern Norway, 9038 Breivika, Tromsø, Norway
[2]Department of Clinical Medicine, University of Tromsø - The Arctic University of Norway, Tromsø, Norway
Full list of author information is available at the end of the article

be adequately adjusted for. Naturally, an interventional trial is impossible to conduct.

Patient's level of education is a known indicator of important factors like physical activity and smoking habits [10], factors that are associated with both increased morbidity and impaired survival after surgery [11].

The aim of this study was to investigate whether major complications after gastro-esophageal and pancreatic surgery for cancer are associated with impaired long-term survival or early mortality only. We also aimed to investigate if such an association was influenced by patient's level of education.

Methods
Cohort identification
A database of surgical procedures, major postoperative complications and survival was extracted from the Norwegian Patient Registry (NPR). The Norwegian Patient Registry enables patients to be tracked from one stay to another, thus allowing for identification of an early complication occurring at a local hospital following transfer from a tertiary hospital where index surgery had been performed. All Norwegian hospitals must submit data to the Norwegian Patient Registry for registry and reimbursement purposes. In the present study, we included data from admissions during 2008–2013. Data on educational level were extracted from Statistics Norway, the Norwegian central bureau of statistics.

We identified all resections of the esophagus, stomach and pancreas in the six-year period from January 1, 2008 to December 1, 2013. Complications within 28 days after

surgery (to the end of 2013) are therefore included in the data material. Data on overall survival until June 30, 2014 were retrieved, thus even the last patient subject to surgery included would have seven months follow-up, if not dying. Operations and reoperations were identified from their Nomesco classification of Surgical Procedures (NCSP) code (2014). NCSP is available for download at http://www.nordclass.se/ncsp.htm.

Only cases with an appropriate cancer diagnosis (ICD-10: C15*, C16* and C25* respectively, where * denotes all sub-codes) applied within eight weeks from surgery were included. Emergency cases were excluded to obtain a cohort of patients that were reasonably fit at index surgery.

Overall survival was defined as survival from index surgery. Major complications were defined as equivalent to Accordion score IV or higher, equaling Clavien-Dindo score IIIb or higher [12, 13], i.e. a re-operation in general anesthesia for a complication, and/or single- or multiple organ failure [12]. We did not attempt to identify less severe complications, as these would be difficult to extract from Norwegian Patient Registry data.

All stays in this database (containing an eligible index operation) were coupled with any subsequent stay at any Norwegian hospital with an admission date within 28 days from discharge from the index stay. Hospital stays (single or coupled) containing one or more major complications were identified. This was done by identification of one of the following procedure codes at index or subsequent stay (NCSP): Reoperation for wound dehiscence (JWA00), for deep infection (JWC00/01), for deep hemorrhage (JWE00/01/02), for anastomotic dehiscence (JWF00/01), reoperation for other causes (JWW96/97/98)

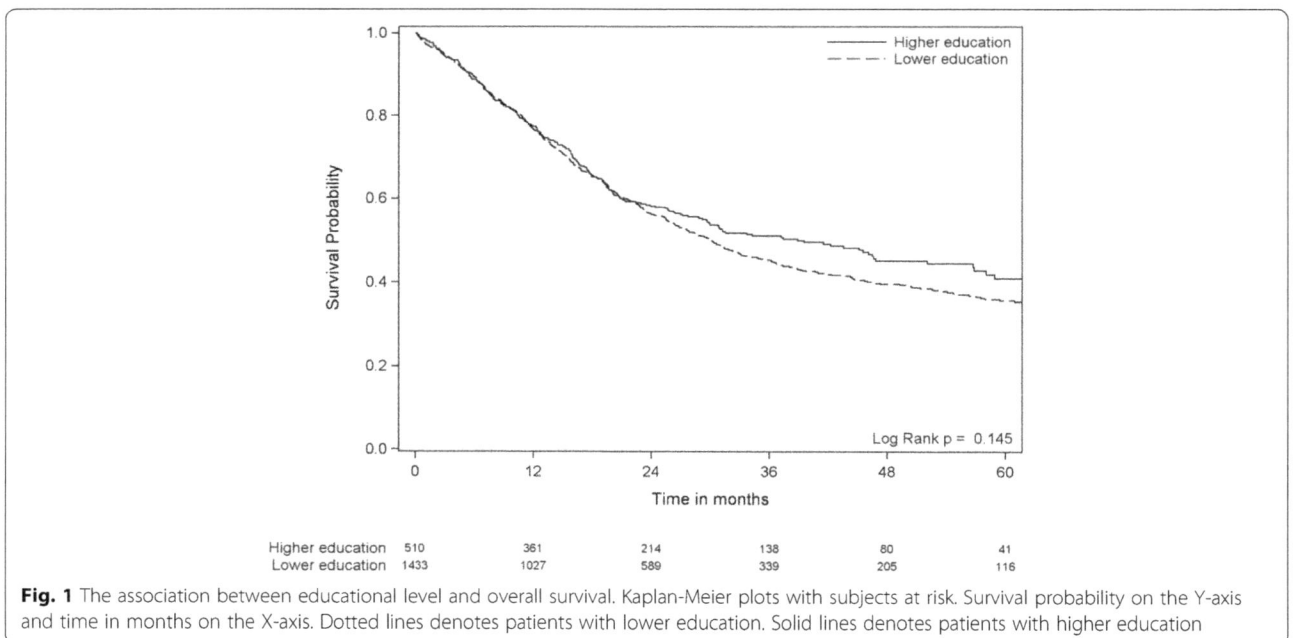

Fig. 1 The association between educational level and overall survival. Kaplan-Meier plots with subjects at risk. Survival probability on the Y-axis and time in months on the X-axis. Dotted lines denotes patients with lower education. Solid lines denotes patients with higher education

or if a tracheostomy was performed (GBB00/03). Also, a major complication was identified from the use of one of the following diagnoses during index or subsequent stays (ICD-10): Bleeding, hematoma or circulatory chock following a procedure (ICD-10: T81.0, T81.1, T81.3).

Validation of algorithm

The algorithms to identify complications were constructed in several wider variations and then validated against hand searched patient files. A tendency to over-score complications (identifying Accordion III or Clavien-Dindo IIIa as "major complications") when using the entire complications section (ICD-10: T81*) was avoided when some sub-codes (ICD-10: T81.2, T81.4, T81.5, T81.6, T81.7, T81.8 and T81.9) were removed from the algorithm. A comparison of the yield from our refined search strings with hand searched patient files in a four-year cohort at our own hospital (150 patients) showed a 100% match in both number of resections and rate of major complications (Accordion IV or higher).

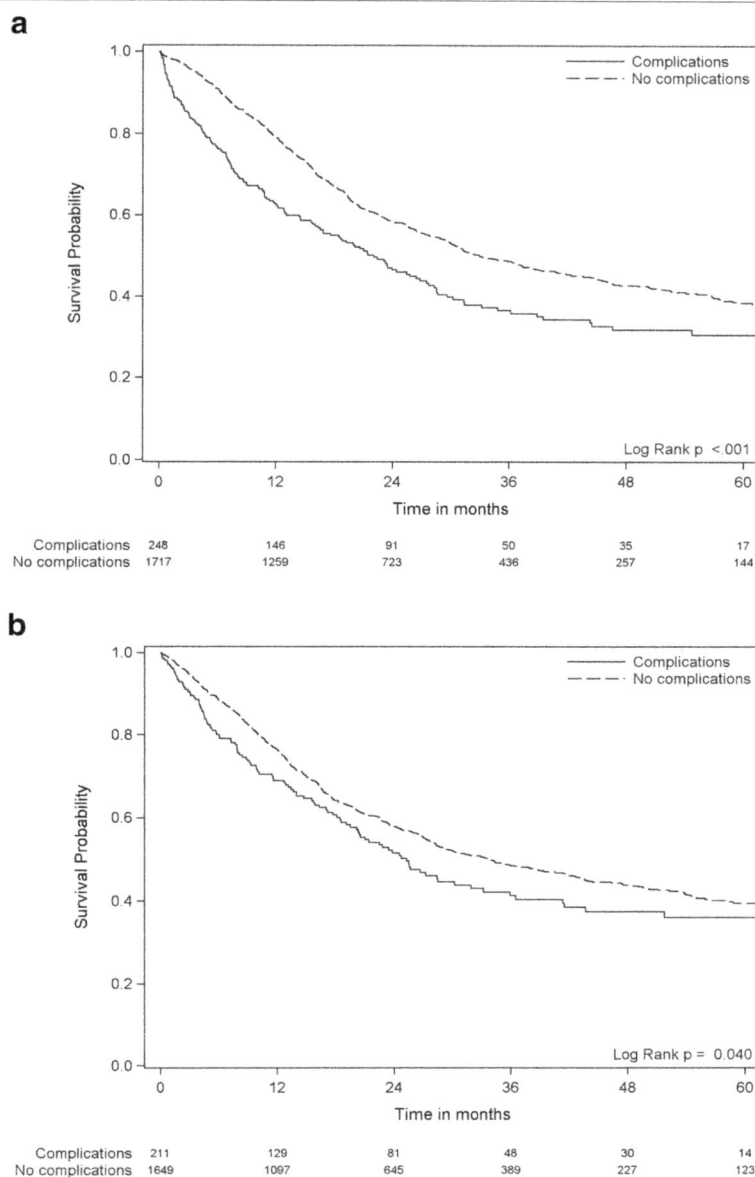

Fig. 2 The association between major postoperative complications and overall survival. Kaplan-Meier plots with subjects at risk. Survival probability on the Y-axis and time in months on the X-axis. Dotted lines denotes patients without any postoperative complications. Solid lines denotes patients who suffered one or more major postoperative complication. **a** All patients included. **b** Patients alive more than 90 days only

Table 1 Cohort characteristics: Number of patients, age, gender, educational level, percentage with complications and estimated median survival according to type of resection

	Esophageal resections	Gastric resections	Pancreatic resections	All patients
Number of patients	331	974	660	1965
Age above 65 years (%)	46.8	67.7	56.4	60.4
Male gender (%)	77.6	62.4	52.7	61.7
Lower educational level (%)	69.5	78.5	68.9	73.7
Complication-rate (%)	17.2	11.1	12.6	12.6
90-day mortality (%)	5.7	6.1	3.9	5.3
Estimated median survival in months	46	36	23	31

Definition of variables

Age at index surgery was analyzed both as a continuous variable and with a cut-off of 65 years. Educational level was divided into higher and lower education. Higher education was defined as education beyond primary and lower secondary school. Surgical resections were stratified into esophageal-, gastric- and pancreatic resections.

Statistics

Statistical analyses were performed with SAS statistics software, SAS Institute, Cary, NC, USA. For comparison of characteristics between different groups and categories, Student t-test for continuous data and Pearson chi-square test for categorical data were used. Logistic regression was used for analyzing associations between age, gender, educational level, type of resection and the risk of a major postoperative complication as well as early (90 days) mortality. Kaplan-Meier survival plots with log-rank test and Cox proportional hazard (PH) regression analysis were used for analysis of overall survival. Both methods were used, as the proportional hazards assumption for Cox regression (constant relative hazards over time) was not met when analyzing the relationships between educational level and survival (Fig. 1) and when analyzing the relationship between complications and survival (Fig. 2). Cox proportional hazard regression analysis using attained age as

the time variable was also used as a supplement, as the proportional hazards assumption was met in this situation. P-values according to the log-rank-test are given in the figures (the Kaplan-Meier survival plots) whereas p-value according to the Cox regression analyses (including the analyses adjusted for possible confounders) in Table 3. P-values <0.05 were considered statistically significant.

Ethics

Centre of Clinical Documentation and Evaluation has concession from the Norwegian Data Protection Authority and confidentiality exemption from the Regional Committee for Medical and Health Research Ethics (REK −Northern chapter). The concession provides access to unique personal data from Norwegian Patient Registry with information about patients treated at Norwegian hospitals in the period 2008–2013. Encrypted patient serial numbers makes it possible to describe patient pathways involving several hospitals and over several years. The concession also includes permission to pair education data from Statistics Norway.

Results

Patient selection and characteristics

A total of 3080 esophageal-, gastric and pancreatic resections were performed between 1January 2008 and

Table 2 Age, gender, educational level and type of resection, and association with major postoperative complications

Variable	Categories	Percentage[a]	OR (95 % CI)[b]	p-value
Age	Above 65 years	12.2	0.91 (0.70–1.20)	0.515
	65 years or less	13.2	1.0	
Gender	Male	13.7	1.29 (0.98–1.72)	0.071
	Female	10.9	1.0	
Educational level	Lower education	13.5	1.41 (1.02–1.95)	0.039
	Higher education	10.0	1.0	
Type of resection	Esophageal	17.2	1.67 (1.18–2.36)	0.004
	Pancreatic	12.6	1.15 (0.85–1.56)	0.358
	Gastric	11.1	1.0	

[a]Percentage that suffered one or more major postoperative complications
[b]Odds ratio, with 95 % confidence interval, for suffering one or more major postoperative complications

Table 3 The association between postoperative complications and overall survival, with hazard ratio (HR) and 95 % confidence interval (95 % CI)

	Unadjusted			Multivariable adjusted for age, gender and type of resection			Multivariable adjusted for age, gender, resection and educational level		
	HR	95 % CI	p-value	HR	95 % CI	p-value	HR	95 % CI	p-value
All patients	1.48	1.24–1.76	<0.001	1.51	1.27–1.79	<0.001	1.50	1.26–1.79	<0.001
Only patients alive >90 days	1.23	1.01–1.50	0.040	1.26	1.03–1.53	0.023	1.26	1.03–1.54	0.022

1December 2013. Of these, 2792 resections were scheduled. Of the 2792 scheduled resections, 1965 were performed for cancer; 331 esophageal resections (16.8 %), 974 gastric resections (49.6 %) and 660 pancreatic resections (33.6 %). Seventy percent of the gastric resections and almost all of the esophageal (99 %) and pancreatic resections (98 %) were performed at the six university hospitals (only four university hospitals perform esophageal resections). Forty percent of esophageal and half of the pancreatic resections were performed at Norway's largest hospital, Oslo University Hospital (OUS). Only 13% of the gastric resections were performed at OUS.

During the follow-up period, 975 (49.6 %) patients died. Median age at index operation was 68 years. A total of 248 patients (12.6 %) suffered one or more major postoperative complication and 37 (14.9 %) of these patients died within 90 days. Consequently, 1717 patients (87.4 %) did not suffer any major complications within 28 days after surgery and 68 (4.0 %) of these patients died within 90 days. Estimated median survival in the entire cohort was 31 months (Table 1) and the estimated five-year survival rate was 37.3 %.

Major postoperative complications

There were no statistically significant linear changes in the rate of complications from 2008 to 2013 ($p = 0.319$). The highest (17.2 %) and lowest (11.1 %) complication rate was seen in esophageal resections and gastric resections, respectively (Table 2). Type of resection and lower educational level (OR = 1.41, 95 % CI = 1.02–1.95, $p = 0.039$) were associated with major postoperative complications. The association with educational level was also present when adjusted for age, gender and type of resection (OR = 1.53, 95 % CI = 1.10–2.13, $p = 0.013$).

Early mortality

One-hundred-and-five (5.3 %) patients died within 90 days after surgery. Suffering one or more postoperative complications was strongly associated with 90-day mortality (OR = 4.25, 95 % CI = 2.78–6.50, $p < 0.001$).

Overall survival

There was no association between educational level and overall survival ($p = 0.145$) (Fig. 1) and this conclusion did not change after multivariable adjustment for age,

gender and type of resection (HR = 1.06, 95 % CI = 0.91–1.23, $p = 0.475$).

Postoperative complications were negatively associated with overall survival both with all patients included (Fig. 2, panel a) ($p < 0.001$) and when the first 90 days of the follow-up period (Fig. 2, panel b) ($p = 0.040$) were excluded. The survival curves (Fig. 2) suggest that the impact of major complications attenuate with time from the index surgery and p-value for interaction with time of follow up was <0.001. The estimated five-year survival rate was 38.2 % in patients who did not suffer any major postoperative complications compared to 30.6 % in patients who did. Major postoperative complications were associated with 23 % higher long term (i.e., excluding early) mortality (HR = 1.23, 95 % CI = 1.01–1.40, $p = 0.040$) (Table 3). Multivariable adjustment for age, gender, type of resection and educational level did not alter the association between major postoperative complications and overall survival (Table 3). Neither did use of attained age (instead of time in study) as the time variable in the Cox regression analysis. There were no significant interaction between type of resection and complications in the survival analysis, i.e., the association between complications and survival were not statistically significantly different according to type of resection. The association between postoperative complications and survival was similar across all types of resections (Fig. 3). Neither hospital volume (OUS vs. other university hospitals; analyzed for esophageal and pancreatic resections) or hospital teaching status (university hospital vs. non-university hospital; analyzed for gastric resections) did affect the association between complications and survival (data not shown).

Discussion

We present a complete national six-year cohort of gastro-esophageal and pancreatic resections for cancer in Norway with major complications and survival. Suffering one or more major postoperative complications was associated with both considerably increased early mortality and statistically significant decreased long-term survival. Educational level did not affect the relationship between complications and survival.

Several studies have demonstrated an association between postoperative complications and decreased survival [5, 6]. This has led to theories suggesting an immune-

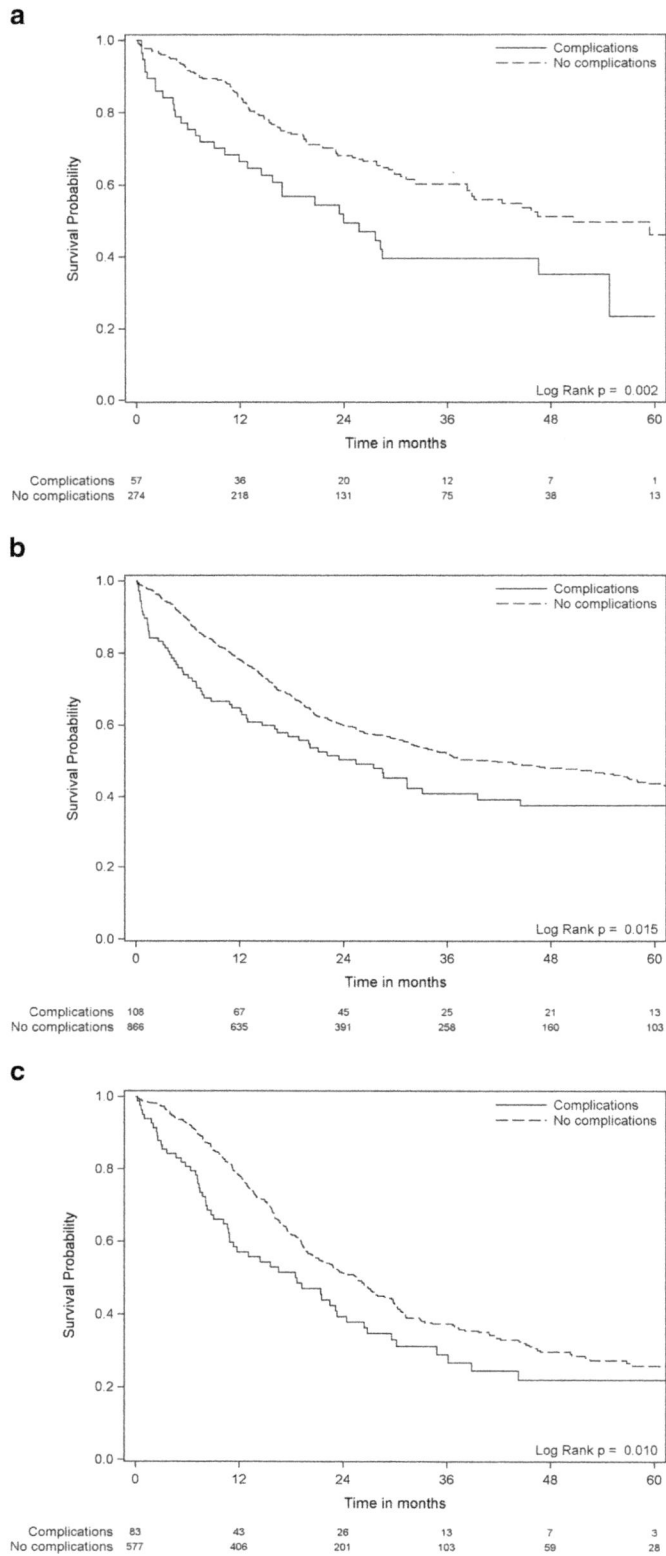

a

| Complications | 57 | 36 | 20 | 12 | 7 | 1 |
| No complications | 274 | 218 | 131 | 75 | 38 | 13 |

b

| Complications | 108 | 67 | 45 | 25 | 21 | 13 |
| No complications | 866 | 635 | 391 | 258 | 160 | 103 |

c

| Complications | 83 | 43 | 26 | 13 | 7 | 3 |
| No complications | 577 | 406 | 201 | 103 | 59 | 28 |

Fig. 3 (See legend on next page.)

(See figure on previous page.)
Fig. 3 The association between major postoperative complications and overall survival. Esophageal, gastric and pancreatic resections analyzed separately. Kaplan-Meier plots with subjects at risk. Survival probability on the Y-axis and time in months on the X-axis. Dotted lines denotes patients without any postoperative complications. Solid lines denotes patients who suffered one or more major postoperative complication. **a** Esophageal resections. **b** Gastric resections. **c** Pancreatic resections

suppressive effect of postoperative complications that might lead to cancer recurrence [5, 8, 9]. A recent meta-analysis reported a hazard ratio (HR) of 1.28 for decreased overall survival after any postoperative complication [6], the cut-offs for early mortality were not reported [6]. We found a similar risk of decreased survival associated with major complications if patients suffering early mortality were excluded (HR = 1.23). In this large, nationwide population-based cohort, we found some evidence to support theories concerning long-standing detrimental effects of complications on survival after gastro-esophageal and pancreatic cancer surgery.

Most studies exploring the issue of postoperative complications and long-term survival have either not used a cut-off at all or a 30-days mortality cut-off to exclude patients with fatal complications [5, 6, 8, 9]. Only a few studies report a cut-off for early mortality of 90-days [7]. Therefore, patients who died later than 30 days, but still arguably as a direct result of their complications may still have been included in the analysis, making it more difficult to address a possible long-standing detrimental effect of non-fatal complications.

Reductions in both overall survival and disease-free survival have been observed in colorectal cancer patients who suffered major complications [7, 8, 14]. In a large study of colon cancer patients, complications were associated with precluded or delayed adjuvant chemotherapy [3]. In the same study, complications were not associated with reduced survival if adjuvant chemotherapy were given within appropriate time-limits [3]. While chemotherapy is an important element to achieve increased survival in resectable stage III and IV colon cancer [15, 16], the effect of adjuvant chemotherapy on long-term survival in gastro-esophageal and pancreatic cancer is variable and less certain [17, 18].

The avoidance of postoperative complications is of utmost importance as complications adversely affect health-related quality of life [1] and survival [5, 6]. Complications may preclude or delay adjuvant chemotherapy [3]. Do complications make patients more susceptible to cancer recurrence and therefore cause decreased longevity? Large prospective registries with detailed information on disease-stage, comorbidity, time of recurrence and cause of death are needed to fully investigate this question. The registries used for our study contain complete national data and a large number of patients but lack information on cancer stage and disease-specific survival.

Conclusions
In a national setting, major postoperative complications are associated with both early mortality and decreased long-term survival after gastro-esophageal and pancreatic cancer surgery. Systematic quality improvement to avoid complications may improve the poor prognosis associated these cancers.

Abbreviations
NPR: Norwegian Patient Registry; NCSP: Nomesco Classification of Surgical Procedures; ICD-10: International Classification of Diseases, 10th edition; OUS: Oslo University Hospital.

Competing interests
The authors declare that they have no competing interests.

Authors' contributions
Study conception and design: EKA, BKJ, KL. Data acquisition: FO and BU. Data analysis: FO, BU, BKJ. Data interpretation and manuscript preparation, editing and final approval: All authors.

Acknowledgements
No additional investigators were involved in this research project.

Funding
This investigation and manuscript preparation received no external funding.

Author details
[1]Department of GI and HPB surgery, University Hospital of Northern Norway, 9038 Breivika, Tromsø, Norway. [2]Department of Clinical Medicine, University of Tromsø - The Arctic University of Norway, Tromsø, Norway. [3]Centre of Clinical Documentation and Evaluation, Northern Norway Regional Health Authority, Tromsø, Norway. [4]Department of Community Medicine, University of Tromsø - The Arctic University of Norway, Tromsø, Norway.

References
1. Brown SR, Mathew R, Keding A, et al. The impact of postoperative complications on long-term quality of life after curative colorectal cancer surgery. Ann Surg. 2014;259(5):916–23.
2. Knechtle WS, Perez SD, Medbery RL, et al. The Association Between Hospital Finances and Complications After Complex Abdominal Surgery: Deficiencies in the Current Health Care Reimbursement System and Implications for the Future. Ann Surg. 2015;262(2):273–9.
3. Krarup PM, Nordholm-Carstensen A, Jorgensen LN, et al. Anastomotic Leak Increases Distant Recurrence and Long-Term Mortality After Curative Resection for Colonic Cancer: A Nationwide Cohort Study. Ann Surg. 2014; 259(5):930–8.

4. Tokunaga M, Tanizawa Y, Bando E, et al. Poor survival rate in patients with postoperative intra-abdominal infectious complications following curative gastrectomy for gastric cancer. Ann Surg Oncol. 2013;20(5):1575–83.

5. Khuri SF, Henderson WG, DePalma RG, et al. Determinants of long-term survival after major surgery and the adverse effect of postoperative complications. Ann Surg. 2005;242(3):326–41.

6. Pucher PH, Aggarwal R, Qurashi M, et al. Meta-analysis of the effect of postoperative in-hospital morbidity on long-term patient survival. Br J Surg. 2014;101(12):1499–508.

7. Artinyan A, Orcutt ST, Anaya DA, et al. Infectious postoperative complications decrease long-term survival in patients undergoing curative surgery for colorectal cancer: a study of 12,075 patients. Ann Surg. 2015; 261(3):497–505.

8. Mavros MN, de Jong M, Dogeas E, et al. Impact of complications on long-term survival after resection of colorectal liver metastases. Br J Surg. 2013; 100(5):711–8.

9. Cho JY, Han HS, Yoon YS, et al. Postoperative complications influence prognosis and recurrence patterns in periampullary cancer. World J Surg. 2013;37(9):2234–41.

10. Isaacs SL, Schroeder SA. Class - the ignored determinant of the nation's health. N Engl J Med. 2004;351(11):1137–42.

11. Frederiksen BL, Osler M, Harling H, et al. The impact of socioeconomic factors on 30-day mortality following elective colorectal cancer surgery: a nationwide study. Eur J Cancer. 2009;45(7):1248–56.

12. Porembka MR, Hall BL, Hirbe M, et al. Quantitative weighting of postoperative complications based on the accordion severity grading system: demonstration of potential impact using the american college of surgeons national surgical quality improvement program. J Am Coll Surg. 2010;210(3):286–98.

13. Strasberg SM, Linehan DC, Hawkins WG. The accordion severity grading system of surgical complications. Ann Surg. 2009;250(2):177–86.

14. Mirnezami A, Mirnezami R, Chandrakumaran K, et al. Increased local recurrence and reduced survival from colorectal cancer following anastomotic leak: systematic review and meta-analysis. Ann Surg. 2011; 253(5):890–9.

15. Gill S, Loprinzi CL, Sargent DJ, et al. Pooled analysis of fluorouracil-based adjuvant therapy for stage II and III colon cancer: who benefits and by how much? J Clin Oncol. 2004;22(10):1797–806.

16. Nordlinger B, Sorbye H, Glimelius B, et al. Perioperative chemotherapy with FOLFOX4 and surgery versus surgery alone for resectable liver metastases from colorectal cancer (EORTC Intergroup trial 40983): a randomised controlled trial. Lancet. 2008;371(9617):1007–16.

17. Bringeland EA, Wasmuth HH, Fougner R, et al. Impact of perioperative chemotherapy on oncological outcomes after gastric cancer surgery. Br J Surg. 2014;101(13):1712–20.

18. Rustgi AK, El-Serag HB. Esophageal carcinoma. N Engl J Med. 2014;371(26): 2499–509.

32

Duodenal intussusception of the remnant stomach after biliopancreatic diversion: a case report

J.-N. Kersebaum[1*] (iD), C. Schafmayer[1], M. Ahrens[1], M. Laudes[2], T. Becker[1] and J. H. Beckmann[1]

Abstract

Background: We present a rare case of an antegrade intussusception of the remnant stomach four years after a biliopancreatic diversion.

Case presentation: A 55-year-old female patient presented with epigastric pain in our emergency room. Laboratory parameters showed an anemia as well as elevated transaminases and hyperbilirubinemia. The CT scan showed an intussusception of the remnant stomach into the duodenum followed by cholestasis. At laparotomy the remnant stomach was resected.

Conclusion: Bowel obstruction and intussusception after bariatric surgery are a rare but often unrecognized complication. Sonography as well as a CT scan should be performed. The exploratory laparoscopy however is the most valuable diagnostic tool in patients with suspected intussusception, due to the high rate of non-specific symptoms and misinterpreted radiographic investigations.

Keywords: Morbid obesity, Scopinaro, Small bowel obstruction, Intussusception

Backround

Bariatric surgery is a suitable treatment of morbid obesity with long term sustainable weight-loss [1, 2]. Surgical procedures are standardized, highly efficient with low rates of complications and mortality. One of the rare long term complications is small bowel obstruction [3], which can be caused by internal hernia or intussusception, with higher risks after procedures involving a Roux-en-Y reconstruction compared with sleeve gastrectomy [4, 5]. A very rare but often unrecognized problem is intussusception, most frequently seen (86%) as a retrograde intussusception of the common channel towards the jejunojejunostomy [6].

Case presentation

The 55-year-old female patient arrived in our emergency room with epigastric for two days.

The patients' prior events are sown on Table 1.

* Correspondence: janniclas.kersebaum@uksh.de
[1]Klinik für Allgemeine, Viszeral-, Transplantations-, Thorax- und Kinderchirurgie, Universitätsklinikum Schleswig- Holstein, Campus Kiel, Arnold-Heller-Str. 3, 24105 Kiel, Germany
Full list of author information is available at the end of the article

Twenty two years before, in 1995, a vertical banded gastroplasty by Mason (Fig. 1, left) was performed (Starting weight 185 kg). After an adequate weight loss of 95 kg in the next years, a rapid weight regain of 87 kg occurred in 2013 due to a gastrogastric fistula. Therefore, the gastroplasty was converted into a biliopancreatic diversion by Scopinaro (Fig. 1, middle). The procedure was started minimal invasively, but had to be converted to open surgery, due to a short jejunal loop. The remnant stomach was not resected. Following the last surgery, an adequate weight loss of 107 kg took place. Starting in early 2017 the patient was regularly admitted to our hospital with tarry stools and iron deficiency anemia despite substitution. Esophagogastroduodenoscopies repeatedly showed a gastrojejunal anastomotic ulcer. At this point, the ulcer appeared to be the cause of the anemia. After interdisciplinary discussion the decision was made to convert the BPD to a Roux-en-Y gastric bypass with resection of the problematical gastrojejunostomy.

On arrival in our emergency room, the blood work showed normal leucocyte counts and a normal CRP value, but elevated transaminases and hyperbilirubinemia. An ultrasound in the emergency room showed a hyperechoic

Table 1 Schematic life-line of the patient including year, weight and event

year	event	weight (kg)	weight change (kg)
1995	Vertical gastroplasty by Mason	185	− 90
2012	Gastrogastric fistula	90	87
2013	Biliopancreatic diversion by Scopinaro	177	−107
early 2017	Anemia; gastrojejunal ulcer in ogd	70	−3
mid 2017	Resection of remnant stomach	67	

mass in the liver hilum and intrahepatic cholestasis. With the epigastric pain continuing, we decided to perform a CT-scan with oral contrastation (Fig. 1a), in which evidence was seen of an intussusception reaching the ligament of Treitz with consecutive intrahepatic cholestasis. A complete antegrade intussusception of the remnant stomach into the duodenum reaching up to the ligament of Treitz (Fig. 2b) was found during surgery. The intussusception was reduced (Fig. 2c-d) and the remnant stomach was resected (Fig. 1, right). The gastrojejunal anastomosis ulcer was resected as a short segment. A new anastomosis was fashioned using a linear stapler. The biliary as well as the common channel remained unchanged with 250 cm and 100 cm respectively. The alimentary channel was shortened to 80 cm.

Following the procedure, no further blood transfusion was needed, and the patient was discharged on the sixth day after surgery. The pathological examination showed a tumor free specimen with chronic antrum gastritis and no indication of malignancy.

Discussion and conclusions

Intussusceptions leading to small bowel obstruction after bariatric surgery are rare. A retrospective single institution study of Zak et al. [7] showed a higher incidence of

repeated operations after Roux-en-Y gastric bypass compared to sleeve gastrectomy. After six years of follow up, 6,9% of 934 patients undergoing RYGB required reoperations for other reasons than cholecystectomy. Non-healing ulcers and intussusception were responsible for 3,7% of these. In their review including 9527 patients, Koppmann et al. [3] described an overall incidence of small bowel obstruction after RYGB of 3,6%. Those complications include internal hernias (due to a Petersen's space hernia, the mesomesenteric defect at the jejunojejunostomy and in the case of a retro colic technique, the mesocolonic defect) in ≤1% in most RYGB studies, an obstruction a the jejunojejunostomy (due to luminal narrowing or acute angulation) in 0.5% and incisional hernias in 0.3% of the cases. In only 10 reported cases included in their review, an intussusception was the cause of the small bowel obstruction. An intussusception can be retrograde or antegrade, but the retrograde intussusception of the common channel is the most common one (86%). Female gender and weight loss are risk factors for intussusception [6]. The most common symptoms are abdominal pain and/or nausea and vomiting. A peritonitis is very uncommon and only 10% of the patients have a palpable mass [8]. Compared to laboratory parameters and physical examination, imaging is much more effective method for diagnostics, with the CT being

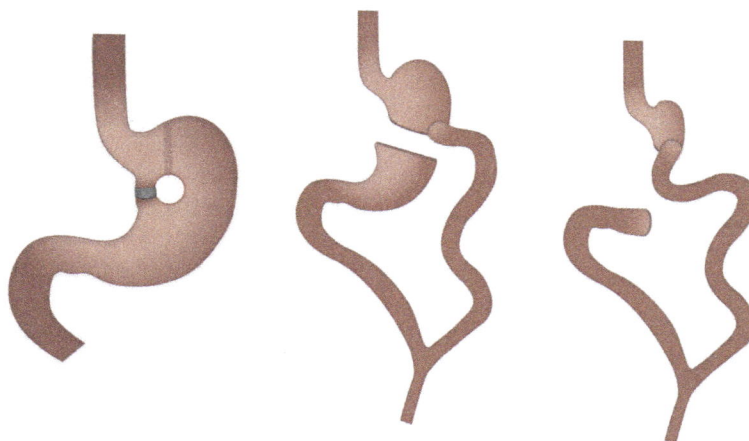

Fig. 1 Vertical gastroplasty by Mason (left). Biliopancreatic Diversion by Scopinaro (middle). Resection of remnant stomach and redone gastrojejunal anastomosis (right)

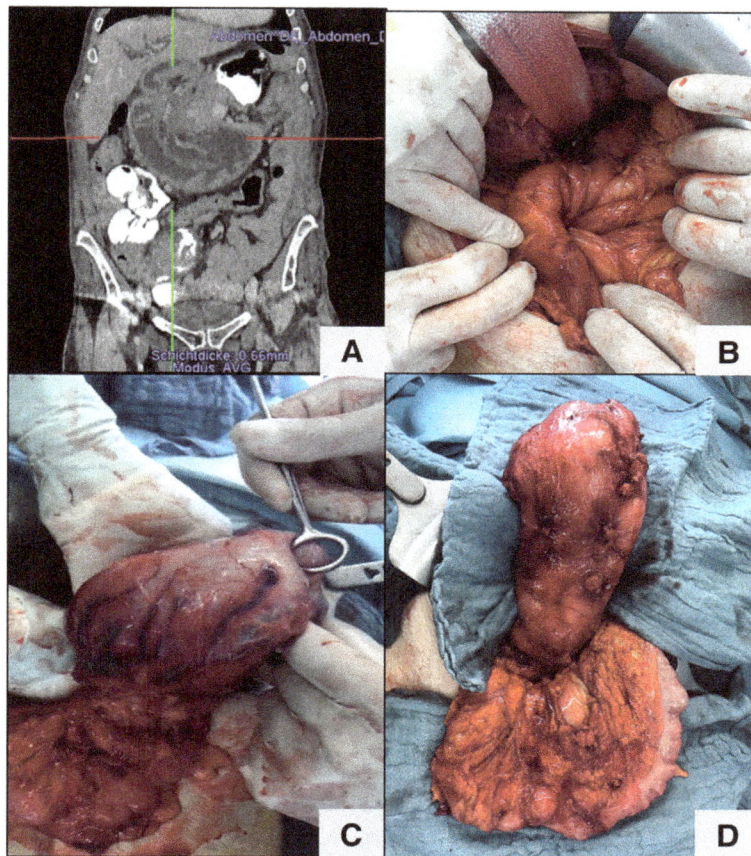

Fig. 2 a Coronal cross section CT with oral contrastation with a target sign. **b** Intraoperative image of the negative lumen of the intussuscepted remnant stomach. **c** Blunt manual reposition of the remnant stomach. **d** Fully repositioned remnant stomach (top) with the transverse colon (bottom) as a size comparison

the technique of choice, with a sensitivity ranging between 64 and 81% [3, 9], but also with its limitations due to a weight limits or the radius of the gantry. An endoscopy might show a stenosis or an ulceration of the upper gastrointestinal tract, but also has its limitations, even with the double-balloon-technique, when trying to reach the remaining stomach. The exploratory laparoscopy is the most valuable diagnostic tool in patients with suspected intussusception, due to the high rate of non-specific symptoms and misinterpreted radiographic investigations. In summary, when presented with a small bowel obstruction after bariatric surgery, the surgeon has to compare the risk of an increase of the patient's mortality in case of a bowel necrosis due to a delay in diagnostics with a relatively minimal morbidity of a negative exploratory laparoscopy.

In conclusion, agreeing with the personal guidelines presented by Bag et al. [6] and Koppmann et al. [3], we strongly emphasis the importance of early imaging diagnostics, preferably the CT and exploratory laparoscopy or even laparotomy in more complex cases.

Abbreviations
BPD: Biliopancreatic diversion; RYGB: Roux-en Y gastric bypass

Authors' contributions
J-NK is the corresponding author, drafted the manuscript and implemented the suggested changes by the reviewer, JB was the surgeon on call and acquired the patients' data and the intraoperative pictures. ML provided the pre-surgical data of the patient and supported her with the nutritional expertise and finalized the visualization of the anatomical changes. CS provided the endoscopic expertise. MA provided the postoperative data, acquired the patient's permission for publication. TB helped structuring and revised the manuscript critically for important intellectual content and provided us with the background information. All authors read and approved the final manuscript.

Competing interests
The authors declare that they have no competing interest.

Author details
[1]Klinik für Allgemeine, Viszeral-, Transplantations-, Thorax- und Kinderchirurgie, Universitätsklinikum Schleswig- Holstein, Campus Kiel, Arnold-Heller-Str. 3, 24105 Kiel, Germany. [2]Klinik für Innere Medizin I, Universitätsklinikum Schleswig- Holstein, Campus Kiel, Kiel, Germany.

References

1. Buchwald H, et al. Bariatric Surgery. JAMA. 2004;292(14):1724.
2. Colquitt JL, Pickett K, Loveman E, Frampton GK. Surgery for weight loss in adults. Cochrane Database of Systematic Reviews. 2014;(8). Art. No.: CD003641. https://doi.org/10.1002/14651858.CD003641.pub4.
3. Koppman JS, Li C, Gandsas A. Small bowel obstruction after laparoscopic roux-En-Y gastric bypass: a review of 9,527 patients. J Am Coll Surg. 2008;206(3):571–84.
4. Daellenbach L, Suter M. Jejunojejunal intussusception after roux-en-Y gastric bypass: a review. Obes Surg. 2011;21(2):253–63.
5. Javanainen M, Penttilä A, Mustonen H, Juuti A, Scheinin T, Leivonen M. A retrospective 2-year follow-up of late complications treated surgically and endoscopically after laparoscopic roux-en-Y gastric bypass (LRYGB) and laparoscopic sleeve gastrectomy (LSG) for morbid obesity. Obes Surg. 2018;28(4):1055-62.
6. Bag H, Karaisli S, Celik SC, Kar H, Tatar F. A rare complication of bariatric surgery: retrograde intussusception. Obes Surg. 2017;27(11):2996–8.
7. Zak Y, Petrusa E, Gee DW. Laparoscopic roux-en-Y gastric bypass patients have an increased lifetime risk of repeat operations when compared to laparoscopic sleeve gastrectomy patients. Surg Endosc Other Interv Tech. 2016;30(5):1833–8.
8. Singla S, Guenthart BA, May L, Gaughan J, Meilahn JE. Intussusception after laparoscopic gastric bypass surgery: an underrecognized complication. Minim Invasive Surg. 2012;2012:464853.
9. Suter M. Reply to 'a Rare Complication of Bariatric Surgery: Retrograde Intussusception. Obes Surg. 2017;27(11):2999–3000.

33

Laparoscopy is an available alternative to open surgery in the treatment of perforated peptic ulcers: a retrospective multicenter study

Antonino Mirabella[1], Tiziana Fiorentini[2], Roberta Tutino[3]* [iD], Nicolò Falco[3], Tommaso Fontana[3], Paolino De Marco[3], Eliana Gulotta[3], Leonardo Gulotta[3], Leo Licari[3], Giuseppe Salamone[3], Irene Melfa[3], Gregorio Scerrino[3], Massimo Lupo[1], Armando Speciale[2] and Gianfranco Cocorullo[3]

Abstract

Background: Perforated peptic ulcers (PPU) remain one of the most frequent causes of death. Their incidence are largely unchanged accounting for 2–4% of peptic ulcers and remain the second most frequent abdominal cause of perforation and of indication for gastric emergency surgery. The minimally invasive approach has been proposed to treat PPU however some concerns on the offered advantages remain.

Methods: Data on 184 consecutive patients undergoing surgery for PPU were collected. Likewise, perioperative data including shock at admission and interval between admission and surgery to evaluate the Boey's score.
It was recorded the laparoscopic or open treatments, the type of surgical procedure, the length of the operation, the intensive care needed, and the length of hospital stay.
Post-operative morbidity and mortality relation with patient's age, surgical technique and Boey's score were evaluated.

Results: The relationship between laparoscopic or open treatment and the Boey's score was statistically significant ($p = 0.000$) being the open technique used for the low-mid group in 41.1% and high score group in 100% and laparoscopy in 58.6% and 0%, respectively. Postoperative complications occurred in 9.7% of patients which were related to the patients' Boey's score, 4.7% in the low-mid score group and 21.4% in the high risk score group ($p = 0.000$). In contrast morbidity was not related to the chosen technique being 12.8% in open technique and 5.3% in laparoscopic one ($p = 0.092$, $p > 0.05$).
30-day post-operative mortality was 3.8% and occurred in the 0.8% of low-mid Boey's score group and in the 10.7% of the high Boey's score group ($p = 0.001$). In respect to the surgical technique it occurred in 6.4% of open procedures and in any case in the Lap one ($p = 0.043$). Finally, there was a statistically significant difference in morbidity and mortality between patients < 70 and > 70 years old ($p = 0.000$; $p = 0.002$).

Conclusions: Laparoscopy tends to be an alternative method to open surgery in the treatment of perforated peptic ulcer. Morbidity and mortality were essentially related to Boey's score. In our series laparoscopy was not used in high risk Boey's score patients and it will be interesting to evaluate its usefulness in high risk patients in large randomized controlled trials.

Keywords: Peptic ulcer perforation, Laparoscopy, Stomach, Aged

* Correspondence: la.tutino@gmail.com
[3]Department of Surgical, Oncological and Stomatological Disciplines, University of Palermo, Palermo, Italy
Full list of author information is available at the end of the article

Background

Perforated gastric ulcers remain one of the most frequent causes of death and disability worldwide.

The use of more tolerable drugs to control hyperacidity (H2 antagonists, proton pump inhibitors) and the treatments for eradication of helicobacter pylori infection (HP) enabled to reduce the rates of acid-reductive surgery (vagotomy, gastric resection) and re-intervention surgery due to recurrences.

The incidence of bleeding ulcers and its related mortality have decreased and its management – mainly guided by endoscopy and interventional radiology - have largely substituted surgery [1].

In contrast the incidence of perforated peptic ulcers (PPU) are largely unchanged, counting 2–4% of peptic ulcers which remain the second most frequent cause of abdominal perforation that requires surgery as well as the most frequent indication for gastric emergency surgery [1–3].

Seventy per cent of deaths from peptic ulcer disease are the result of perforation [3] and these should probably be attributed to the increasing use of anti-inflammatory drugs (NSAIDs) especially among aged patients with considerable co-morbidities for whom unchanged high morbidity rate (up to 50%) and mortality rate (up to 25%) still occur [4].

The minimal invasive approach has been proposed to treat PPU as well as other surgical emergencies, increasing the ability to tolerate the treatment among patients. In most centers the rate of laparoscopic management has gradually increased along with the improvement of technical skills [1–15].

Methods

This study has assessed 184 consecutive patients undergoing surgery for PPU from 2006 to 2016 in three of the four major emergency surgery centers of Palermo (700.000 inhabitants), the Emergency and General Surgery O.U. of the University Hospital, the Emergency and General Surgery O.U. of "Villa Sofia" Hospital and the Emergency and General Surgery O.U. of "Cervello" Hospital.

The patients were identified by the diagnostic code on admission of ICD-9: 531.1, 531.5, 532.1, 532.5, 533.1, 533.5, recording demographical data including age, sex and ASA.

The analysis included the perioperative data including "shock at admission" and "time between admission and surgery" to evaluate the Boey's score.

Also recorded the surgical procedures used, laparoscopic (Lap) or open, the type of surgical procedure, the length of the operation, the intensive care unit (ICU) needed and the lengths of hospital stay.

Post-operative morbidity and mortality were examined, while their relation with patient's age, surgical technique and Boey's score evaluated.

Statistical analysis

Descriptive data are presented as percentage, mean ± standard deviation [SD] for parametric data and median, range and/or 95% confidence interval (CI) for non-parametric data.

The relationship between post-operative complications and mortality with age, Boey's score and surgical technique were analyzed using the Pearson's chi-square test or Fisher's exact test. A p-value of $< 0,05$ was considered to be statistically significant.

Statistical analysis was conducted using SPSS software (SPSS, Chicago, Illinois, USA).

Results

One hundred and eighty-four patients (61 female [range 22–91; mean 62 years], 123 male [range 21–88; mean age 59 years], M/F 3.1/1) underwent abdominal surgery for PPU between 2006 and 2016.

The estimated incidence in our district was 0.003%.

Median ASA score was 3. Shock at admission was reported in 64 patients (34.7%) while the time between the manifestation of symptoms and surgery was > to 24 h in 56 patients (30.4%).

One hundred twenty-eight patients showed a Boey's score of 0–2 (low-mid), while 56 of 3(high) (Table 1).

Open surgery was performed in 109 patients (59%) while 75 patients (41%) underwent laparoscopic surgery.

Contraindications to laparoscopy were Boey's score > 2, multiple laparotomies, inadequate surgical skills.

No age restriction to Lap was adopted being Lap performed in patients that range between 35 and 79 years old.

Patients underwent ulcorraphy, ulcorraphy and omental patch or omental patch according to the diameter of the perforation (> or < 1 cm) and to the friability of the tissue surrounding the ulcer (Table 2).

Median length of the surgical procedure was 70 (50–125) minutes for Lap technique and 52 (38–80) minutes for the open one.

Conversion rate was 26% (20 patients) and was due to adhesions or diffuse peritonitis.

ICU admission was required for 30 pts. (16%).

The mean length of hospital stay was 9 ± 4 days.

Table 1 Patients' Boey's score

Boey's score	Open	Lap
0–2	53	75
3	56	0

Table 2 Patients' surgical management

Surgical treatment	Open	Lap
Ulcorraphy	86	64
ulcorraphy and omental patch	20	9
omental patch only	3	2
Tot.	109	75

The relationship between Lap and Open to the different Boey's scores was analyzed and there was a statistically difference between the two independent binomial proportions being open technique used for the low-mid group and high score group in 41.4% and 100%, respectively, while lap technique was used in 58.6% and 0% ($p = 0.000$).

Postoperative complications occurred in 18 patients (9.7%) (Table 3).

The relationship between patients' Boey's score and morbidity revealed that 6 patients (4.7%) in the low-mid score group and 12 patients (21.4%) in the high risk score group had post-operative complications. A statistically significant difference in proportions of .167, $p = 0.000$ was found.

Morbidity was 12.8% (14/109) in open technique while 5.3% (4/75) in lap approach and the difference between the two independent binomial proportions was not statistically significant ($p = 0.092$, $p > 0.05$).

30-day post-operative mortality was 3.8% and causes arise from gastrointestinal bleeding to myocardial

infarction (IMA) and septic shock with multiorgan failure (MOF) (Table 4).

In respect to mortality low-mid Boey's score group showed 0.8% (1/128) while high Boey's score group showed 10.7% (6/56) and there was a statistically significant difference in proportions of .099, $p = 0.001$.

Mortality was 6.4% (7/109) in open technique conversely no deaths occurred in the Lap one. Due to small sample size, Fisher's exact test was run. There was a statistically significant difference between the two independent binomial proportions ($p = 0.043$).

Patients older than 70 years were 9% (18 pts.), among them complications arose in 39% (7 pts.) and 30-day mortality was 22% (4pts.). There was a statistically significant difference in morbidity and mortality between patients < 70 and > 70 years old ($p = 0.000$; $p = 0.002$).

Discussion

PPU diagnosis is based on clinical history, clinical findings and instrumental exams.

The reported estimated incidence is 1.5–3%, with a lifetime prevalence of 5% and a mortality rate ranging from 1.3 to 20% [16]. We considered patients operated in three of the four major hospitals of the district and our estimated incidence has been lower than reported data being 0.003%.

CT scan of the abdomen tends to be the most reliable exam in hemodynamically stable patients allowing also the identification of the perforation site [17, 18].

Table 3 Post-operative complications and related outcomes

	Type of surgery	Post-operative complications (10%)	Complication Treatment	Outcome
1	Lap	Acute pulmonary edema	ICU admission	Good
2	Lap	Fistula (low output)	Conservative	Good
3	Lap	Fistula (low output)	Conservative	Good
4	Lap	Fistula (high output)	Surgery	Good
5	Open	bronchopulmonary infection	ICU admission	Good
6	Open	bronchopulmonary infection	Conservative	Good
7	Open	IMA	ICU admission	Exitus
8	Open	gastric hemorrhage	Endoscopic	Good
9	Open	gastric hemorrhage	ICU admission	Exitus
10	Open	Septic Shock, MOF	ICU admission	Exitus
11	Open	bronchopulmonary infection	Conservative	Good
12	Open	bronchopulmonary infection	Conservative	Good
13	Open	IMA	ICU admission	Good
14	Open	bronchopulmonary infection	Conservative	Good
15	Open	IMA	ICU admission	Exitus
16	Open	Septic Shock	ICU admission	Exitus
17	Open	Septic Shock, MOF	ICU admission	Exitus
18	Open	Septic Shock, MOF	ICU admission	Exitus

Table 4 Post-operative mortality

Cases	Type of surgery	Post-operative days	Age (years)	Cause
1	Open	I	87	septic shock, MOF
2	Open	II	68	septic shock, MOF
3	Open	V	60	septic shock, MOF
4	Open	VIII	75	Gastric hemorrhage
5	Open	VIII	67	IMA
6	Open	X	83	IMA
7	Open	XV	79	septic shock, MOF

Several predictive scores were proposed over time for PPU even if most of them, as the Mannheim Peritonitis Index, are general scores often needing operative data.

The Boey's score, a specific PPU score, due to its simplicity and high predictive value was largely used, with the following three parameters: state of shock on admission (systolic blood pressure < 90 mmHg), ASA III–V (presence of severe comorbidities), and duration of symptoms (> 24 h) [19, 20].

While many papers reported a relation between the Boey's score and mortality only [1, 18, 21–23], Lohsiriwat reported a progressive increase in both morbidity and mortality related to increasing Boey's score (11%, 47%, 75% and 77% for morbidity and of 1%,8%,33% and 38% for mortality) [19].

We analyzed the relationship between morbidity and mortality and low-mid (0–2) or high (3) Boey's score showing a statistically significant relation between those ($p = 0.000$; $p = 0.001$). Morbidity was in our series 4.7% for Boey's score 0–2 and 21.4% for Boey's score 3 while mortality was 0.8% and 10.7%, respectively. Our morbidity rates were inferior to those reported by Lohsiriwat, this could be due to exclusion of wound infections from the outcomes that in this type of contamined or dirty operation can reach 15–40%.

Laparoscopy in the management of PPU has increased also due to the large diffusion of adequate skills among surgeons, as it happened to other surgical procedures that are actually mainly managed by minimal invasive approach [24, 25].

A recent Italian survey on the laparoscopic technique in the acute abdomen, published in 2016, shows that about 70% of the participant centers have modified the management of duodenal perforation in recent years comparing to the data from a 2012 Italian consensus (SICE-ACOI-SIC-SICUT-SICOP-EAES). Actually, more than 50% of gastro-duodenal perforations are treated by laparoscopy [25, 26].

A Cochrane review on the use of laparoscopic repair for PPU including three RCTs have found no statistically significant differences between laparoscopic and open surgery in the proportion of abdominal septic complications, pulmonary complications and number of septic abdominal complications. Authors stated that laparoscopic surgery results are not clinically different from those of open surgery [2, 4, 27, 28].

Contraindication to the laparoscopic approach were shock at admission, high Boey's score, concomitant other ulcers complications, large perforations, technical difficulties, previous upper abdominal operations and serious associated cardiopulmonary diseases [28].

We valued as contraindication to laparoscopy: Boey's score > 2, multiple laparotomies and inadequate surgical skills.

According to Berteleff, the choice of the surgical technique depends on lesion characteristics: if margins are edematous, friable, and/or difficult to mobilize, the repair can be limited to an omental patch, eventually associated with one or more sealant devices, while margins tend to be easily brought together without tension, direct suturing can be sufficient with or without omentoplasty [4].

Siu found 21.5% of conversion and causes of conversion: ulcers > 1 cm, technical difficulties and unidentifiable perforations [29].

In our series, main causes of conversion were adhesions and diffuse peritonitis while, on the basis of the diameter of the ulcer, the surgical repair was tailored looking at the dimension not necessarily as a reason to convert as suggested by Berteleff [4].

Lau demonstrated that laparoscopic repair of PPU confers short-term benefits in terms of postoperative pain and wound morbidity and that it is safe and effective as open repair [28].

In this regards our data showed that patients operated with open technique have higher morbidity rates (12.8% vs 5.3%) even if not statistically significant difference was proved ($p = 0.092$, $p > 0.05$). However, in our opinion this high rate of morbidity should be correlated to the inclusion in the open group of patients with higher Boey's score who were not managed laparoscopically.

These data were confirmed by our patient's mortality rate that were 6.4% in open surgery while 0% in laparoscopic surgery with a statistically significant difference ($p = 0.043$).

The progressive increase of elderly population suffering from PPU often with frank peritonitis may represent an obstacle to a more rapid discharge and to an immediate resumption of normal activities [29].

In our series no age restriction to Lap was adopted, it was actually performed in patients with ages ranged between 35 and 79 years old and our data showed a statistically significant difference in morbidity and mortality between patients < 70 and > 70 years old ($p = 0.000$; $p = 0.002$) irrespective of the used technique.

Conclusions

In conclusion findings show that laparoscopy could be a possible alternative to open surgery when treating perforated peptic ulcer, and literature data don't show a statistically significant difference from open surgery.

Morbidity and mortality resulted statistically related to Boey's score, while only mortality was statistically related to the surgical technique being laparoscopy not used in high risk Boey's score patients.

In this regard, it would be interesting to evaluate the safety and usefulness of laparoscopic surgery in high risk patients.

However, there would be the need of large RCTs to verify those outcomes.

Abbreviations
ASA: American society of anestesiologists; HP: helicobacter pylori infection; ICD: international classification of diseases; ICU: intensive care unit; IMA: myocardial infarction; Lap: laparoscopy; MOF: multiorgan failure; NSAIDs: anti-inflammatory drugs; PPU: perforated peptic ulcers

Acknowledgements
We thank Dr. Sahara Seidita for the English language revision.

Authors' contributions
AM, TF, AS, ML and GC gave substantial contribution to the conception of the work. RT, NF, TF, LL, GS1, LG, EG, GS2, IM, PDM gave substantial contribution to the acquisition, analysis and interpretation of data. AS, ML and GC revised critically the work for important intellectual contents. All authors gave their final approval of the version to be published.

Competing interests
The authors declare that they have no competing interest.

Author details
[1]O.U. of Emergency and General Surgery of "Villa Sofia" Hospital, Palermo, Italy. [2]O.U. of Emergency and General Surgery of "Cervello" Hospital, Palermo, Italy. [3]Department of Surgical, Oncological and Stomatological Disciplines, University of Palermo, Palermo, Italy.

References
1. Thorsen K, Søreide JA, Søreide K. Scoring systems for outcome prediction in patients with perforated peptic ulcer. Scand J Trauma Resus. 2013;21(1):25.
2. Sanabria AE, Morales CH, Villegas MI. Laparoscopic repair for perforated peptic ulcer disease. Cochrane Db Syst Rev. 2005;(4):CD004778.
3. Lagoo S, Mc Mahon RL, Kalkharu M, et al. The sixth decision regarding perforated duodenal ulcer. JSLS. 2002;6(4):359–68.
4. Bertleff M, Lange JF. Laparoscopic correction of perforated peptic ulcer: first choice? A review of literature. Surg Endosc. 2010;24(6):1231–9.
5. Pappas TN, Lagoo SA. Laparoscopic repair for perforated peptic ulcer. Ann Surg. 2002;235(3):320.
6. Matsuda M, Nishiyama M, Hanai T, et al. Laparoscopic omental patch repair for perforated peptic ulcer. Ann Surg. 1995;221(3):236.
7. Lui FY, Davis KA. Gastroduodenal perforation: maximal or minimal intervention? Scand J Surg. 2010;99(2):73–7.
8. Mouret J, Francois Y, Vignal J, et al. Laparoscopic treatment of perforated duodenal ulcer. Brit J Surg. 1990;77(9):1006.
9. Nathanson LK, Easter DW, Cuschieri A. Laparoscopic repair peritoneal toilette of perforated duodenal ulcer. Surg Endosc. 1990;4(4):232–3.
10. Cocorullo G, Tutino R, Falco N, et al. Three-port colectomy: reduced port laparoscopy for general surgeons. A single center experience. Ann Ital Chir. 2016;87:350–5.
11. Cocorullo G, Mirabella A, Falco N, et al. An investigation of bedside laparoscopy in the ICU for cases of non-occlusive mesenteric ischemia. World J Emerg Surg. 2017;12:4.
12. Cocorullo G, Falco N, Tutino R, et al. Open versus laparoscopic approach in the treatment of abdominal emergencies in elderly population. G Chir. 2016;37(3):108–12.
13. Cocorullo G, Falco N, Fontana T, et al. Update in laparoscopic approach to acute mesenteric ischemia. In: emergency laparoscopy. Cham: Springer; 2016. p. 179–84.
14. Cocorullo G, Tutino R, Falco N, et al. Surgical emergencies in Crohn's disease. In: Crohn's disease. Cham: Springer; 2016. p. 153–7.
15. Cocorullo G, Tutino R, Falco N, et al. Laparoscopic ileocecal resection in acute and chronic presentations of Crohn's disease. A single center experience. G Chir. 2017;37(5):220–3.
16. Chou NH, Mok KT, Chang HT, et al. Risk factors of mortality in perforated peptic ulcer. Eur J Surg. 2000;166(2):149–53.
17. Di Saverio S, Bassi M, Smerieri N, et al. Diagnosis and treatment of perforated or bleeding peptic ulcer s: 2013 WSES position paper. World J Emerg Surg. 2014;9:45.
18. Thorsen K, Glomsaker TB, von Meer A, et al. Trends in diagnosis and surgical management of patients with perforated peptic ulcer. J Gastrointest Surg. 2011;15(8):1329–35.
19. Lohsiriwat V, Prapasrivorakul S, Lohsiriwat D. Perforated peptic ulcer: clinical presentation, surgical outcomes, and the accuracy of the Boey scoring system in predicting postoperative morbidity and mortality. World J Surg. 2009;33(1):80–5.
20. Boey J, Choi SK, Poon A, et al. Risk stratification in perforated duodenal ulcers. A prospective validation of predictive factors. Ann Surg. 1987; 205(1):22.
21. Moller MH, Adamsen S, Thomsen RW, et al. Multicentre trial of a perioperative protocol to reduce mortality in patients with peptic ulcer perforation. Brit J Surg. 2011;98(6):802–10.
22. Møller MH, Engebjerg MC, Adamsen S, et al. The peptic ulcer perforation (PULP) score: a predictor of mortality following peptic ulcer perforation. A cohort study. Acta Anaesth Scand. 2012;56(5):655–62.
23. Thorsen K, Søreide JA, Søreide K. What is the best predictor of mortality in perforated peptic ulcer disease? A population-based, multivariate regression analysis including three clinical scoring systems. J Gastrointest Surg. 2014;18(7):1261–8.
24. Conzo G, Gambardella C, Candela G, et al. Single center experience with laparoscopic adrenalectomy on a large clinical series. BMC Surg. 2018;18(1):2.
25. Agresta F, Ansaloni L, Baiocchi GL, et al. Laparoscopic approach to acute abdomen from the Consensus Development Conference of the Società Italiana di Chirurgia Endoscopica e nuove tecnologie (SICE), Associazione Chirurghi Ospedalieri Italiani (ACOI), Società Italiana di Chirurgia (SIC), Società Italiana di Chirurgia d'Urgenza e del Trauma (SICUT), Società Italiana di Chirurgia nell'Ospedalità Privata (SICOP), and the European Association for Endoscopic Surgery (EAES). Surg Endosc. 2012;26(8):2134–64.
26. Agresta F, Campanile FC, Podda M, et al. Current status of laparoscopy for acute abdomen in Italy: a critical appraisal of 2012 clinical guidelines from two consecutive nationwide surveys with analysis of 271,323 cases over 5 years. Surg Endosc. 2017;31(4):1785–95.
27. Siu WT, Leong HT, Law BKB, et al. Laparoscopic repair for perforated peptic ulcer: a randomized controlled trial. Ann Surg. 2002;235(3):313.
28. Lau H. Laparoscopic repair of perforated peptic ulcer. A meta-analysis. Surg Endosc. 2004;18(7):1013–21.

34

Gastric leiomyosarcoma and diagnostic pitfalls: a case report

Anis Hasnaoui[1*], Raja Jouini[2], Dhafer Haddad[1], Haithem Zaafouri[1], Ahmed Bouhafa[1], Anis Ben Maamer[1] and Ehsen Ben Brahim[2]

Abstract

Background: Since the advent of immunohistochemistry for the diagnosis of stromal tumours, the incidence of leiomyosarcomas has significantly decreased. Nowadays, gastric leiomyosarcoma is an exceptionally rare tumour. We report the second case in the English literature of gastric leiomyosarcoma revealed with massive bleeding and hemodynamic instability and diagnostic pitfalls that we encountered.

Case presentation: A 63-year-old woman, with 2 years' history of dizziness and weakness probably related to an anaemic syndrome, presented to the emergency room with hematemesis, melena and hemodynamic instability. On examination, she had conjunctival pallor with reduced general condition, blood pressure of 90/45 mmHg and a pulse between 110 and 120 beats per minute. On digital rectal examination, she had melena. Laboratory blood tests revealed a haemoglobin level at 38 g/L.
The patient was admitted to the intensive care department. After initial resuscitation, transfusion and intravenous Omeprazole continuous infusion, her condition was stabilized. She underwent upper gastrointestinal endoscopy showing a tumour of the cardia, protruding in the lumen with mucosal ulceration and clots in the stomach. Biopsies were taken. Histological examination showed interlacing bundles of spindle cells, ill-defined cell borders, elongated hyperchromatic nuclei with marked pleomorphism and paranuclear vacuolization. Immunohistochemistry showed positivity for Vimentine, a strong and diffuse immunoreactivity for smooth muscle actin (SMA). Immunoreactivities for KIT and DOG1 were doubtful.
Computed tomography scan revealed a seven-cm tumour of the cardia, without adenopathy or liver metastasis.
The patient underwent laparotomy. A total gastrectomy was performed without lymphadenectomy. Post-operative course was uneventful.
Histological examination of the tumour specimen found the same features as preoperative biopsies with negative margins. We solicited a second opinion of an expert in a reference centre for sarcomas in France, who confirmed the diagnosis of a high grade gastric leiomyosarcoma.

Conclusion: Gastric leiomyosarcoma is a rare tumour. Diagnosis is based on histological examination with immunohistochemistry, which could be sometimes confusing like in our case. The validation of a pathological expert is recommended.

Keywords: Leiomyosarcoma, Gastric, Bleeding, H-caldesmon, KIT, DOG1, GIST

* Correspondence: hasnaouianis001@gmail.com
[1]Department of General Surgery, Habib Thameur Hospital, Tunis El Manar University, Ali Ben Ayed Street 2037 Montfleury, Tunis, Tunisia
Full list of author information is available at the end of the article

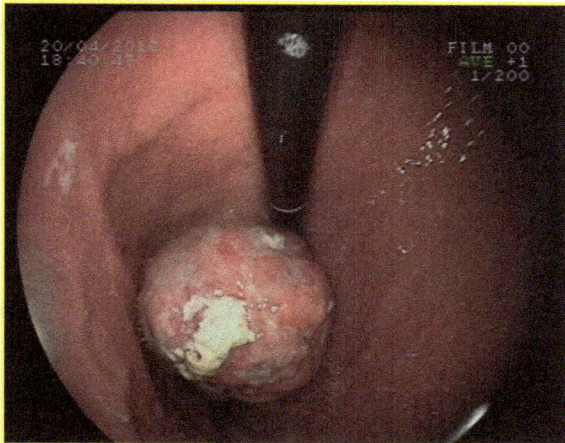

Fig. 1 Tumour of the cardia protruding in the gastric lumen

Background

Gastrointestinal stromal tumours (GISTs) were considered to be of smooth muscle origin. They were misdiagnosed as leiomyomas and leiomyosarcomas. Since the advent of immunohistochemistry for the diagnosis of stromal tumours, the incidence of leiomyosarcomas has significantly decreased. Nowadays, gastric leiomyosarcoma is an exceptionally rare tumour [1]. Discovery of this tumour is generally made at a late stage as its growth is often insidious. Diagnosis relies on accurate histological examination with immunohistochemistry, as treatment and prognosis differ widely between different types of mesenchymal tumours.

We present the case of a gastric leiomyosarcoma revealed by a massive upper gastrointestinal bleeding and diagnostic pitfalls that we encountered.

Case presentation

A 63-year-old woman, with 2 years' history of dizziness and weakness probably related to an anaemic syndrome, presented to the emergency room with hematemesis, melena and hemodynamic instability. There was no history of chronic liver disease, dyspepsia, ulcer disease, nonsteroidal anti-inflammatory drugs or aspirin use.

On examination, she had conjunctival pallor with reduced general condition, blood pressure of 90/45 mmHg and a pulse between 110 and 120 beats per minute. On digital rectal examination, she had melena. There were no abdominal wall varices, no hepatomegaly, and no palpable mass or adenopathy.

Laboratory blood tests revealed a haemoglobin level at 38 g/l with haematocrit at 13.4%. The mean corpuscular volume was in the normal range.

The patient was admitted to the intensive care department. After initial resuscitation, transfusion and intravenous Omeprazole continuous infusion, her condition was stabilized. She underwent upper gastrointestinal endoscopy showing a tumour of the cardia, protruding in the lumen with mucosal ulceration and clots in the stomach (Fig. 1). Biopsies were taken. Histological examination showed interlacing bundles of spindle cells, ill-defined cell borders, elongated hyperchromatic nuclei with marked pleomorphism and numerous mitoses. Immunohistochemistry showed positivity for Vimentine, a strong and diffuse immunoreactivity for SMA. Immunoreactivities for KIT and DOG1 were doubtful.

Computed tomography (CT) scan revealed a seven-cm tumour of the cardia, without adenopathy or liver metastasis (Fig. 2).

After multidisciplinary meeting, we suspected the diagnosis of stromal tumour of the cardia with high risk of re-bleeding and we decided to perform a total gastrectomy.

The patient underwent laparotomy. There was a nine-cm tumour of the cardia and the fundus, and no sign of peritoneal seeding or liver metastasis. A total gastrectomy was performed without lymphadenectomy (Fig. 3). Post-operative course was uneventful.

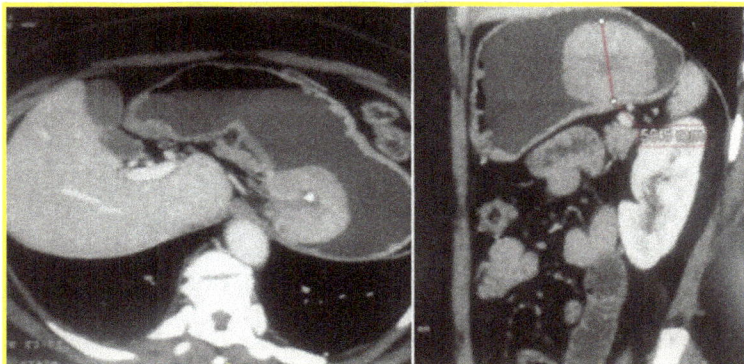

Fig. 2 CT scan showing the tumour in the cardia

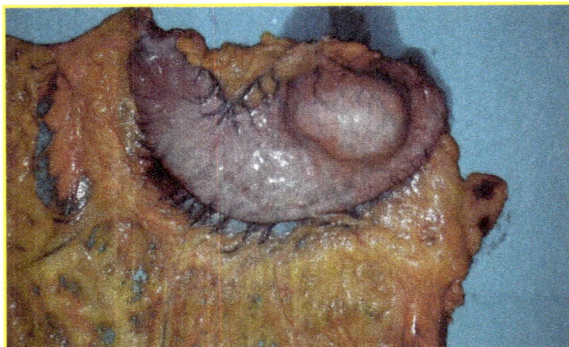

Fig. 3 Resection specimen: Total gastrectomy with a nine-cm tumour of the cardia and fundus

Histological examination of the tumour specimen found the same features as preoperative biopsies with negative margins (Fig. 4). We solicited a second opinion of an expert in a reference centre for sarcomas in France. Immunohistochemistry showed the following: DOG1 staining was focally positive for some normal cells of Cajal. Otherwise, neoplastic cells were DOG1 -, c Kit - (Fig. 5), CD34 -, smooth muscle actin + and h-caldesmon + (Fig. 6). In conclusion, it was in favour of a high grade gastric leiomyosarcoma.

Discussion and conclusion

Before the late 90's, GISTs were misdiagnosed as leiomyomas and leiomyosarcomas [2]. Advances in immunohistochemistry led to the decrease of the incidence of

gastric leiomyosarcomas to 1% of all malignant gastric tumours [1, 3, 4]. We report a case of this rare sarcoma with some particularities.

First, gastric leiomyosarcomas are generally insidious since they have a predominant extraluminal component [5]. It may be revealed by gastric outlet obstruction, perforation [6] or bleeding like in our case. Bleeding generally occurs when the tumour erodes the mucosa causing a chronic anaemia. Massive bleeding is not very common. To our knowledge, this is the second case in the literature of gastric leiomyosarcoma with massive bleeding and hemodynamic instability [4].

Second, arising between the muscularis propria and muscularis mucosa layers, diagnosis of leiomyosarcomas relies on histological examination of deep biopsies. Conventional endoscopy usually yields superficial and normal mucosa. Endoscopic ultrasonography, on the other hand, has been proved to be of great sensitivity, up to 97% [1], in the diagnosis of these tumours. It may be required to obtain deep biopsies. In our establishment, this technique was not available. Nevertheless, we succeeded to obtain an adequate sampling with conventional endoscopy. This is may be due to the endoluminal growth of the tumour and mucosal ulceration.

Third, histological examination was not evident. In the first and second pathology reports, based respectively on endoscopic biopsies and resection specimen, we had doubts about the positivity of KIT and DOG1 immunoreactivities. These two markers present the basis for the diagnosis of GISTs. Miettinen et al. declared that sensitivities of DOG1 and KIT were nearly

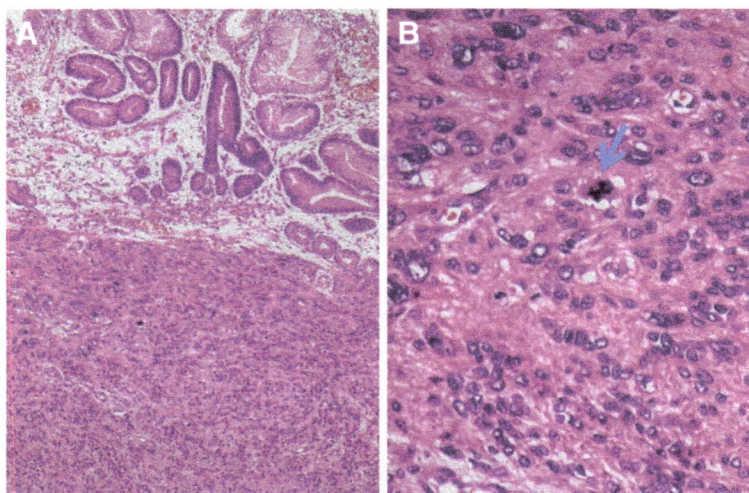

Fig. 4 Gastric fusocellular proliferation (**a**) with marked atypia and numerous mitoses (**b**). Arrow shows an abnormal mitotic figure (Haematoxylin and eosin stain)

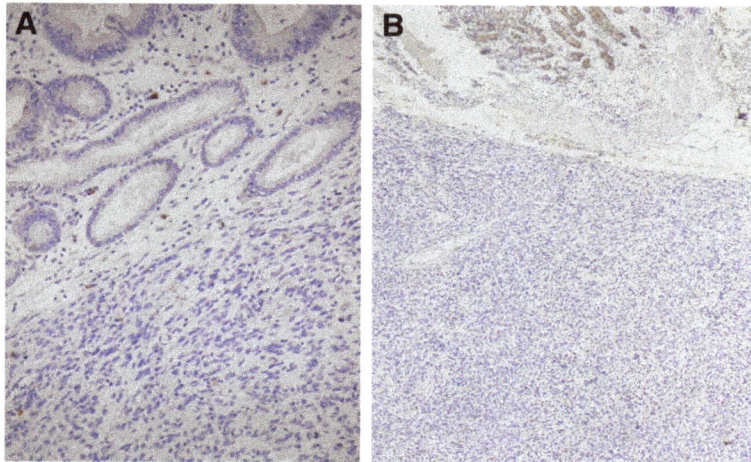

Fig. 5 Immunohistochemically, tumor cells are KIT negative, only mast cells are positive (**a**). Tumor cells are also DOG 1 negative (**b**), with normal positivity in gastric epithelium

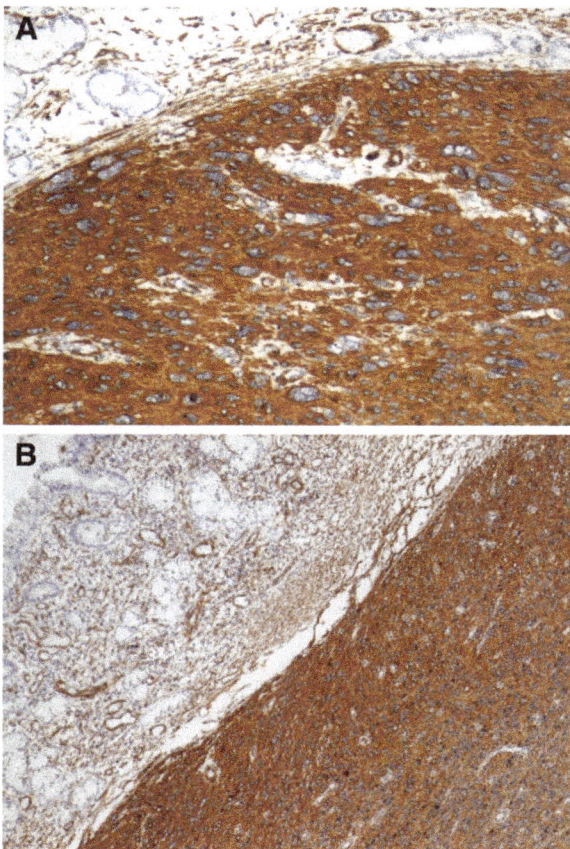

Fig. 6 Immunohistochemically, tumor cells express SMA (**a**) and h-caldesmon (**b**)

identical: 94.4% and 94.7% [7]. DOG1 is considered the best marker for GISTs with better specificity [8, 9]. More recent studies showed that DOG1 positivity could be detected in neoplastic tissues other than GISTs [10–12]. But, there were no cases of gastric leiomyosarcoma with positive DOG1 staining like ours. In our case, positivity of DOG1 markers resulted in diagnostic confusion, especially that postoperative therapeutic approach will differ depending on whether it is a stromal tumour or not. In such cases, based on Ray-Coquard et al. study [13], the European Society for Medical Oncology (ESMO) recommends the validation of a pathological expert "when the original diagnosis was made outside a reference centre/network" [14]. So, we requested another opinion from an expert in France to confirm the diagnosis.

Finally, the localization of the tumour in the cardia is exceptional and presents a challenge for the surgeon especially if adjacent structures, such as the aorta, are invaded. In fact, surgery is the only curative option for leiomyosarcomas. The type of surgery depends on the size and localization of the tumour [15]. It ranges from a wedge resection to a total gastrectomy with en bloc resection if adjacent organs are invaded. In March 2018, Sato et al. first published a case of a small gastric leiomyosarcoma treated with endoscopic submucosal dissection [16]. Resection margins affect directly the prognosis. Systematic lymphadenectomy is not recommended as leiomyosarcoma have predilection for hematogenous spread and lymph node involvement is rare [6]. In our case, a total gastrectomy was performed rather than partial resection due to the size and localization of the tumour.

In conclusion, gastric leiomyosarcoma is a rare tumour. Diagnosis is based on histological examination with immunohistochemistry, which could be sometimes confusing like in our case. The validation of a pathological expert is recommended. Treatment depends on surgery with a very little place reserved for chemotherapy and radiotherapy in advanced cases [17, 18]. Prognosis is still very poor [1, 4, 19].

Abbreviations

CT: Computed tomography; ESMO: European Society for Medical Oncology; GIST: Gastrointestinal stromal tumours; SMA: Smooth muscle actin

Acknowledgements

The authors are pleased to acknowledge professor Jean-François Emile (Department of Histopathology in Ambroise Paré Hospital, France), who contributed to the diagnostic study.

Authors' contributions

Conception and design of study: HA, ZH, BMA, BA. Acquisition of data: HA, JR, HD. Data analysis and interpretation: JR, BBE, HD, HA. Drafting of manuscript: HA, ZH. Critical analysis and approval of final version of manuscript: BMA, BA. All authors read and approved the final manuscript.

Competing interests

The authors declare that they have no competing interests.

Author details

[1]Department of General Surgery, Habib Thameur Hospital, Tunis El Manar University, Ali Ben Ayed Street 2037 Montfleury, Tunis, Tunisia. [2]Department of Histopathology and Cytology, Habib Thameur Hospital, Tunis El Manar University, Tunis, Tunisia.

References

1. Karila-Cohen P, Petit T, Kotobi H, Merran S. Léiomyosarcome gastrique. J Radiol. 2004;85:1993–7.
2. Bazin P, Cabanne F, Feroldi J, Martin JF. Tumeurs myoides intra-murales de l'estomac: considérations microscopiques à propos de 6 cas. Ann Anat Path. 1960;5:484–97.
3. Miettinen M, Fetsch JF. Evaluation of biological potential of smooth muscle tumours. Histopathology. 2006;48(1):97–105.
4. Soufi M, Errougani A, Chekkof RM. Primary gastric leiomyosarcoma in young revealed by a massive hematemesis. J Gastrointest Cancer. 2009; 40(1–2):69–72.
5. Beyrouti MI, Beyrouti R, Ben Amar M, Frikha F, et al. Sarcomes gastriques. Presse Med. 2008;37:60–6.
6. Weledji EP, Enoworock G, Ngowe MN. Gastric leiomyosarcoma as a rare cause of gastric outlet obstruction and perforation: a case report. BMC Res Notes. 2014;7:479.
7. Miettinen M, Wang ZF, Lasota J. DOG1 antibody in the differential diagnosis of gastrointestinal stromal tumors: a study of 1840 cases. Am J Surg Pathol. 2009;33(9):1401–8.
8. Robert BW, Christopher LC, Xin C, Brian PR, Subbaya S, Kelli M, et al. The novel marker, DOG1, is expressed ubiquitously in gastrointestinal stromal tumors irrespective of KIT or PDGFRA mutation status. Am J Pathol. 2004; 165(1):107–13.
9. González-Cámpora R, Delgado MD, Amate AH, Gallardo SP, León MS, Beltrán AL. Old and new immunohistochemical markers for the diagnosis of gastrointestinal stromal tumors. Anal Quant Cytol Histol. 2011;33(1):1–11.
10. Swalchick W, Shamekh R, Bui MM. Is DOG1 Immunoreactivity specific to gastrointestinal stromal tumor? Cancer Control. 2015;22(4):498–504.
11. Sah SP, McCluggage WG. DOG1 immunoreactivity in uterine leiomyosarcomas. J Clin Pathol. 2013;66(1):40–3.
12. So Jung L, Chung SH, Ahrong K, Kyungbin K, Kyung UC. Gastrointestinal tract spindle cell tumors with interstitial cells of Cajal: prevalence excluding gastrointestinal stromal tumors. Oncol Lett. 2016;12(2):1287–92.
13. Ray-Coquard I, Montesco MC, Coindre JM, et al. Sarcoma: concordance between initial diagnosis and centralized expert review in a population-based study within three European regions. Ann Oncol. 2012;23:2442–9.
14. The ESMO/European Sarcoma Network Working Group. Soft tissue and visceral sarcomas: ESMO clinical practice guidelines for diagnosis, treatment and follow-up. Ann Oncol. 2014;25(3):102–12.
15. Piso P, Schlitt HJ, Klempnauer J. Stromal sarcoma of the stomach: therapeutic considerations. Eur J Surg. 2000;166(12):954–8.
16. Sato T, Akahoshi K, Tomoeda N, Kinoshita N, Kubokawa M, Yodoe K, et al. Leiomyosarcoma of the stomach treated by endoscopic submucosal dissection. Clin J Gastroenterol. 2018;11:1–6.
17. Grant CS, Kim CH, Farrugia G, Zinsmeister A, Goellner JR. Gastric Leiomyosarcoma. Prognostic factors and surgical management. Arch Surg. 1991;126:985–90.
18. O'Hanlon DM, Griffin SM. Management of other oesophageal and gastric neoplasms. In upper gastrointestinal surgery. A companion to specialist surgical practice. Edited by Michael griffin S, Raimes SA. London, NW1 7DX. WB Saunders Company Ltd: England; 2000.
19. Hsieh CC, Shih CS, Wu YC, et al. Leiomyosarcoma of the gastric cardia and fundus. Zhonghua Yi Xue Za Zhi. 1999;62:418–24.

Permissions

List of Contributors

Klaus T von Trotha, Marcel Binnebösel, Son Truong and Ulf P Neumann
Department of Surgery, University Hospital of the RWTH Aachen, Germany

Florian F Behrendt
Department of Diagnostic Radiology, University Hospital of the RWTH Aachen, Germany

Hermann E Wasmuth
Department of Medicine III, University Hospital of the RWTH Aachen, Germany

Marc Jansen
Department of Surgery, HELIOS Hospital Emil von Behring Berlin, Germany

Jie Wu, Qi-Xun Chen, Xing-Ming Zhou and Wei-Ming Mao
Department of Thoarcic Surgery, Zhejinang Cancer Hospital, 38 Guangji Road, Hangzhou 310022, China

Mark J Krasna
Meridian Cancer Care, Jersey Shore University Medical Center, Neptune, New Jersey, USA

IM Luppino
Gastroenterology and Endoscopy Unit, T. Campanella Oncological Foundation, Catanzaro, Italy

B Amato
General Surgery Unit, Dept of General Surgery, Geriatric and Endoscopy, University Federico II, Naples, Italy

G Silecchia
General Surgery Unit, Dept of Medical and Surgical Biotechnology and Sciences, University la Sapienza, Roma, Italy

G Orlando, MA Lerose, R Gervasi and A Puzziello
Endocrinosurgery Unit, Dept of Medical and Surgical Sciences, University Magna Graecia, Catanzaro, Italy

Hyasinta Jaka
Department of Internal Medicine, Catholic University of Health and Allied Sciences- Bugando, Mwanza, Tanzania

Endoscopic unit, Bugando Medical Center, Mwanza, Tanzania

Mabula D Mchembe
Department of Surgery, Muhimbili University of Health and Allied Sciences, Dar Es Salaam, Tanzania

Peter F Rambau
Department of Pathology, Catholic University of Health and Allied Sciences- Bugando, Mwanza, Tanzania

Phillipo L Chalya
Department of Surgery, Catholic University of Health and Allied Sciences- Bugando, Mwanza, Tanzania

Jodok Matthias Grueneberger, Goran Marjanovic and Simon Kuesters
Department of General and Visceral Surgery, University of Freiburg, Hugstetter Strasse 55, 79106 Freiburg, Germany

Iwona Karcz-Socha and Krystyna Zwirska-Korczala
Department of Physiology, Silesian Medical University, Katowitz, Poland

Katharina Schmidt and W Konrad Karcz
Department of General Surgery, University of Schleswig-Holstein, Campus Lübeck, Lübeck, Germany

Nicole Pech, Thomas Manger and Christine Stroh
Department of General, Abdominal and Pediatric Surgery, Municipal Hospital Gera, Strasse des Friedens 122, Gera 07548, Germany

Frank Meyer and Hans Lippert
Department of General, Abdominal and Vascular Surgery, University Hospital, Magdeburg, Germany

Antanas Mickevicius, Rytis Markelis, Audrius Parseliunas, Mindaugas Kiudelis, Zilvinas Endzinas and Almantas Maleckas
Department of Surgery, Lithuanian University of Health Sciences, Eiveniu Str. 2, Kaunas LT-50009, Lithuania

Povilas Ignatavicius and Zilvinas Dambrauskas
Laboratory of Surgical Gastroenterology, Institute for Digestive System Research, Lithuanian University of Health Sciences, Eivenių str. 2, Kaunas LT-50009, Lithuania

Dainora Butkute
Department of Oncology, Lithuanian University of Health Sciences, Eivenių str. 2, Kaunas LT-50009, Lithuania

Catharina Ruf, Oliver Thomusch, Matthias Goos, Frank Makowiec and Guenther Ruf
Department of Surgery, University of Freiburg, Universitätsklinikum, Hugstetterstr. 55, D-79106 Freiburg, Germany

Gerald Illerhaus
Department of Oncology, University of Freiburg, Freiburg, Germany

Shailesh Puntambekar, Sanjay Kumar, Saurabh Joshi, Geetanjali Agarwal, Sunil Reddy and Jainul Mallik
Galaxy Care Laparoscopy Institute, Opposite Garware College, 25-A, Ayurvedic Rasashala Premises, Karve Road, Pune, Maharashtra 411004, India

Rahul Kenawadekar
Galaxy Care Laparoscopy Institute, Opposite Garware College, 25-A, Ayurvedic Rasashala Premises, Karve Road, Pune, Maharashtra 411004, India
Department of Surgery, JNMC, KLE University, Belgaum, India

Ana M Ramos-Levi, Lucio Cabrerizo, Pilar Matía and Miguel A Rubio
Department of Endocrinology and Nutrition, Hospital Clínico San Carlos, Instituto de Investigación Sanitaria San Carlos (IdISSC), Facultad de Medicina, Complutense University, Madrid, Spain

Andrés Sánchez-Pernaute and Antonio J Torres
Department of Surgery, Hospital Clínico San Carlos, Instituto de Investigación Sanitaria San Carlos (IdISSC), Facultad de Medicina, Complutense University, Madrid, Spain

Gintare Jakstaite, Narimantas Evaldas Samalavicius and Giedre Smailyte
Clinic of Oncosurgery of Oncology Institute, Clinic of Internal Diseases, Family Medicine and Oncology of Medical Faculty, Vilnius University, 1 Santariskiu Street, Vilnius LT-08660, Lithuania

Raimundas Lunevicius
Liver, Renal and Surgery Department, King's College Hospital NHS Foundation Trust, King's Health Partners Academic Health Sciences Centre, Denmark Hill, London SE5 9RS, UK

Xuewei Ding, Han Liang, Qiang Xue and Xishan Hao
Department of Gastrointestinal Oncology, National Clinical Research Center for Cancer, Tianjin Cancer Institute and Hospital, Tianjin Medical University, Huanhuxi Road, Ti-Yuan-Bei, Hexi District, Tianjin 300060, P. R. China

Fang Yan
Department of Pediatrics, Division of Gastroenterology, Hepatology and Nutrition, Vanderbilt University Medical Center, Nashville, TN, USA
Department of Immunology, Key Laboratory of Cancer Prevention and Therapy, National Clinical Research Center for Cancer, Tianjin Cancer Institute and Hospital, Tianjin Medical University, Tianjin, P. R. China

Hui Li and Xiubao Ren
Department of Immunology, Key Laboratory of Cancer Prevention and Therapy, National Clinical Research Center for Cancer, Tianjin Cancer Institute and Hospital, Tianjin Medical University, Tianjin, P. R. China

Kuo Zhang
Department of Laboratory Animal Science, Peking University Health Science Center, Beijing, P. R. China

Mu-Sheng Zeng
State Key Laboratory of Oncology in South China, Cancer Center, Sun Yet-Sen University, No.651, Dongfeng Road East, Guangzhou, China

You-Fang Chen, Zhi-Liang Huang and Zhe-Sheng Wen
State Key Laboratory of Oncology in South China, Cancer Center, Sun Yet-Sen University, No.651, Dongfeng Road East, Guangzhou, China
Department of Thoracic Oncology, Cancer Center, Sun Yet-Sen University, No.651, Dongfeng Road East, Guangzhou, China

Gang Ma and Xun Cao
State Key Laboratory of Oncology in South China, Cancer Center, Sun Yet-Sen University, No.651, Dongfeng Road East, Guangzhou, China

Department of Critical Care Medicine, Cancer Center, Sun Yet-Sen University, No.651, Dongfeng Road East, Guangzhou, China

Rong-Zhen Luo and Jie-Hua He
State Key Laboratory of Oncology in South China, Cancer Center, Sun Yet-Sen University, No.651, Dongfeng Road East, Guangzhou, China
Department of Pathology, Cancer Center, Sun Yet-Sen University, No.651, Dongfeng Road East, Guangzhou, China

Li-Ru He
State Key Laboratory of Oncology in South China, Cancer Center, Sun Yet-Sen University, No.651, Dongfeng Road East, Guangzhou, China
Department of Radiation Oncology, Cancer Center, Sun Yet-Sen University, No.651, Dongfeng Road East, Guangzhou, China

Lois Haruna, Ahmed Aber, Farhan Rashid and Marco Barreca
Department of General Surgery, Luton and Dunstable Hospital, Lewsey Road, Luton, Bedfordshire LU4 ODZ, UK

Haruhiko Cho, Takaki Yoshikawa and Akira Tsuburaya
Department of Gastrointestinal Surgery, Kanagawa Cancer Center, 1-1-2 Nakao, Asahi, 241-0815 Yokohama, Kanagawa, Japan

Takanobu Yamada, Tsutomu Hayashi, Toru Aoyama, Junya Shirai and Hirohito Fujikawa
Department of Gastrointestinal Surgery, Kanagawa Cancer Center, 1-1-2 Nakao, Asahi, 241-0815 Yokohama, Kanagawa, Japan
Department of Surgery, Yokohama City University, Yokohama, Japan

Yasushi Rino and Munetaka Masuda
Department of Surgery, Yokohama City University, Yokohama, Japan

Hideki Taniguchi
Department of Anesthesiology, Kanagawa Cancer Center, 1-1-2 Nakao, Asahi, 241-0815 Yokohama, Kanagawa, Japan

Ryoji Fukushima
Department of Surgery, Teikyo University School of Medicine, 2-11-1 Kaga, 173-8605 Itabashi, Tokyo, Japan

Luigi Marano, Bartolomeo Braccio, Michele Schettino, Giuseppe Izzo, Angelo Cosenza, Michele Grassia, Raffaele Porfidia, Gianmarco Reda, Marianna Petrillo, Giuseppe Esposito and Natale Di Martino
Institution: VIII General and Gastrointestinal Surgery (Chief Prof. N. Di Martino) - School of Medicine - Second University of Naples - Piazza Miraglia 2, 80138 Naples, Italy

Jia-Qin Cai, Ke Chen, Yi-Ping Mou, Yu Pan, Xiao-Wu Xu, Yu-Cheng Zhou and Chao-Jie Huang
Department of General Surgery, Sir Run Run Shaw Hospital, School of Medicine, Zhejiang University, 3 East Qingchun Road, Hangzhou 310016, Zhejiang Province, China

Rimantas Bausys, Augustinas Bausys and Eugenijus Stratilatovas
Department of Abdominal Surgery and Oncology, National Cancer Institute, Santariskiu str. 1, Vilnius 08660, Lithuania
Faculty of Medicine, Vilnius University, Ciurlionio str. 21, Vilnius 03101, Lithuania

Kazimieras Maneikis and Dalius Klimas
Faculty of Medicine, Vilnius University, Ciurlionio str. 21, Vilnius 03101, Lithuania

Kestutis Strupas
Faculty of Medicine, Vilnius University, Ciurlionio str. 21, Vilnius 03101, Lithuania
Center of Abdominal surgery, Vilnius University Hospital Santaros Klinikos, Santariskiu str. 2, Washington 08661, USA

Indre Vysniauskaite
School of Medicine, Georgetown University, Washington, D.C., USA

Martynas Luksta
Center of Abdominal surgery, Vilnius University Hospital Santaros Klinikos, Santariskiu str. 2, Washington 08661, USA

Masashi Takeuchi, Kenjiro Ishii, Hiroaki Seki, Nobutaka Yasui, Michio Sakata, Akihiko Shimada and Hidetoshi Matsumoto
Department of Surgery, Keiyu Hospital, 3-7-3 Minatomirai, Nishi-ku, Yokohama-shi, Kanagawa 220-8521, Japan

Ke Chen, Yu Pan, Shu-ting Zhai, Jun-hai Pan, Wei-hua Yu, Ding-wei Chen, Jia-fei Yan and Xian-fa Wang
Department of Gastrointestinal Surgery, Sir Run Run Shaw Hospital, School of Medicine, Zhejiang University, 3 East Qingchun Road, Hangzhou 310016, Zhejiang Province, China

Francesco Cavallin, Rita Alfieri, Marco Scarpa, Matteo Cagol, Ermanno Ancona and Carlo Castoro
Esophageal and Digestive Tract Surgical Unit, Regional Centre for Esophageal Disease, Veneto Institute of Oncology IOV IRCCS, Padova, Italy

Alberto Ruol
3rd Surgical Clinic, Azienda Ospedaliera di Padova, Padova, Italy

Matteo Fassan and Massimo Rugge
Department of Medicine (DIMED), Surgical Pathology and Cytopathology Unit, University of Padova, Padova, Italy

Lars Fischer, Anna-Laura Wekerle, Markus W. Büchler and Beat P. Müller-Stich
Department of General, Visceral and Transplantation Surgery, University of Heidelberg, Im Neuenheimer Feld 110, 69120 Heidelberg, Germany

Markus K. Diener
Department of General, Visceral and Transplantation Surgery, University of Heidelberg, Im Neuenheimer Feld 110, 69120 Heidelberg, Germany
Study Centre of the German Surgical Society (SDGC), University of Heidelberg, Im Neuenheimer Feld 110, 69120 Heidelberg, Germany

Thomas Bruckner
Institute of Medical Biometry and Informatics, University of Heidelberg, Im Neuenheimer Feld 305, 69120 Heidelberg, Germany

Inga Wegener
Study Centre of the German Surgical Society (SDGC), University of Heidelberg, Im Neuenheimer Feld 110, 69120 Heidelberg, Germany

Moritz V. Frankenberg
Salem Hospital, Zeppelinstraße 11 – 33, 69121 Heidelberg, Germany

Daniel Gärtner and Michael R. Schön
Department of General and Visceral Surgery, Städtisches Krankenhaus Karlsruhe, Moltkestraße 90, 76133 Karlsruhe, Germany

Matthias C. Raggi and Emre Tanay
Department of General and Visceral Surgery, Agaplesion Bethesda Krankenhaus Stuttgart, Hohenheimer Straße 21, 70184 Stuttgart, Germany

Rainer Brydniak and Norbert Runkel
Department of General and Visceral Surgery, Schwarzwald- Baar Klinikum, Klinikstraße 11, 78052 Villingen-Schwenningen, Germany

Corinna Attenberger
Department of Surgery, Caritas-Krankenhaus St. Josef, Landshuter Straße 65, 93053 Regensburg, Germany

Min-Seop Son and Andreas Türler
Department of General and Visceral Surgery, Johanniter Krankenhaus, Johanniter GmbH, Johanniterstraße 3, 53113 Bonn, Germany

Rudolf Weiner
Department of Bariatric Surgery and Metabolic Surgery, Sana Klinikum Offenbach GmbH, Starkenburgring 66, 63069 Offenbach, Germany

Kamleshsingh Shadhu
Department of General Surgery, Jiangsu Province Hospital, First Affiliated hospital of Nanjing Medical University, Guangzhou Road, 300, Gulou District, Nanjing 210029, Jiangsu Province, People's Republic of China
Pancreas Center, Jiangsu Province Hospital, First Affiliated hospital of Nanjing Medical University, Guangzhou Road, 300, Gulou District, Nanjing 210029, Jiangsu Province, People's Republic of China

Dadhija Ramlagun
Department of General Surgery, Jiangsu Province Hospital, First Affiliated hospital of Nanjing Medical University, Guangzhou Road, 300, Gulou District, Nanjing 210029, Jiangsu Province, People's Republic of China
Department of Breast Surgery, Jiangsu Province Hospital, First Affiliated hospital of Nanjing Medical University, Guangzhou Road, 300, Gulou District, Nanjing 210029, Jiangsu Province, People's Republic of China

Xiaochun Ping
Department of General Surgery, Jiangsu Province Hospital, First Affiliated hospital of Nanjing Medical University, Guangzhou Road, 300, Gulou District, Nanjing 210029, Jiangsu Province, People's Republic of China

Department of Gastric Surgery, Jiangsu Province Hospital, First Affiliated hospital of Nanjing Medical University, Guangzhou Road, 300, Gulou District, Nanjing 210029, Jiangsu Province, People's Republic of China

Ji-Hyun Kim, Kyong-Hwa Jun and Hyung-Min Chin
Department of Surgery, St. Vincent's Hospital, College of Medicine, The Catholic University of Korea, Seoul, Republic of Korea

Aneesh Shrihari Dhorepatil, Daniel Cottam, Amit Surve, Walter Medlin, Hinali Zaveri, Christina Richards and Austin Cottam
Bariatric Medicine Institute, 1046 East 100 South, Salt Lake City, UT 84102, USA

Chihoko Nobori, Kenjiro Kimura, Go Ohira, Ryosuke Amano, Sadaaki Yamazoe, Hiroaki Tanaka, Kosei Hirakawa and Masaichi Ohira
Department of Surgical Oncology, Osaka City University Graduate School of Medicine, 1-4-3 Asahi-machi, Abeno-ku, Osaka, Japan

Kentaro Naito and Toshihiro Takami
Department of Neurosurgery, Osaka City University Graduate School of Medicine, 1-4-3 Asahi-machi, Abeno-ku, Osaka, Japan

Mamoru Morimoto, Tetsushi Hayakawa, Hidehiko Kitagami and Moritsugu Tanaka
Department of Surgery, Kariya Toyota General Hospital, Kariya, Japan

Yoichi Matsuo and Hiromitsu Takeyama
Department of Gastroenterological Surgery, Nagoya City University Graduate School of Medical Sciences, Kawasumi 1, Mizuho-cho, Mizuhoku, Nagoya 467-8601, Japan

Song Soo Yang and Yeong Cheol Im
Department of Surgery, Ulsan University Hospital, University of Ulsan College of Medicine, 877, Bangeojinsunhwando-ro, Dong-gu, Ulsan 44033, Republic of Korea

Haithem Zaafouri, Anis Hasnaoui, Dhafer Haddad, Ahmed Bouhafa and Anis Ben Maamer
Department of General Surgery Habib Thameur Hospital, Ali Ben Ayed Street's 2037 Montfleury, Tunis, Tunisia

Sonia Essghaeir
Department of Radiology Habib Thameur Hospital, Tunis, Tunisia

Meriam Sabbah and Jamel Kharrat
Department of Gastroenterology Habib Thameur Hospital, Tunis, Tunisia

Ke Chen, Yang He, Jia-Qin Cai, Yu Pan, Di Wu, Ding-Wei Chen, Jia-Fei Yan, Hendi Maher and Yi-Ping Mou
Department of General Surgery, Sir Run Run Shaw Hospital, School of Medicine, Zhejiang University, 3 East Qingchun Road, Hangzhou 310016Zhejiang Province, China

Tsutomu Namikawa, Yasuhiro Kawanishi, Eri Munekage, Masaya Munekage, Takahito Sugase, Hiroyuki Kitagawa and Kazuhiro Hanazaki
Department of Surgery, Kochi Medical School, Kohasu, Oko-cho, Nankoku, Kochi 783-8505, Japan

Kazune Fujisawa and Makoto Hiroi
Department of Pathology, Kochi Medical School, Kochi, Japan

Hiromichi Maeda
Cancer Treatment Center, Kochi Medical School Hospital, Kochi, Japan

Michiya Kobayashi
Cancer Treatment Center, Kochi Medical School Hospital, Kochi, Japan
Department of Human Health and Medical Sciences, Kochi Medical School, Kochi, Japan

Tatsuya Kumon
Department of Surgery, Noichi Central Hospital, Kochi, Japan

Eirik Kjus Aahlin and Kristoffer Lassen
Department of GI and HPB surgery, University Hospital of Northern Norway, 9038 Breivika, Tromsø, Norway
Department of Clinical Medicine, University of Tromsø - The Arctic University of Norway, Tromsø, Norway

Frank Olsen and Bård Uleberg
Centre of Clinical Documentation and Evaluation, Northern Norway Regional Health Authority, Tromsø, Norway

Bjarne K. Jacobsen
Centre of Clinical Documentation and Evaluation, Northern Norway Regional Health Authority, Tromsø, Norway
Department of Community Medicine, University of Tromsø - The Arctic University of Norway, Tromsø, Norway

J.-N. Kersebaum, C. Schafmayer, M. Ahrens, T. Becker and J. H. Beckmann
Klinik für Allgemeine, Viszeral-, Transplantations-, Thorax- und Kinderchirurgie, Universitätsklinikum Schleswig- Holstein, Campus Kiel, Arnold-Heller-Str. 3, 24105 Kiel, Germany

M. Laudes
Klinik für Innere Medizin I, Universitätsklinikum Schleswig- Holstein, Campus Kiel, Kiel, Germany

Antonino Mirabella and Massimo Lupo
O.U. of Emergency and General Surgery of "Villa Sofia" Hospital, Palermo, Italy

Tiziana Fiorentini and Armando Speciale
O.U. of Emergency and General Surgery of "Cervello" Hospital, Palermo, Italy

Roberta Tutino, Nicolò Falco, Tommaso Fontana, Paolino De Marco, Eliana Gulotta, Leonardo Gulotta, Leo Licari, Giuseppe Salamone, Irene Melfa, Gregorio Scerrino and Gianfranco Cocorullo
Department of Surgical, Oncological and Stomatological Disciplines, University of Palermo, Palermo, Italy

Anis Hasnaoui, Dhafer Haddad, Haithem Zaafouri, Ahmed Bouhafa and Anis Ben Maamer
Department of General Surgery, Habib Thameur Hospital, Tunis El Manar University, Ali Ben Ayed Street 2037 Montfleury, Tunis, Tunisia

Raja Jouini and Ehsen Ben Brahim
Department of Histopathology and Cytology, Habib Thameur Hospital, Tunis El Manar University, Tunis, Tunisia

Index

www.ingramcontent.com/pod-product-compliance
Lightning Source LLC
Chambersburg PA
CBHW061250190326
41458CB00011B/3630